Drug Abuse
SOURCEBOOK

SIXTH EDITION

Health Reference Series

Drug Abuse
SOURCEBOOK

SIXTH EDITION

Basic Consumer Health Information about the Abuse of Cocaine, Club Drugs, Marijuana, Inhalants, Heroin, Hallucinogens, and Other Illicit Substances and the Misuse of Prescription and Over-the-Counter Medications

Along with Facts and Statistics about Drug Use and Addiction, Treatment and Recovery, Drug Testing, Drug-Abuse Prevention and Intervention, Glossaries of Related Terms, and Directories of Resources for Additional Help and Information

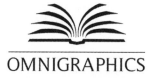

OMNIGRAPHICS
615 Griswold, Ste. 901, Detroit, MI 48226

Copyright © 2019 Omnigraphics

ISBN 978-0-7808-1683-1

E-ISBN 978-0-7808-1684-8

Library of Congress Cataloging-in-Publication Data

Title: Drug abuse sourcebook: basic consumer health information about the abuse of cocaine, club drugs, marijuana, inhalants, heroin, hallucinogens, and other illicit substances and the misuse of prescription and over-the-counter medications; along with facts and statistics about drug use and addiction, treatment and recovery, drug testing, drug abuse prevention and intervention, glossaries of related terms, and directories of resources for additional help and information / Angela Williams, managing editor.

Description: Sixth edition. | Detroit, MI: Omnigraphics, [2019] | Includes bibliographical references and index.

Identifiers: LCCN 2018057794 | ISBN 9780780816831 (hard cover: alk. paper) | ISBN 9780780816848 (ebook)

Subjects: LCSH: Drug abuse--Prevention--Handbooks, manuals, etc. | Drug abuse--Treatment--Handbooks, manuals, etc. | Drug addiction--Treatment--Handbooks, manuals, etc.

Classification: LCC HV5801.D724 2019 | DDC 362.29--dc23

LC record available at https://lccn.loc.gov/2018057794

Table of Contents

Part III: Drugs of Abuse

Part IV: The Causes and Consequences of Drug Abuse and Addiction

Part V: Drug-Abuse Treatment and Recovery

Part VI: Drug-Abuse Testing and Prevention

Part VII: Additional Help and Information

Preface

About This Book

Drug abuse remains a growing problem in the United States. A survey conducted by the Substance Abuse and Mental Health Services Administration (SAMHSA) found that an estimated 24.6 million Americans ages 12 or older—9.4 percent of the population—had used an illicit drug or abused a prescription medication. This figure represented an increase from previous years mainly due to the widespread prevalence of marijuana use and increasing prescription drug misuse. There are spots of good news, however. The same survey also found that the abuse of other illicit drugs, such as heroin and cocaine, had decreased in recent years. Nevertheless, the medical, social, and familial costs of substance use are enormous—nearly $740 billion a year according to the U.S. Department of Justice (DOJ).

Drug Abuse Sourcebook, Sixth Edition provides updated information about the abuse of illegal drugs and the misuse of prescription and over-the-counter medications. It offers facts and statistics related to U.S. drug-using populations and presents details about specific drugs of abuse, including their health-related consequences, addiction potential, and other harms to individuals, their families, and communities. Drug treatment and recovery options are discussed, along with information on drug testing and drug-use prevention strategies for parents, employers, individuals, and others seeking help for themselves or a loved one. The book concludes with glossaries of terms related to drug abuse and directories of resources for additional help and information.

How to Use This Book

This book is divided into parts and chapters. Parts focus on broad areas of interest. Chapters are devoted to single topics within a part.

Part I: Facts and Statistics about Drug Abuse in the United States presents core data regarding the drug abuse problem, detailing the prevalence of drug abuse and the costs to society in terms of medical care, hospitalization, social consequences, and treatment outcomes. It also discusses federal regulation of prescriptions, laws pertaining to illegal and legal drugs, and the current debate over medical and legalized marijuana.

Part II: Drug Abuse and Specific Populations describes drug use initiation and the effects of drug abuse on various groups of people, including children, adolescents, and women. It also addresses different social factors affecting drug abuse, such as socioeconomic or employment status, and it considers drug use in inmate, veteran, senior, and disabled populations.

Part III: Drugs of Abuse provides facts about illicit and misused substances, such as performance enhancers, cannabinoids, inhalants, hallucinogens, narcotics, sedatives, and stimulants, including anabolic steroids, marijuana, Rohypnol, ecstasy (MDMA), LSD, heroin, hydrocodone, cocaine, methamphetamine, and many others. The part concludes with information about new and emerging drugs of abuse.

Part IV: The Causes and Consequences of Drug Abuse and Addiction explains the science behind addiction and what is known about the risk factors that can lead to drug dependency. Concerns related to coexisting alcohol problems or multidrug use are addressed, and the medical, legal, financial, and social ramifications of drug abuse are discussed. The part also looks at the connection between substance abuse and infectious diseases, and it addresses related mental-health issues, including suicide ideation.

Part V: Drug-Abuse Treatment and Recovery offers suggestions for recognizing the existence of a drug problem and options for taking steps toward achieving and maintaining a healthy lifestyle, including first aid, intervention, and detoxification. It provides details about various treatment approaches and reports on strategies for sustaining recovery. The part also discusses the legal rights of those in recovery and concerns related to the criminal-justice system.

Part VI: Drug-Abuse Testing and Prevention lays the groundwork for responses to drug abuse—in society, in schools, and especially in the home. It discusses the influence of parents on their children's choices related to drug abuse, and it addresses concerns about preventing drug abuse in the workplace. Drug testing is discussed in detail, and federal drug-abuse prevention campaigns are described.

Part VII: Additional Help and Information provides resources for readers seeking further assistance. It includes a glossary of terms related to drug abuse and a listing of street terms for common drugs of abuse. It concludes with directories of state substance abuse agencies and other organizations providing resources on drug abuse and addiction.

Bibliographic Note

This volume contains documents and excerpts from publications issued by the following U.S. government agencies: Centers for Disease Control and Prevention (CDC); Centers for Medicare & Medicaid Services (CMS); DEA Diversion Control Division; Federal Bureau of Investigation (FBI); Get Smart About Drugs; Just Think Twice; National Cancer Institute (NCI); National Institute of Justice (NIJ); National Institutes of Health (NIH); National Institute on Drug Abuse (NIDA); National Institute on Drug Abuse (NIDA) for Teens; Office of Disease Prevention and Health Promotion (ODPHP); Office on Women's Health (OWH); Substance Abuse and Mental Health Services Administration (SAMHSA); U.S. Department of Health and Human Services (HHS); U.S. Drug Enforcement Administration (DEA); and U.S. Food and Drug Administration (FDA).

About the Health Reference Series

The *Health Reference Series* is designed to provide basic medical information for patients, families, caregivers, and the general public. Each volume takes a particular topic and provides comprehensive coverage. This is especially important for people who may be dealing with a newly diagnosed disease or a chronic disorder in themselves or in a family member. People looking for preventive guidance, information about disease warning signs, medical statistics, and risk factors for health problems will also find answers to their questions in the *Health Reference Series*. The *Series*, however, is not intended to serve as a tool for diagnosing illness, in prescribing treatments, or as a substitute for the physician/patient relationship. All people concerned about medical symptoms or the possibility of disease are encouraged to seek professional care from an appropriate healthcare provider.

A Note about Spelling and Style

Health Reference Series editors use *Stedman's Medical Dictionary* as an authority for questions related to the spelling of medical terms and the *Chicago Manual of Style* for questions related to grammatical structures, punctuation, and other editorial concerns. Consistent adherence is not always possible, however, because the individual volumes within the *Series* include many documents from a wide variety of different producers, and the editor's primary goal is to present material from each source as accurately as is possible. This sometimes means that information in different chapters or sections may follow other guidelines and alternate spelling authorities. For example, occasionally a copyright holder may require that eponymous terms be shown in possessive forms (Crohn's disease vs. Crohn disease) or that British spelling norms be retained (leukaemia vs. leukemia).

Medical Review

Omnigraphics contracts with a team of qualified, senior medical professionals who serve as medical consultants for the *Health Reference Series*. As necessary, medical consultants review reprinted material for currency and accuracy. Citations including the phrase "Reviewed (month, year)" indicate material reviewed by this team. Medical consultation services are provided to the *Health Reference Series* editors by:

Dr. Vijayalakshmi, MBBS, DGO, MD
Dr. Senthil Selvan, MBBS, DCH, MD
Dr. K. Sivanandham, MBBS, DCH, MS (Research), PhD

Our Advisory Board

We would like to thank the following board members for providing initial guidance on the development of this series:

- Dr. Lynda Baker, Associate Professor of Library and Information Science, Wayne State University, Detroit, MI

- Nancy Bulgarelli, William Beaumont Hospital Library, Royal Oak, MI

- Karen Imarisio, Bloomfield Township Public Library, Bloomfield Township, MI

- Karen Morgan, Mardigian Library, University of Michigan-Dearborn, Dearborn, MI

- Rosemary Orlando, St. Clair Shores Public Library, St. Clair Shores, MI

Health Reference Series *Update Policy*

The inaugural book in the *Health Reference Series* was the first edition of *Cancer Sourcebook* published in 1989. Since then, the *Series* has been enthusiastically received by librarians and in the medical community. In order to maintain the standard of providing high-quality health information for the layperson the editorial staff at Omnigraphics felt it was necessary to implement a policy of updating volumes when warranted.

Medical researchers have been making tremendous strides, and it is the purpose of the *Health Reference Series* to stay current with the most recent advances. Each decision to update a volume is made on an individual basis. Some of the considerations include how much new information is available and the feedback we receive from people who use the books. If there is a topic you would like to see added to the update list, or an area of medical concern you feel has not been adequately addressed, please write to:

Managing Editor
Health Reference Series
Omnigraphics
615 Griswold, Ste. 901
Detroit, MI 48226

Part One

Facts and Statistics about Drug Abuse in the United States

Chapter 1

Prevalence of Drug Abuse in the United States

Although progress has been made in substantially lowering rates of substance abuse in the United States, the use of mind- and behavior-altering substances continues to take a major toll on the health of individuals, families, and communities nationwide.

Substance abuse—involving drugs, alcohol, or both—is associated with a range of destructive social conditions, including family disruptions, financial problems, lost productivity, failure in school, domestic violence, child abuse, and crime. Moreover, both social attitudes and legal responses to the consumption of alcohol and illicit drugs make substance abuse one of the most complex public-health issues. Estimates of the total overall costs of substance abuse in the United States, including lost productivity and health- and crime-related costs, exceed $600 billion annually.

This chapter contains text excerpted from the following sources: Text in this chapter begins with excerpts from "Substance Abuse," Office of Disease Prevention and Health Promotion (ODPHP), U.S. Department of Health and Human Services (HHS), July 20, 2018; Text under the heading "Facts and Statistics on Substance Use in the United States" is excerpted from "DrugFacts: Nationwide Trends," National Institute on Drug Abuse (NIDA), June 2015. Reviewed January 2019.

Facts and Statistics on Substance Use in the United States

The Substance Abuse and Mental Health Services Administration (SAMHSA) conducts the annual National Survey on Drug Use and Health (NSDUH), a major source of information on substance use, abuse, and dependence among Americans age 12 years and older. Survey respondents report whether they have used specific substances ever in their lives (lifetime), over the past year, and over the past month (also referred to as "current use"). Most analyses focus on past-month use.

The following are facts and statistics on substance use in the United States in 2013, the most recent year for NSDUH survey results. Approximately 67,800 people responded to the survey in 2013.

Illicit-Drug Use

Illicit-drug use in the United States has been increasing. In 2013, an estimated 24.6 million Americans age 12 or older—9.4 percent of the population—had used an illicit drug in the month prior to when the survey was conducted. This number is up from 8.3 percent in 2002. The increase mostly reflects a rise in use of marijuana, the most commonly used illicit drug.

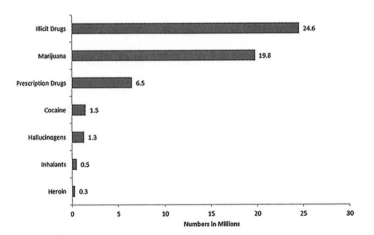

Figure 1.1. *Illicit-Drug Use 2013*

Marijuana use has increased since 2007. In 2013, there were 19.8 million current users—about 7.5 percent of people age 12 or older—up from 14.5 million (5.8%) in 2007.

Use of most drugs other than marijuana has stabilized over the past decade or has declined. In 2013, 6.5 million Americans age 12 or older (or 2.5%) had used prescription drugs nonmedically in the previous month. Prescription drugs include pain relievers, tranquilizers, stimulants, and sedatives. And 1.3 million Americans (0.5%) had used hallucinogens (a category that includes ecstasy and LSD (lysergic acid diethylamide)) in the past month.

Cocaine use has decreased in the last few years. In 2013, the number of current users age 12 or older was 1.5 million. This number is lower than in 2002 to 2007 (ranging from 2.0 to 2.4 million).

Methamphetamine use was higher in 2013, with 595,000 current users, compared with 353,000 users in 2010.

Most people use drugs for the first time when they are teenagers. There were just over 2.8 million new users of illicit drugs in 2013, or about 7,800 new users per day. Over half (54.1%) were under 18 years of age.

More than half of new illicit-drug users begin with marijuana. Next most common are prescription pain relievers, followed by inhalants (which is most common among younger teens).

Drug use is highest among people in their late teens and twenties. In 2013, 22.6 percent of 18- to 20-year-olds reported using an illicit drug in the past month.

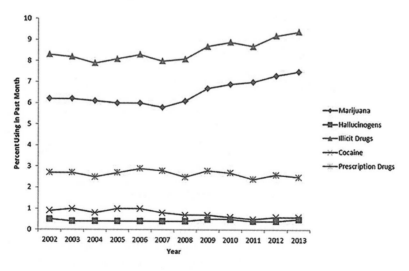

Figure 1.2. *Use of Selected Illicit Drugs*

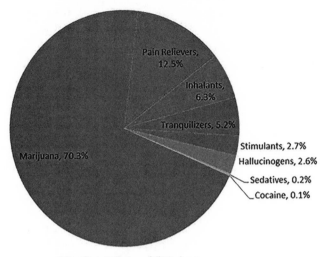

2.8 million initiates of illicit drugs

Figure 1.3. *First Specific Drugs Associated with Initiation of Illicit-Drug Use 2013*

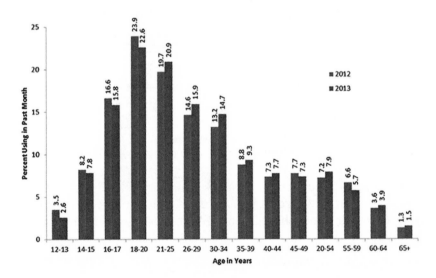

Figure 1.4. *Illicit-Drug Use by Age 2012 and 2013*

Drug use is increasing among people in their fifties and early sixties. This increase is, in part, due to the aging of the baby boomers, whose rates of illicit-drug use have historically been higher than those of previous generations.

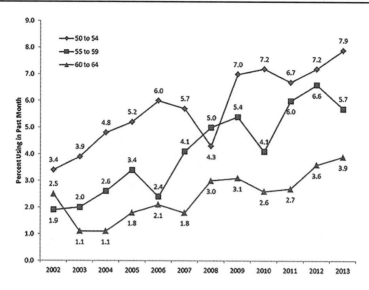

Figure 1.5. *Illicit-Drug Use among Adults Age 50 to 64*

Alcohol

Drinking by underage persons (ages 12 to 20) has declined. Current alcohol use by this age group declined from 28.8 to 22.7 percent between 2002 and 2013, while binge drinking declined from 19.3 to 14.2 percent and the rate of heavy drinking went from 6.2 to 3.7 percent.

Binge and heavy drinking are more widespread among men than women. In 2013, 30.2 percent of men and 16.0 percent of women 12 and older reported binge drinking in the past month. And 9.5 percent of men and 3.3 percent of women reported heavy alcohol use.

Driving under the influence of alcohol has also declined slightly. In 2013, an estimated 28.7 million people, or 10.9 percent of persons age 12 or older, had driven under the influence of alcohol at least once in the past year, down from 14.2 percent in 2002. Although this decline is encouraging, any driving under the influence remains a cause for concern.

Note: Binge drinking is five or more drinks on the same occasion. Heavy drinking is binge drinking on at least five separate days in the past month.

Tobacco

Fewer Americans are smoking. In 2013, an estimated 55.8 million Americans age 12 or older, or 21.3 percent of the population, were current cigarette smokers. This reflects a continual but slow downward trend from 2002, when the rate was 26 percent.

Teen smoking is declining more rapidly. The rate of past-month cigarette use among 12- to 17-year-olds went from 13 percent in 2002 to 5.6 percent in 2013.

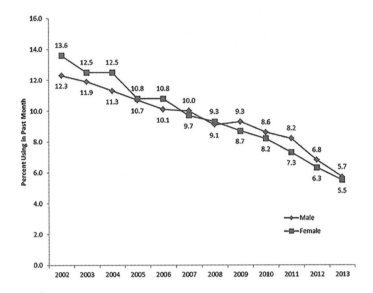

Figure 1.6. *Cigarette Use among Youth Age 12 to 17 by Gender*

Substance Dependence/Abuse and Treatment

Rates of alcohol dependence/abuse declined from 2002 to 2013. In 2013, 17.3 million Americans (6.6% of the population) were

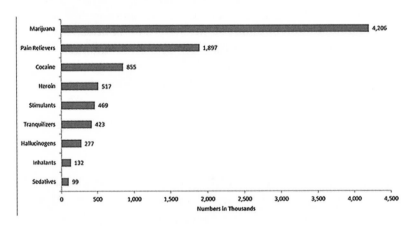

Figure 1.7. *Specific Illicit-Drug Dependence or Abuse in 2013*

dependent on alcohol or had problems related to their alcohol use (abuse). This is a decline from 18.1 million (or 7.7%) in 2002.

After alcohol, marijuana has the highest rate of dependence or abuse among all drugs. In 2013, 4.2 million Americans met clinical criteria for dependence or abuse of marijuana in the past year—more than twice the number for dependence/abuse of prescription pain relievers (1.9 million) and nearly five times the number for dependence/abuse of cocaine (855,000).

There continues to be a large "treatment gap" in this country. In 2013, an estimated 22.7 million Americans (8.6%) needed treatment for a problem related to drugs or alcohol, but only about 2.5 million people (0.9%) received treatment at a specialty facility.

Chapter 2

Drugs: Abuse and Addiction

Chapter Contents

Section 2.1

What Is Drug Abuse?

This section contains text excerpted from the following sources:
Text in this section begins with excerpts from "Drug Abuse,"
MedlinePlus, National Institutes of Health (NIH), December
28, 2016; Text under the heading "How Drug Abuse Starts and
Progresses" is excerpted from "Preventing Drug Use among
Children and Adolescents (In Brief)," National Institute
on Drug Abuse (NIDA), October 2003. Reviewed January 2019.

Drug abuse is a serious public-health problem that affects almost every community and family in some way. Each year drug abuse causes millions of serious illnesses or injuries among Americans. Abused drugs include:

- Methamphetamine
- Anabolic steroids
- Club drugs
- Cocaine
- Heroin
- Inhalants
- Marijuana
- Prescription drugs, including opioids

Drug abuse also plays a role in many major social problems, such as drugged driving, violence, stress, and child abuse. Drug abuse can lead to homelessness, crime, and missed work or problems with keeping a job. It harms unborn babies and destroys families. There are different types of treatment for drug abuse. But the best approach is to prevent drug abuse in the first place.

How Drug Abuse Starts and Progresses

Studies such as the National Survey on Drug Use and Health (NSDUH), formally called the National Household Survey on Drug Abuse (NHSDA), reported by the Substance Abuse and Mental Health Services Administration (SAMHSA), indicate that some children are already abusing drugs at age 12 or 13, which likely means that some begin even earlier. Early abuse often includes such substances as tobacco, alcohol, inhalants, marijuana, and prescription drugs such as sleeping pills and antianxiety medicines. If drug abuse persists into later adolescence, abusers typically become more heavily involved with marijuana and then advance to other drugs, while continuing their abuse of tobacco and alcohol. Studies have also shown that abuse of drugs in late childhood and early adolescence is associated with greater drug involvement. It is important to note that most youth, however, do not progress to abusing other drugs.

Scientists have proposed various explanations for why some individuals become involved with drugs and then escalate to abuse. One explanation points to a biological cause, such as having a family history of drug or alcohol abuse. Another explanation is that abusing drugs can lead to affiliation with drug-abusing peers, which, in turn, exposes the individual to other drugs.

Researchers have found that youth who rapidly increase their substance abuse have high levels of risk factors with low levels of protective factors. Gender, race, and geographic location can also play a role in how and when children begin abusing drugs.

Section 2.2

What Is Drug Addiction?

This section includes text excerpted from "Drugs, Brains, and Behavior: The Science of Addiction," National Institute on Drug Abuse (NIDA), July 2018.

Addiction is defined as a chronic, relapsing disorder characterized by compulsive drug seeking and use despite adverse consequences. It is considered a brain disorder, because it involves functional changes to brain circuits involved in reward, stress, and self-control, and those changes may last a long time after a person has stopped taking drugs.

Addiction is a lot like other diseases, such as heart disease. Both disrupt the normal, healthy functioning of an organ in the body, both have serious harmful effects, and both are, in many cases, preventable and treatable. If left untreated, they can last a lifetime and may lead to death.

Note: The term "addiction" as used in this section, is equivalent to a severe substance use as defined in the fifth edition of the Diagnostic and Statistical Manual of Mental Disorders *(DSM-5, 2013).*

Why Do People Take Drugs?

In general, people take drugs for a few reasons:

- **To feel good.** Drugs can produce intense feelings of pleasure. This initial euphoria is followed by other effects, which differ with the type of drug used. For example, with stimulants such as cocaine, the high is followed by feelings of power, self-confidence, and increased energy. In contrast, the euphoria caused by opioids such as heroin is followed by feelings of relaxation and satisfaction.

- **To feel better.** Some people who suffer from social anxiety, stress, and depression start using drugs to try to feel less anxious. Stress can play a major role in starting and continuing drug use as well as relapse (a return to drug use) in patients recovering from addiction.

- **To do better.** Some people feel pressure to improve their focus in school or at work or their abilities in sports. This can play a role in trying or continuing to use drugs, such as prescription stimulants or cocaine.

- **Curiosity and social pressure.** In this respect, teens are particularly at risk because peer pressure can be very strong. Teens are more likely than adults to act in risky or daring ways in an effort to impress their friends and show their independence from parents and social rules.

If Taking Drugs Makes People Feel Good or Better, What's the Problem?

When they first use a drug, people may perceive what seem to be positive effects. They also may believe they can control their use. But drugs can quickly take over a person's life. Over time, if drug use continues, other pleasurable activities become less pleasurable, and the person has to take the drug just to feel "normal." They have a hard time controlling their need to take drugs even though it causes many problems for themselves and their loved ones. Some people may start to feel the need to take more of a drug or take it more often, even in the early stages of their drug use. These are the tell-tale signs of an addiction.

Even relatively moderate drug use poses dangers. Consider how a social drinker can become intoxicated, get behind the wheel of a car, and quickly turn a pleasurable activity into a tragedy that affects many lives. Occasional drug use, such as misusing an opioid to get high, can have similarly disastrous effects, including overdose and dangerously impaired driving.

Do People Freely Choose to Keep Using Drugs?

The initial decision to take drugs is typically voluntary. But with continued use, a person's ability to exert self-control can become seriously impaired; this impairment in self-control is the hallmark of addiction.

Brain-imaging studies of people with addiction show physical changes in areas of the brain that are critical to judgment, decision-making, learning and memory, and behavior control. These changes help explain the compulsive nature of addiction.

Why Do Some People Become Addicted to Drugs, While Others Do Not?

As with other diseases and disorders, the likelihood of developing an addiction differs from person to person, and no single factor determines whether a person will become addicted to drugs. In general, the more risk factors a person has, the greater the chance that taking drugs will lead to drug use and addiction. Protective factors, on the other hand, reduce a person's risk. Risk and protective factors may be either environmental or biological.

Table 2.1. Risk and Protective Factors

Risk Factors	Protective Factors
Aggressive behavior in childhood	Good self-control
Lack of parental supervision	Parental monitoring and support
Poor social skills	Positive relationships
Drug experimentation	Good grades
Availability of drugs at school	School antidrug policies
Community poverty	Neighborhood resources

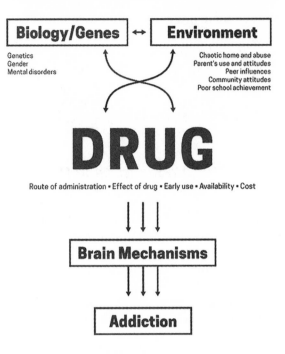

Figure 2.1. *Risk Factors for Drug Addiction*

What Biological Factors Increase Risk of Addiction

Biological factors that can affect a person's risk of addiction include their genes, stage of development, and even gender or ethnicity. Scientists estimate that genes, including the effects environmental factors have on a person's gene expression, called epigenetics, account for between 40 and 60 percent of a person's risk of addiction. Also, teens and people with mental disorders are at greater risk of drug use and addiction than others.

What Environmental Factors Increase the Risk of Addiction

Environmental factors are those related to the family, school, and neighborhood. Factors that can increase a person's risk include the following:

- **Home and family.** The home environment, especially during childhood, is a very important factor. Parents or older family members who use drugs or misuse alcohol, or who break the law, can increase children's risk of future drug problems.

- **Peer and school.** Friends and other peers can have an increasingly strong influence during the teen years. Teens who use drugs can sway even those without risk factors to try drugs for the first time. Struggling in school or having poor social skills can put a child at further risk for using or becoming addicted to drugs.

What Other Factors Increase the Risk of Addiction

Besides the factors mentioned above there are a few other factors too that increase the risk of addiction. They are:

- **Early use.** Although taking drugs at any age can lead to addiction, research shows that the earlier a person begins to use drugs, the more likely he or she is to develop serious problems. This may be due to the harmful effect that drugs can have on the developing brain. It also may result from a mix of early social and biological risk factors, including lack of a stable home or family, exposure to physical or sexual abuse, genes, or mental illness. Still, the fact remains that early use is a strong indicator of problems ahead, including addiction.

- **How the drug is taken.** Smoking a drug or injecting it into a vein increases its addictive potential. Both smoked and injected drugs enter the brain within seconds, producing a powerful rush of pleasure. However, this intense high can fade within a few minutes. Scientists believe this starkly felt contrast drives some people to repeated drug taking in an attempt to recapture the fleeting pleasurable state.

The Adolescent Brain

The brain continues to develop into adulthood and undergoes dramatic changes during adolescence. One of the brain areas still maturing during adolescence is the prefrontal cortex—the part of the brain that allows people to assess situations, make sound decisions, and keep emotions and desires under control. The fact that this critical part of a teen's brain is still a work in progress puts them at increased risk for making poor decisions, such as trying drugs or continuing to take them. Introducing drugs during this period of development may cause brain changes that have profound and long-lasting consequences.

Chapter 3

How Drugs Impact Brain

The human brain is the most complex organ in the body. This three-pound mass of gray and white matter sits at the center of all human activity—you need it to drive a car, to enjoy a meal, to breathe, to create an artistic masterpiece, and to enjoy everyday activities. The brain regulates your body's basic functions, enables you to interpret and respond to everything you experience, and shapes your behavior. In short, your brain is you—everything you think and feel, and who you are.

How Does the Brain Work?

The brain is often likened to an incredibly complex and intricate computer. Instead of electrical circuits on the silicon chips that control our electronic devices, the brain consists of billions of cells, called "neurons," which are organized into circuits and networks. Each neuron acts as a switch controlling the flow of information. If a neuron receives enough signals from other neurons connected to it, it "fires," sending its own signal on to other neurons in the circuit.

The brain is made up of many parts with interconnected circuits that all work together as a team. Different brain circuits are responsible for coordinating and performing specific functions. Networks of neurons send signals back and forth to each other and among different

This chapter includes text excerpted from "Drugs, Brains, and Behavior: The Science of Addiction," National Institute on Drug Abuse (NIDA), July 2018.

parts of the brain, the spinal cord, and nerves in the rest of the body (the peripheral nervous system).

To send a message, a neuron releases a neurotransmitter into the gap (or synapse) between it and the next cell. The neurotransmitter crosses the synapse and attaches to receptors on the receiving neuron, like a key into a lock. This causes changes in the receiving cell. Other molecules, called "transporters," recycle neurotransmitters (that is, bring them back into the neuron that released them), thereby limiting or shutting off the signal between neurons.

How Do Drugs Work in the Brain?

Drugs interfere with the way neurons send, receive, and process signals via neurotransmitters. Some drugs, such as marijuana and heroin, can activate neurons because their chemical structure mimics that of a natural neurotransmitter in the body. This allows the drugs to attach onto and activate the neurons. Although, these drugs mimic the brain's own chemicals, they don't activate neurons in the same way as a natural neurotransmitter, and they lead to abnormal messages being sent through the network.

Other drugs, such as amphetamine or cocaine, can cause the neurons to release abnormally large amounts of natural neurotransmitters or prevent the normal recycling of these brain chemicals by interfering with transporters. This too amplifies or disrupts the normal communication between neurons.

What Parts of the Brain Are Affected by Drug Use?

Drugs can alter important brain areas that are necessary for life-sustaining functions and can drive the compulsive drug use that marks addiction. Brain areas affected by drug use include:

- **The basal ganglia**, which play an important role in positive forms of motivation, including the pleasurable effects of healthy activities like eating, socializing, and sex, and are also involved in the formation of habits and routines. These areas form a key node of what is sometimes called the brain's "reward circuit." Drugs overactivate this circuit, producing the euphoria of the drug high; but with repeated exposure, the circuit adapts to the presence of the drug, diminishing its sensitivity and making it hard to feel pleasure from anything besides the drug.

- **The extended amygdala** plays a role in stressful feelings like anxiety, irritability, and unease, which characterize withdrawal after the drug high fades and thus motivates the person to seek the drug again. This circuit becomes increasingly sensitive with increased drug use. Over time, a person with substance-use disorder uses drugs to get temporary relief from this discomfort rather than to get high.

- **The prefrontal cortex** powers the ability to think, plan, solve problems, make decisions, and exert self-control over impulses. This is also the last part of the brain to mature, making teens most vulnerable. Shifting balance between this circuit and the reward and stress circuits of the basal ganglia and extended amygdala makes a person with a substance-use disorder seek the drug compulsively with reduced impulse control.

Some drugs, such as opioids, also affect other parts of the brain, such as the brain stem, which control basic functions critical to life, such as heart rate, breathing, and sleeping, which helps explain why overdoses can cause depressed breathing and death.

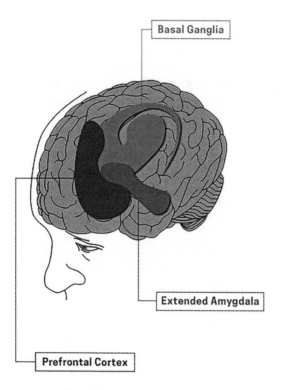

Figure 3.1. *Parts of the Brain* (Source: Facing Addiction in America: The Surgeon General's Report on Alcohol, Drugs, and Health)

How Do Drugs Produce Pleasure?

Pleasure or euphoria—the high from drugs—is still poorly understood, but probably involves surges of chemical signaling compounds including the body's natural opioids (endorphins) and other neurotransmitters in parts of the basal ganglia (the reward circuit). When some drugs are taken, they can cause surges of these neurotransmitters much greater than the smaller bursts, naturally produced in association with healthy rewards like eating, music, creative pursuits, or social interaction.

It was once thought that surges of the neurotransmitter dopamine produced by drugs directly caused the euphoria, but scientists now think dopamine has more to do with getting us to repeat pleasurable activities (reinforcement) than with producing pleasure directly.

How Does Dopamine Reinforce Drug Use?

Our brains are wired to increase the odds that we will repeat pleasurable activities. The neurotransmitter dopamine is central to this. Whenever the reward circuit is activated by a healthy,

A pleasurable experience, a burst of dopamine signals that something important is happening that needs to be remembered. This dopamine signal causes changes in neural connectivity that make it easier to repeat the activity again and again without thinking about it, leading to the formation of habits.

Just as drugs produce intense euphoria, they also produce much larger surges of dopamine, powerfully reinforcing the connection between consumption of the drug, the resulting pleasure, and all the external cues linked to the experience. Large surges of dopamine "teach" the brain to seek drugs at the expense of other, healthier goals and activities.

Cues in a person's daily routine or environment that have become linked with drug use because of changes to the reward circuit can trigger uncontrollable cravings whenever the person is exposed to these cues, even if the drug itself is not available. This learned "reflex" can last a long time, even in people who haven't used drugs in many years. For example, people who have been drug-free for a decade can experience cravings when returning to an old neighborhood or house where they used drugs. As with riding a bike, the brain remembers.

Why Are Drugs More Addictive than Natural Rewards?

For the brain, the difference between normal rewards and drug rewards can be likened to the difference between someone whispering into your ear and someone shouting into a microphone. Just as we turn down the volume on a radio that is too loud, the brain of someone who misuses drugs adjusts by producing fewer neurotransmitters in the reward circuit, or by reducing the number of receptors that can receive signals. As a result, the person's ability to experience pleasure from naturally rewarding (i.e., reinforcing) activities is also reduced.

This is why a person who misuses drugs eventually feels flat, without motivation, lifeless, and/or depressed, and is unable to enjoy things that were previously pleasurable. Now, the person needs to keep taking drugs to experience even a normal level of reward—which only makes the problem worse, like a vicious cycle. Also, the person will often need to take larger amounts of the drug to produce the familiar high—an effect known as tolerance.

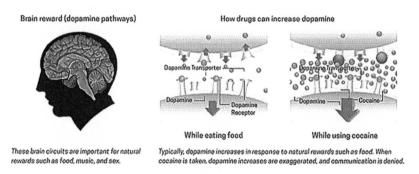

Brain reward (dopamine pathways)

How drugs can increase dopamine

While eating food

While using cocaine

These brain circuits are important for natural rewards such as food, music, and sex.

Typically, dopamine increases in response to natural rewards such as food. When cocaine is taken, dopamine increases are exaggerated, and communication is denied.

Figure 3.2. *Some Drugs Target the Brain's Pleasure Center*

Chapter 4

Genetics and Epigenetics of Addiction

Why do some people become addicted while others don't?

Family studies that include identical twins, fraternal twins, adoptees, and siblings suggest that as much as half of a person's risk of becoming addicted to nicotine, alcohol, or other drugs depends on his or her genetic makeup. Pinning down the biological basis for this risk is an important avenue of research for scientists trying to solve the problem of drug addiction.

Genes—functional units of deoxyribonucleic acid (DNA) that make up the human genome—provide the information that directs a body's basic cellular activities. Research on the human genome has shown that, on average, the DNA sequences of any two people are 99.9 percent the same. However, that 0.1 percent variation is profoundly important—it's still three million differences in the nearly three billion base pairs of DNA sequence! These differences contribute to visible variations, such as height and hair color, and invisible traits, such as increased risk for or protection from certain diseases such as heart attack, stroke, diabetes, and addiction.

Some diseases, such as sickle cell anemia (SCA) or cystic fibrosis (CF), are caused by an error, known as a mutation, in a single gene. Some mutations, such as the *BRCA1* and *2* mutations that are linked to a much higher risk of breast and ovarian cancer, have become critical

This chapter includes text excerpted from "Genetics and Epigenetics of Addiction," National Institute on Drug Abuse (NIDA), February 2016.

medical tools in evaluating a patient's risk for serious diseases. Medical researchers have had striking success at unraveling the genetics of these single-gene disorders, though finding treatments or cures have not been as simple. Most diseases, including addiction, are complex, and variations in many different genes contribute to a person's overall level of risk or protection. The good news is that scientists are actively pursuing many more paths to treatment and prevention of these more complex illnesses.

Linking Genes to Health: Genome-Wide Association Studies

The advances in DNA analysis are helping researchers untangle complex genetic interactions by examining a person's entire genome all at once. Technologies such as genome-wide association studies (GWAS), whole genome sequencing, and exome sequencing (looking at just the protein-coding genes) identify subtle variations in DNA sequence called single-nucleotide polymorphisms (SNPs). SNPs are differences in just a single letter of the genetic code from one person to another. If an SNP appears more often in people with a disease than those without, it is thought to either directly affect susceptibility to that disease or be a marker for another variation that does.

GWAS and sequencing are extremely powerful tools because they can find a connection between a known gene or genes and a disorder, and can identify genes that may have been overlooked or were previously unknown.

Through these methods, scientists can gather more evidence from affected families or use animal models and biochemical experiments to verify and understand the link between a gene and the risk of addiction. These findings would then be the basis for developing new treatment and intervention approaches.

The Role of the Environment in Diseases Such as Addiction

That old saying "nature or nurture" might be better phrased "nature and nurture" because research shows that a person's health is the result of dynamic interactions between genes and the environment. For example, both genetics and lifestyle factors—such as diet, physical activity, and stress—affect high blood pressure risk. National Institute on Drug Abuse (NIDA) research has led to discoveries about how a person's surroundings affect drug use in particular.

For example, a community that provides healthy after-school activities has been shown to reduce vulnerability to drug addiction, and available data show that access to exercise can discourage drug-seeking behavior, an effect that is more pronounced in males than in females.

In addition, studies suggest that an animal's drug use can be affected by that of its cage mate, showing that some social influences can enhance risk or protection. In addition, exposure to drugs or stress in a person's social or cultural environment can alter both gene expression and gene function, which, in some cases, may persist throughout a person's life. Research also suggests that genes can play a part in how a person responds to his or her environment, placing some people at higher risk for disease than others.

Epigenetics: Where Genes Meet the Environment

Epigenetics is the study of functional, and sometimes inherited, changes in the regulation of gene activity and expression that are not dependent on gene sequence. "Epi-" itself means "above" or "in addition to." Environmental exposures or choices people make can actually "mark"—or remodel—the structure of DNA at the cell level or even at the level of the whole organism. So, although each cell type in the human body effectively contains the same genetic information, epigenetic regulatory systems enable the development of different cell types (e.g., skin, liver, or nerve cells) in response to the environment. These epigenetic marks can affect health and even the expression of the traits passed to children. For example, when a person uses cocaine, it can mark the DNA, increasing the production of proteins common in addiction. Increased levels of these altered proteins correspond with drug-seeking behaviors in animals.

Histones, as another example, are like protein spools that provide an organizational structure for genes. Genes coil around histones, tightening or loosening to control gene expression. Drug exposure can affect specific histones, modifying gene expression in localized brain regions. Science has shown that manipulation of histone-modifying enzymes and binding proteins may have promise in treating substance-use disorders.

The development of multidimensional data sets that include and integrate genetic and epigenetic information provides unique insights into the molecular genetic processes underlying the causes and consequences of drug addiction. Studying and using these data types to identify biological factors involved in substance abuse is increasingly important because technologic advances have improved the ability of researchers to single out individual genes or brain processes that may inform new prevention and treatment interventions.

Genetics and Precision Medicine

Clinicians often find substantial variability in how individual patients respond to treatment. Part of that variability is due to genetics. Genes influence the numbers and types of receptors in people's brain, how quickly their bodies metabolize drugs, and how well they respond to different medications. Learning more about the genetic, epigenetic, and neurobiological bases of addiction will eventually advance the science of addiction.

Scientists will be able to translate this knowledge into new treatments directed at specific targets in the brain or to treatment approaches that can be customized for each patient—called pharmacogenomics. This emerging science, often called precision medicine, promises to harness the power of genomic information to improve treatments for addiction by tailoring the treatment to the person's specific genetic makeup. By knowing a person's genomic information, healthcare providers will be better equipped to match patients with the most suitable treatments and medication dosages, and to avoid or minimize adverse reactions.

Chapter 5

Drug Abuse and Related Hospitalization Costs

Chapter Contents

Section 5.1

Substance Abuse Cost to Society

This section contains text excerpted from the following sources: Text under the heading "Costs of Substance Abuse" is excerpted from "Trends and Statistics," National Institute on Drug Abuse (NIDA), April 2017; Text under the heading "Overview of Study Findings" is excerpted from "Excessive Drinking Is Draining the U.S. Economy," National Institute for Occupational Safety and Health (NIOSH), Centers for Disease Control and Prevention (CDC), July 13, 2018.

Costs of Substance Abuse

Abuse of tobacco, alcohol, and illicit drugs is costly to the nation, exacting more than $740 billion annually in costs related to crime, lost work productivity, and healthcare.

Table 5.1. Costs of Substance Abuse

	Healthcare	Overall	Year Estimate Based On
Tobacco	$168 billion	$300 billion	2010
Alcohol	$27 billion	$249 billion	2010
Illicit Drugs	$11 billion	$193 billion	2007
Prescription Opioids	$26 billion	$78.5 billion	2013

Overview of Study Findings

The cost of excessive alcohol use in the United States rose to almost a quarter trillion dollars in 2010. Implementing effective community-based interventions can reduce excessive drinking and its costs.

Excessive alcohol use is known to kill about 88,000 people in the United States each year, but a Centers for Disease Control and Prevention (CDC) study suggests it is also a drain on the American economy, mostly due to losses in workplace productivity.

Total Cost

The cost of excessive alcohol use in the United States reached $249 billion in 2010, or about $2.05 per drink. Most (77%) of these costs were due to binge drinking. Binge drinking is defined as drinking four or more alcoholic beverages per occasion for women or five or more drinks per occasion for men. Further, two of every five dollars were paid by federal, state, and local governments, demonstrating that we are all paying for excessive alcohol use.

State Costs

Excessive alcohol use cost states and the District of Columbia (DC) a median of $3.5 billion in 2010, ranging from $488 million in North Dakota to $35 billion in California. DC had the highest cost per person ($1,526, compared to the $807 national average), and New Mexico had the highest cost per drink ($2.77, compared to the $2.05 national average).

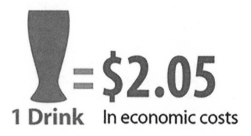

1 Drink In economic costs

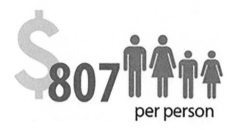

per person

Figure 5.1. *Cost of Drinking*

Cost Breakout

The researchers found that the cost of this dangerous behavior impacts many aspects of the drinker's life and the lives of those around them. However, most of the costs resulted from losses in workplace productivity (72% of the total cost), healthcare expenses for treating problems caused by excessive drinking (11% of total), law enforcement and other criminal justice expenses (10%), and losses from motor vehicle crashes related to excessive alcohol use (5%).

These estimates update two previous CDC studies that found excessive drinking cost the U.S. $223.5 billion and cost states and DC a median of $2.9 billion in 2006. The researchers believe that the study still underestimates the cost of excessive drinking because information on alcohol is often underreported or unavailable, and the study did not include other costs, such as pain and suffering due to alcohol-related injuries and diseases.

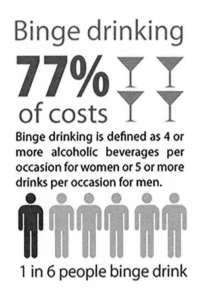

Figure 5.2. *Cost of Binge Drinking*

How Excessive Alcohol Consumption Can Be Prevented and Reduce Its Economic Costs

Communities can use effective interventions to prevent excessive drinking and related harms and costs. These include:

- Implementing pricing strategies to increase the price of alcohol

- Regulating the number and location of outlets at which alcohol is sold (outlet density)

- Holding alcohol retailers liable for injuries or damages caused by their intoxicated or underage customers

- Avoiding moving from state-controlled alcohol sales to commercial alcohol sales (privatization)

Section 5.2

Drug-Related Hospital Emergency Room Visits

This section includes text excerpted from "Drug-Related Hospital Emergency Room Visits," National Institute on Drug Abuse (NIDA), May 2011. Reviewed January 2019.

National estimates on drug-related visits to hospital emergency departments (ED) are obtained from the Drug Abuse Warning Network (DAWN), a public health surveillance system managed by the Substance Abuse and Mental Health Services Administration (SAMHSA), U.S. Department of Health and Human Services (HHS). DAWN data are based on a national sample of general, nonfederal hospitals operating 24-hour emergency departments (EDs). Information is collected for all types of drugs—including illegal drugs, inhalants, alcohol—and abuse of prescription and over-the-counter (OTC) medications and dietary supplements.

Highlights from the 2009 Drug Abuse Warning Network

In 2009, there were nearly 4.6 million drug-related ED visits nationwide. These visits included reports of drug abuse, adverse reactions to drugs, or other drug-related consequences. Almost 50 percent were attributed to adverse reactions to pharmaceuticals taken as prescribed, and 45 percent involved drug abuse. DAWN estimates that of the 2.1 million drug abuse visits:

- 27.1 percent involved nonmedical use of pharmaceuticals (i.e., prescription or OTC medications, dietary supplements)

- 21.2 percent involved illicit drugs

- 14.3 percent involved alcohol, in combination with other drugs

ED visits involving nonmedical use of pharmaceuticals (either alone or in combination with another drug) increased 98.4 percent between 2004 and 2009, from 627,291 visits to 1,244,679, respectively. ED visits involving adverse reactions to pharmaceuticals increased 82.9 percent between 2005 and 2009, from 1,250,377 to 2,287,273 visits, respectively.

The majority of drug-related ED visits were made by patients 21 or older (80.9%, or 3,717,030 visits). Of these, slightly less than half involved drug abuse. Patients age 20 or younger accounted for 19.1 percent (877,802 visits) of all drug-related visits in 2009; about half of these visits involved drug abuse.

Illicit Drugs

In 2009, almost one million visits involved an illicit drug, either alone or in combination with other types of drugs. DAWN estimates that:

- Cocaine was involved in 422,896 ED visits.

- Marijuana was involved in 376,467 ED visits.

- Heroin was involved in 213,118 ED visits.

- Stimulants, including amphetamines and methamphetamine, were involved in 93,562 ED visits.

- Other illicit drugs—such as phencyclidine (PCP), ecstasy, and gamma-hydroxybutyrate (GHB)—were involved much less frequently than any of the drug types mentioned above.

The rates of ED visits involving cocaine, marijuana, and heroin were higher for males than for females. Rates for cocaine were highest among individuals age 35 to 44, rates for heroin were highest among individuals age 21 to 24, stimulant use was highest among those 25 to 29, and marijuana use was highest for those age 18 to 20.

Alcohol and Other Drugs

Approximately 32 percent (658,263) of all drug abuse ED visits in 2009 involved the use of alcohol, either alone or in combination with another drug. DAWN reports alcohol-related data when it is used alone among individuals under the age of 21 or in combination with other drugs among all groups, regardless of age. Because DAWN does not account for ED visits involving alcohol use alone in adults, the actual number of ED visits involving alcohol among the general population is thought to be significantly higher than what is reported in DAWN.

In 2009, DAWN estimated 519,650 ED visits related to the use of alcohol in combination with other drugs. Alcohol was most frequently combined with:

- Central nervous system (CNS) agents (e.g., analgesics, stimulants, sedatives) (229,230 visits)

- Cocaine (152,631 visits)

- Marijuana (125,438 visits)

- Psychotherapeutic agents (e.g., antidepressants and antipsychotics) (44,217 visits)

- Heroin (43,110 visits)

While alcohol use is illegal for individuals under age 21, DAWN estimates that in 2009 there were 199,429 alcohol-related ED visits among individuals under age 21; 76,918 ED visits were reported among those age 12 to 17, and 120,853 alcohol-related ED visits were reported among those age 18 to 20.

Nonmedical Use of Pharmaceuticals

In 2009, 1.2 million ED visits involved the nonmedical use of pharmaceuticals or dietary supplements. The most frequently reported drugs in the nonmedical use category of ED visits were opiate/opioid analgesics, present in 50 percent of nonmedical-use ED visits; and psychotherapeutic agents, (commonly used to treat anxiety and sleep disorders), present in more than one-third of nonmedical ED visits. Included among the most frequently reported opioids were single-ingredient formulations (e.g., oxycodone) and combination forms (e.g., hydrocodone with acetaminophen). Methadone, together with single-ingredient and combination forms of oxycodone and hydrocodone, was also included under the most frequently reported opioids classification:

- Hydrocodone (alone or in combination) in 104,490 ED visits

- Oxycodone (alone or in combination) in 175,949 ED visits

- Methadone in 70,637 ED visits

Increases in Drug-Related ED Visits over Time

The total number of drug-related ED visits increased 81 percent from 2004 (2.5 million) to 2009 (4.6 million). ED visits involving nonmedical use of pharmaceuticals increased 98.4 percent over the same period, from 627,291 visits to 1,244,679.

The largest pharmaceutical increases were observed for oxycodone products (242.2% increase), alprazolam (148.3% increase), and hydrocodone products (124.5%). Among ED visits involving illicit drugs, only those involving ecstasy increased more than 100 percent from 2004 to 2009 (123.2% increase).

For patients age 20 or younger, ED visits resulting from nonmedical use of pharmaceuticals increased 45.4 percent between 2004 and 2009 (116,644 and 169,589 visits, respectively). Among patients age 21 or older, there was an increase of 111.0 percent.

ED visits involving adverse reactions to pharmaceuticals increased 82.9 percent between 2005 and 2009, from 1,250,377 visits to 2,287,273. The majority of adverse reaction visits were made by patients 21 or older, particularly among patients 65 or older; the rate increased 89.2 percent from 2005 to 2009 among this age group.

Section 5.3

Increase in Emergency Room Visits Related to Ecstasy

This section includes text excerpted from "Ecstasy-Related Emergency Department Visits by Young People Increased between 2005 and 2011; Alcohol Involvement Remains a Concern," Substance Abuse and Mental Health Services Administration (SAMHSA), December 3, 2013. Reviewed January 2019.

MDMA (3,4-methylenedioxymethamphetamine), also known as Ecstasy or Molly, is an illicit drug that has both stimulant and hallucinogenic properties. Ecstasy is usually taken by mouth, but can also be snorted or smoked. Ecstasy produces feelings of increased energy, euphoria, and distorts the user's senses and perception of time.

Abuse of ecstasy can produce a variety of undesirable health effects such as anxiety and confusion. These effects can last one week or longer after using the drug. Also, serious health risks such as becoming dangerously overheated, high blood pressure, and kidney and heart failure are associated with ecstasy abuse. When ecstasy is mixed with alcohol, the stimulating effects of ecstasy cause the user to be less aware of alcohol intoxication. This mixture can lead to poor decision making and bodily harm. The ecstasy–alcohol mixture also causes a longer lasting euphoria than ecstasy or alcohol alone, which could increase the potential for abuse.

According to the Drug Abuse Warning Network (DAWN), the estimated number of emergency department (ED) visits involving ecstasy in patients younger than 21 years old increased 128 percent, from 4,460 visits in 2005 to 2010, 176 visits in 2011. In each year from 2005 to 2011, an average of 33 percent of ED visits among those younger than 21 that involved ecstasy also involved alcohol. The increase in ED visits involving ecstasy in this population is a cause for concern due to the serious health risks involved with ecstasy use and the higher potential for abuse when ecstasy is mixed with alcohol.

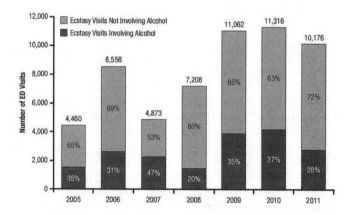

Figure 5.3. *Emergency Department (ED) Visits Involving Ecstasy in Patients Younger than 21, by Alcohol Involvement: 2005 to 2011.*

Section 5.4

Deaths from Drug Overdoses

This section includes text excerpted from "U.S. Drug Overdose Deaths Continue to Rise; Increase Fueled by Synthetic Opioids," Centers for Disease Control and Prevention (CDC), March 29, 2018.

An in-depth analysis of 2016 U.S. drug overdose data shows that America's overdose epidemic is spreading geographically and increasing across demographic groups. The report, from researchers at the

Centers for Disease Control and Prevention (CDC), appeared in an issue of Morbidity and Mortality Weekly Report (MMWR).

Drug overdoses killed 63,632 Americans in 2016. Nearly two-thirds of these deaths (66%) involved a prescription or illicit opioid. Overdose deaths increased in all categories of drugs examined for men and women, people ages 15 and older, all races and ethnicities, and across all levels of urbanization.

The CDC's analysis confirms that recent increases in drug overdose deaths are driven by continued sharp increases in deaths involving synthetic opioids other than methadone, such as illicitly manufactured fentanyl (IMF).

"No area of the United States is exempt from this epidemic—we all know a friend, family member, or loved one devastated by opioids," said CDC Principal Deputy Director Anne Schuchat, M.D. "All branches of the federal government are working together to reduce the availability of illicit drugs, prevent deaths from overdoses, treat people with substance-use disorders, and prevent people from starting using drugs in the first place."

The CDC's analysis, based on 2015 to 2016 data from 31 states and Washington, DC, showed:

- Across demographic categories, the largest increase in opioid overdose death rates was in males between the ages of 25 to 44.

- Overall drug overdose death rates increased by 21.5 percent.

- The overdose death rate from synthetic opioids (other than methadone) more than doubled, likely driven by illicitly manufactured fentanyl (IMF).

- The prescription opioid-related overdose death rate increased by 10.6 percent.

- The heroin-related overdose death rate increased by 19.5 percent.

- The cocaine-related overdose death rate increased by 52.4 percent.

- The psychostimulant-related overdose death rate increased by 33.3 percent.

IMF is mixed into counterfeit opioid and benzodiazepine pills, heroin, and cocaine, likely contributing to increases in overdoses involving these other substances.

Overdose Death Rates Differ by State

Opioid death rates differed across the states examined in this study:

- Death rates from overdoses involving synthetic opioids increased in 21 states, with 10 states doubling their rates from 2015 to 2016.

- New Hampshire, West Virginia, and Massachusetts had the highest death rates from synthetic opioids.

- Fourteen states had significant increases in death rates involving heroin, with Washington DC, West Virginia, and Ohio having the highest rates.

- Eight states had significant increases in death rates involving prescription opioids. West Virginia, Maryland, Maine, and Utah had the highest rates.

- Sixteen states had significant increases in death rates involving cocaine, with Washington DC, Rhode Island, and Ohio having the highest rates.

- Fourteen states had significant increases in death rates involving psychostimulants; the highest death rates occurred primarily in the Midwest and Western regions.

"Effective, synchronized programs to prevent drug overdoses will require coordination of law enforcement, first responders, mental health/substance-abuse providers, public health agencies, and community partners," said the report's lead author, Puja Seth, Ph.D.

How to Coordinate the Public-Health and Public-Safety Responses to Overdose Deaths

The CDC's report highlights the continued need for public health and law enforcement to work together in preventing overdose deaths and taking action to:

- Protect people with opioid-use disorder (OUD) by expanding treatment capacity and naloxone distribution

- Support programs that reduce the harms of injecting opioids, including programs offering screening for human immunodeficiency virus (HIV) and hepatitis B and C in combination with referral to treatment

- Improve coordination among law enforcement and public-health agencies to reduce and improve detection of the illicit opioid supply

- Improve opioid prescribing to reduce unnecessary exposure to opioids and prevent addiction by training providers and implementing CDC's *Guideline for Prescribing Opioids for Chronic Pain*

- Improve access to and use of prescription drug monitoring programs

Chapter 6

Understanding the Legal Use of Controlled Substances

Chapter Contents

Section 6.1

Prescriptions for Controlled Substances

This section includes text excerpted from "Drug Diversion
Toolkit: Controlled Substance Integrity—Documentation From
Drop-Off to Pickup," Centers for Medicare & Medicaid
Services (CMS), February 2016.

Abuse of Controlled Substances

The abuse of controlled substances in the United States and their
diversion to individuals for whom they were not prescribed is a seemingly uphill battle for healthcare professionals, law enforcement, and
policymakers. The crisis extends beyond our country's borders. The
Global Burden of Disease (GBD) Study 2010 is the first of its kind to
assess the worldwide burden of disease attributable to illicit-drug use
and dependence. The study demonstrated that opioid dependence was
the primary contributor to illicit drug-related deaths worldwide. In
addition, the United States was one of the top four countries in the
world with the highest rate of burden. From 1999 to 2010, opioid-related deaths in the United States dramatically increased in number,
according to the Centers for Disease Control and Prevention (CDC).
The number of deaths parallels the 300 percent increase in sales of
opioid prescriptions during that same time.

While pharmacists routinely use their professional judgment when
determining whether to fill prescriptions for controlled substances,
added scrutiny is required to prevent diversion to the illicit drug market. Pharmacists are responsible for dispensing prescription drugs
appropriately while intercepting prescriptions that are not issued by
authorized prescribers for lawful medicinal purposes. As the primary
gatekeepers between prescriptions and access to controlled substances,
pharmacists are strategically positioned to ensure that all requirements are met in order to comply with State and Federal regulations.

Drop-Off
Patient Identification

Verification that a prescription was issued to a valid patient is one
of the first steps to ensure the integrity of a prescription for a controlled
substance. Patient identification is an important dispensing consideration, so identification issues may occur at drop-off, at pickup, or
both. It is good practice for a patient to provide identification when the

pharmacy staff does not know the patient. This practice will help prevent fraud, waste, and abuse in the pharmacy, including, for example, the fraudulent use of another's identity to obtain drugs under a false claim for a Federal benefit. Medicaid law requires that the pharmacist make a reasonable effort to obtain, record, and maintain identifying information on individuals receiving prescription drug benefits under the program. The U.S. Drug Enforcement Administration's (DEA) Office of Diversion Control explains that pharmacists must require "every purchaser of a controlled substance not known to him or her to furnish suitable identification" when dispensing controlled substances that are not prescription drugs. Half of all States go a step further—as of June 30, 2013, 25 States required or allowed pharmacists to request patient identification prior to dispensing a prescription for any controlled substance. Individual pharmacies may choose to establish a policy requiring photo identification as well. Examples of typically acceptable forms of identification include a valid driver's license or similar State-issued photo identification card, a military identification card, or a passport.

A prescription drug monitoring program (PDMP, or just PMP) is a State-sponsored prescription drug database that provides a unified system for sharing patients' prescription information between healthcare practitioners, pharmacists, and members of law enforcement who are authorized to use the system. In addition, some States that require pharmacies to record a patient's proof of identity and other personally identifiable information in the State's PDMP. How PDMPs are used, when they must be queried, what information is recorded, and who may access the information varies from State to State as do the reporting requirements.

As of January 2016, 30 States are participating members in the National Association of Boards of Pharmacy's (NABP) PMP Inter-Connect, which allows those with access to a State's PDMP to search other member States' PDMPs for patients who may be doctor shopping across State lines.

In addition to verification of a patient's identity, pharmacy personnel should exercise professional judgment regarding the type of information provided by the patient prior to filling the prescription. According to the DEA, common characteristics of a drug abuser include:

- Patient provides vague or evasive answers for medical history or allergies

- Patient claims to be from out of town

- Patient claims to have no regular doctor

- Patient claims to have no health insurance
- Patient has an unusually high level of knowledge of controlled substances and
- Patient claims that only a particular medication is effective

Pharmacy technicians and interns should document any of the above information on the prescription hard copy when a customer drops off the prescription. Pharmacists should review this information to determine if there needs to be further investigation.

Prescription Requirements

Performing a thorough inspection of the prescription hard copy is essential to ensure controlled substance integrity. This step may help identify a photocopied or altered prescription. October 1, 2008, Federal law has required that printed prescriptions issued to Medicaid patients have these three tamper-resistant characteristics:

1. One or more industry-recognized features designed to prevent unauthorized copying of a completed or blank prescription form;

2. One or more industry-recognized features designed to prevent the erasure or modification of information written on the prescription pad by the prescriber; and

3. One or more industry-recognized features designed to prevent the use of counterfeit prescription forms.

In addition to ensuring that a prescription is issued on a tamper-resistant prescription blank for Medicaid patients and that the prescription has not been altered or tampered with, pharmacy personnel should ensure that the prescription contains all required information. A valid prescription for a controlled substance must contain all of the following:

- Patient's full name and address
- Drug name, strength, dosage form
- Quantity or amount prescribed
- Directions for use
- Practitioner's name and address and
- Practitioner's DEA registration number
- Number of refills authorized; Schedule II (C-II) prescriptions may not be refilled

Federal law mandates that a prescriber sign and date a prescription for a controlled substance on the day he or she issues it. There is no Federal limit on when a written C-II prescription expires. However, some States, such as Louisiana, have established expiration rules on such prescriptions. Even though U.S. Code does not allow refill of C-II prescriptions, the DEA generally allows a provider to issue multiple subsequent prescriptions for C-II substances.

Prescribing Authority

In addition to verifying that the prescription blank appears valid and contains all required information, the pharmacist should recognize whether the practitioner has authority to prescribe the controlled substance in the State where the prescription was written. A June 2013 report released by the U.S. Department of Health and Human Services (HHS), Office of Inspector General (HHS-OIG) found that in 2009, tens of thousands of prescriptions (including 29,212 prescriptions for controlled substances) were inappropriately ordered nationwide by individuals who did not have the authority to prescribe medications and were paid for under Medicare Part D. This finding was based on a comparison of prescriptions found in Centers for Medicare & Medicaid Services (CMS) prescription drug event (PDE) database with the qualifications of prescribers as reflected in CMS' National Plan and Provider Enumeration System (NPPES) database. Using this data, HHS-OIG identified the top four types of providers that had prescribed Part D drugs without authority: dietitians and nutritionists; audiologists or other hearing- and speech-related service providers; massage therapists; and athletic trainers. In its comments on the report, CMS noted that "the instances identified by OIG are likely due to administrative data input and maintenance issues affecting database accuracy and reliability." While there is some question about the extent of prescribing without authority, CMS and HHS-OIG agree that guidance is needed to identify and investigate apparent instances of prescribing without authority.

Effective June 1, 2010, mid-level practitioners received Federal prescribing authority. Mid-level practitioners provide care to patients while working under the supervision of a physician and may include physician assistants, nurse practitioners, and nurse anesthetists just to name a few. A mid-level practitioner may be authorized to prescribe controlled substances depending on the regulations of the State in which he or she practices. To ensure that a practitioner is prescribing within the scope of practice designated by Federal and State law, pharmacy technicians and pharmacists should be familiar with the prescribing scope of all practitioners, including mid-level practitioners in their State.

Pharmacy personnel should be familiar with 21 C.F.R. Section 1306.04, which states that a pharmacist has the corresponding responsibility to ensure that a prescription for a controlled substance is issued in the "usual course" of business for the prescriber and for a "legitimate medical purpose."

Electronic Prescribing

A Federal rule to allow for e-prescribing of controlled substances became effective June 1, 2010. Prescribers have the choice of writing prescriptions for controlled substances manually or electronically, and pharmacies may receive, dispense, and store electronic prescriptions electronically; however, not all States have authorized e-prescribing for controlled substances, especially C-II drugs. Pharmacists and technicians should be familiar with their State's e-prescribing regulatory requirements. The DEA requires registrants to comply with all State and Federal laws. When State laws are more restrictive than Federal laws, registrants must comply with the more stringent State requirements.

Multiple Schedule II Prescriptions

In certain instances, a prescriber may determine that it is appropriate to issue multiple prescriptions for C-II substances to a patient. Federal law permits a prescriber to issue "multiple prescriptions authorizing the patient to receive a total of up to a 90-days supply." The prescriber must date and sign each sequential prescription on the day he or she issues it and must indicate the earliest date that each prescription may be filled by annotating a "dispense after" date on each prescription blank. To ensure compliance, pharmacy personnel should make certain not to fill any prescription that contains a "dispense after" notation until the date designated on the C-II prescription.

The November 2007 Final Rule related to the issuance of multiple C-II prescriptions conflicted with previous regulations with respect to permissible changes to C-II prescriptions by pharmacists. Until the DEA resolves this matter, pharmacists should exercise professional judgment and comply with State and Federal regulations regarding changes that may be made to C-II prescriptions.

Changes to Controlled Substance Prescriptions by Pharmacists

Perform a careful inspection of the controlled substance prescription to ensure it does not contain any errors or require further clarification prior to filling. Only the following information may be changed on a Schedule III to V controlled substance prescription after consultation with the prescriber:

- Patient's address

- Drug strength

- Quantity to be dispensed

- Directions for use

- Issue date

- Dosage form, and

- Generic substitution

Pharmacists are prohibited from making any changes to the patient's name, the controlled substance prescribed (except for generic substitution), or the prescriber's signature. If any of the required information for a controlled substance is missing, or if the prescriber must be contacted to obtain or clarify any information prior to filling the prescription, the information should be documented on the prescription hard copy. A good practice is to record the date the information was obtained, the name of the prescriber or authorized agent (if applicable) who provided the required information, and the initials of the dispensing pharmacist on the prescription hard copy. When clarifying an electronic prescription for a controlled substance, pharmacists should print a hard copy on which to record the required information, rescan the prescription, and store the hard copy in a manner that complies with Federal requirements.

Drug Utilization Review

Prior to dispensing any prescription, a pharmacist should perform a drug utilization review of the patient's medication history. Pay particular attention to duplicate therapies, early refills, filling of drugs with antagonistic effects, and multiple prescribers for controlled substances. Also, be aware of drugs commonly misused for "bridging." In the outpatient setting, bridging may involve the

47

inappropriate use of prescription drugs by an abuser to reduce the severity of physiologic withdrawal symptoms associated with the abused substance of choice until the abuser can achieve the next high. Although bridging is more traditionally associated with the pharmaceutical management of patients residing in substance-abuse treatment centers, bridging in the outpatient setting may be considered misuse. Substances commonly involved in bridging may include methadone, buprenorphine, buprenorphine/naloxone, gabapentin, and tramadol. In addition, performing a routine review of previously documented patient notes and a review of the patient's medication history may alert the pharmacist to prior suspicious activity. This may include things such as a history of frequent early refill requests, lost or spilled medication, or corresponding follow-up communication notes with prescribers.

Controlled Substance Inventory Records and Dispensing

The *Pharmacist's Manual* states:

Every pharmacy must maintain complete and accurate records on a current basis for each controlled substance purchased, received, stored, distributed, dispensed, or otherwise disposed of. These records are required to provide accountability of all controlled substances from the manufacturing process through the dispensing pharmacy and to the ultimate user.

In addition, maintain C-II controlled substance records and inventories separately from all other records. Many pharmacies maintain a separate perpetual inventory system for C-II controlled substances. To ensure accuracy and accountability of those drugs, use a log book to record each time inventory is received, dispensed, recalled, or outdated and sent to a third party reverse distributor for destruction. Although the laws do not require every pharmacy to follow an identical process to manage controlled substance inventory and records, pharmacy personnel must ensure that the processes in place comply with all Federal and State requirements.

For purposes of accuracy and safety, implement a process to double count all controlled substance prescriptions prior to dispensing. The filling technician or pharmacist should verify the quantity to be dispensed, count the medication twice to ensure accuracy, circle the quantity verified, and document their initials on the prescription label.

Partial Fills

Federal law permits partial filling of Schedule III, IV, and V controlled substance prescriptions. In addition, the number of times the prescription is refilled may exceed the originally authorized number of refills so long as the total quantity of medication dispensed does not exceed the total quantity authorized on the original prescription. Record documentation of each partial filling of Schedules III, IV, and V prescriptions in the same manner as a refill.

Partial filling of C-II controlled substances is also permitted in certain situations. For example, a partial filling is permissible if the pharmacy is unable to supply the full quantity to the patient at the time the prescription is presented or called in for an emergency. The dispensing pharmacist must document the date, time, and partial quantity dispensed on the original C-II prescription hard copy. Federal law stipulates that any unfilled balance of the C-II prescription may be dispensed to the patient only within 72 hours of the first partial filling. If the remaining balance is either not filled or unable to be filled within 72 hours, the pharmacist must notify the prescriber, the remaining balance on the prescription must be forfeited, and no further quantities may be dispensed to the patient without a new prescription.

A partial filling of a C-II prescription is also permitted when the patient either resides in a long-term care facility or has been medically diagnosed with a terminal illness. A prescription that meets either of these criteria is valid for a maximum of 60 days from the date the prescriber issued it, and the medication may be dispensed in single units.

To be in compliance, ensure that evidence of terminal illness or residency in a long-term-care facility is documented on the original prescription hard copy. According to the Code of Federal Regulations (CFR): "For each partial filling, the dispensing pharmacist shall record on the back of the prescription (or on another appropriate record, uniformly maintained, and readily retrievable) the date of the partial filling, quantity dispensed, remaining quantity authorized to be dispensed, and the identification of the dispensing pharmacist."

Controlled Substance Refill Requests

In 2012, the DEA issued a letter of clarification to the legal counsel for Omnicare, Inc., (Omnicare) regarding the practice of sending refill reminders to prescribers on behalf of a patient for a controlled substance. The DEA determined that Omnicare was not complying with the Controlled Substances Act (CSA) because it was utilizing refill reminder notification forms that were prepopulated with all information, and only a prescriber's signature was required to make the prescription valid. In the letter, the DEA explicitly states that the intent of the CSA is to ensure that "every prescription for a controlled substance must be predicated on a determination by an individual practitioner that the dispensing of the controlled substance is for a legitimate medical purpose by a practitioner acting in the usual course of professional practice." In this instance, the DEA determined that Omnicare had acted as an unauthorized "agent" for the physician and the subsequent submission of such requests was a violation of the CSA. Although the Federal law has not changed, the $50 million settlement agreement that Omnicare reached with the DEA for this and other violations caught the attention of pharmacists, pharmacies, State pharmacy boards, and pharmacy associations nationwide. Retail and long-term care pharmacies may not submit a refill request to a practitioner for a controlled substance prescription that is in the format of a partially or fully prepopulated prescription template because the pharmacy is not an authorized "agent" of the prescriber. A reminder notification that contains a blank prescription template that the prescriber must complete is acceptable. Pharmacy personnel should assess controlled substance refill request procedures to ensure that the process and any associated forms comply with the CSA.

Pickup
Patient Counseling

Section 4401 of the Omnibus Budget Reconciliation Act of 1990 (OBRA '90) dramatically impacted the delivery of pharmaceutical care and the interaction between patient and pharmacist. OBRA '90 was initially established to improve therapeutic outcomes of Medicaid recipients and includes three key pharmaceutical components:

1. A prospective drug review of the patient's profile;

2. Maintenance of essential patient and drug therapy information;

3. Provision of medication counseling for all Medicaid patients.

To ensure compliance and as a condition of receiving Federal Medicaid funds, each State was required to establish standards. According to the National Association of Boards of Pharmacy (NABP), as of 2012, all 50 States and the District of Columbia (DC) require patient counseling or an offer to counsel for Medicaid beneficiaries. In addition, almost all States require pharmacies to maintain patient profiles. Although

OBRA '90 was initially established to improve the therapeutic outcomes of Medicaid patients, the application of State-mandated patient counseling requirements was extended to non-Medicaid patients in most States. All patients are entitled to the same standard of care with regard to patient counseling.

OBRA '90 patient counseling standards include:

- Name of the drug (brand name, generic, or other descriptive information)

- Intended use and expected action

- Route, dosage form, dosage, and administration schedule

- Common severe side effects or adverse effects or interactions and therapeutic contraindications that may be encountered, including how to avoid them and the action required if they occur

Techniques for self-monitoring of drug therapy:

- Proper storage

- Potential drug–drug interactions or drug-disease contraindications

- Prescription refill information, and

- Action to be taken in the event of a missed dose

Many States have unique requirements for: counseling when the patient is not in the pharmacy; the distribution of supplemental written materials; and notification to the patient when a generic substitution has been made. Pharmacy personnel are responsible for compliance with all patient counseling regulations in the States in which they practice. Patient counseling is an important part of healthcare delivery, especially since pharmacists have a "corresponding responsibility" to monitor patient use of prescription medications, especially controlled substances. Unfortunately, pharmacy counseling rates are consistently below 50 percent in surveys of the practice.

Documentation at the time a prescription is picked up is an important final step to ensure integrity when prescriptions for controlled substances are dispensed. Pharmacists and pharmacy technicians have a responsibility to ensure positive patient identification when prescriptions for a controlled substance are picked up. This measure helps prevent fraud, waste, and abuse, such as identity theft to obtain drugs under a false claim for a Federal benefit. State identification requirements and PDMP reporting requirements may vary. Pharmacists and pharmacy technicians should familiarize themselves with the regulations established by the State and corresponding compliance.

Signature Logs

Signature logs serve an important purpose in retail pharmacy. From the billing standpoint, they provide documentation of the delivery and receipt of services to patients. From the patient counseling standpoint, signature logs aid pharmacies with documenting that patient counseling was offered. A "yes" or "no" checkbox next to the signature can be marked by the patient or patient's agent when the prescription is picked up to document whether counseling was accepted or declined. A process should be established to ensure that prescriptions that are not picked up in the store (in other words, delivered or mailed) also comply with documentation requirements. Because signature logs are tools that may be utilized to demonstrate a pharmacy's compliance with billing, dispensing, and patient counseling requirements, they should be retained and stored in an organized manner in a secure location to facilitate retrieval in the event of a pharmacy audit.

Key Points

Pharmacists, pharmacy interns, and pharmacy technicians should integrate the following aspects when handling prescriptions for controlled substances:

- Confirm the patient's identity
- Verify that the prescription contains all required information
- Confirm the prescriber has authority to prescribe the medication
- Document any changes made to the original prescription as permitted by law
- Perform a drug utilization review
- Properly document full or partial dispensing(s)
- Verify that refill request forms comply with Federal and State requirements

- Comply with patient counseling requirements
- Collect patient signature to record the pickup of the medication
- Report required information to the state PDMP.

Section 6.2

Is Marijuana Medicine?

This section includes text excerpted from "Marijuana as Medicine," National Institute on Drug Abuse (NIDA), June 2018.

What Is Medical Marijuana?

The term *medical marijuana* refers to using the whole, unprocessed marijuana plant or its basic extracts to treat symptoms of illness and other conditions. The U.S. Food and Drug Administration (FDA) has not recognized or approved the marijuana plant as medicine.

However, scientific study of the chemicals in marijuana, called cannabinoids, has led to two FDA-approved medications that contain cannabinoid chemicals in pill form.

Because the marijuana plant contains chemicals that may help treat a range of illnesses and symptoms, many people argue that it should be legal for medical purposes. In fact, a growing number of states have legalized marijuana for medical use.

Why Isn't the Marijuana Plant an U.S. Food and Drug Administration-Approved Medicine?

The FDA requires carefully conducted studies (clinical trials) in hundreds to thousands of human subjects to determine the benefits and risks of a possible medication. So far, researchers haven't conducted enough large-scale clinical trials that show that the benefits of the marijuana plant (as opposed to its cannabinoid ingredients) outweigh its risks in patients it's meant to treat.

Some studies have suggested that medical marijuana legalization might be associated with decreased prescription opioid use and overdose deaths, but researchers don't have enough evidence yet to confirm this finding. For example, one study found that Medicare Part D prescriptions filled for all opioids decreased in states with medical marijuana laws. Another study examined Medicaid prescription data and found that medical marijuana laws and adult-use marijuana laws were associated with lower opioid prescribing rates (5.88 percent and 6.88 percent lower, respectively).

Additionally, one National Institute on Drug Abuse (NIDA)-funded study suggested a link between medical marijuana legalization and fewer overdose deaths from prescription opioids. These studies, however, are population-based and can't show that medical marijuana legalization caused the decrease in deaths or that pain patients changed their drug-taking behavior. A more detailed NIDA-funded analysis showed that legally protected medical marijuana dispensaries, not just medical marijuana laws, were also associated with a decrease in the following:

- Opioid prescribing

- Self-reports of opioid misuse

- Treatment admissions for opioid addiction

Additionally, some data suggests that medical marijuana treatment may reduce the opioid dose prescribed for pain patients, while another National Institutes of Health (NIH)-funded study suggests that *Cannabis* use appears to increase the risk of developing and opioid-use disorder. NIDA is funding additional studies to determine the link between medical marijuana use and the use or misuse of opioids for specific types of pain, and also its possible role for treatment of opioid-use disorder.

What Are Cannabinoids?

Cannabinoids are chemicals related to *delta-9-tetrahydrocannabinol* (THC), marijuana's main mind-altering ingredient that makes people "high." The marijuana plant contains more than 100 cannabinoids. Scientists as well as illegal manufacturers have produced many cannabinoids in the lab. Some of these cannabinoids are extremely powerful and have led to serious health effects when misused.

The body also produces its own cannabinoid chemicals. They play a role in regulating pleasure, memory, thinking, concentration, body movement, awareness of time, appetite, pain, and the senses (taste, touch, smell, hearing, and sight).

How Might Cannabinoids Be Useful as Medicine?

Currently, the two main cannabinoids from the marijuana plant that are of medical interest are THC and cannabidiol (CBD).

THC can increase appetite and reduce nausea. THC may also decrease pain, inflammation (swelling and redness), and muscle control problems. Unlike THC, CBD is a cannabinoid that doesn't make people "high." These drugs aren't popular for recreational use because they aren't intoxicating. It may be useful in reducing pain and inflammation, controlling epileptic seizures, and possibly even treating mental illness and addictions. Many researchers, including those funded by the National Institutes of Health (NIH), are continuing to explore the possible uses of THC, CBD, and other cannabinoids for medical treatment.

For instance, animal studies have shown that marijuana extracts may help kill certain cancer cells and reduce the size of others. Evidence from one cell culture study with rodents suggests that purified extracts from whole-plant marijuana can slow the growth of cancer cells from one of the most serious types of brain tumors. Research in mice showed that treatment with purified extracts of THC and CBD, when used with radiation, increased the cancer-killing effects of the radiation.

Scientists are also conducting preclinical and clinical trials with marijuana and its extracts to treat symptoms of illness and other conditions, such as:

- Diseases that affect the immune system, including:
- Human immunodeficiency virus (HIV)/ acquired immunodeficiency syndrome (AIDS)
- Multiple sclerosis (MS), which causes a gradual loss of muscle control
- Inflammation
- Pain
- Seizures
- Substance-use disorders
- Mental disorders

Are People with Health- and Age-Related Problems More Vulnerable to Marijuana Risks?

State-approved medicinal use of marijuana is a fairly new practice. For that reason, marijuana's effects on people who are weakened because of age or illness are still relatively unknown. Older people and those suffering from diseases such as cancer or AIDS could be more vulnerable to the drug's harmful effects, but more research is needed.

Using Medical Marijuana during and after Pregnancy

Some women report using marijuana to treat severe nausea they have during pregnancy. But there's no research that shows that this practice is safe, and doctors generally don't recommend it.

Pregnant women shouldn't use medical marijuana without first checking with their healthcare provider. Animal studies have shown that moderate amounts of THC given to pregnant or nursing women could have long-lasting effects on the child, including abnormal patterns of social interactions and learning issues.

Chapter 7

Regulations Regarding Controlled Substances

Chapter Contents

Section 7.1

The Controlled Substances Act and the Schedule Classifications

This section includes text excerpted from "Drugs of Abuse," U.S. Drug Enforcement Administration (DEA), June 15, 2017.

Controlling Drugs or Other Substances through Formal Scheduling

The Controlled Substances Act (CSA) places all substances which were in some manner regulated under existing federal law into one of five schedules. This placement is based upon the substance medical use, potential for abuse, and safety or dependence liability. The Act also provides a mechanism for substances to be controlled (added to or transferred between schedules) or decontrolled (removed from control). The procedure for these actions is found in Section 201 of the Act (21 U.S.C. §811).

Proceedings to add, delete, or change the schedule of a drug or other substance may be initiated by the U.S. Drug Enforcement Administration (DEA), the U.S. Department of Health and Human Services (HHS), or by petition from any interested party, including:

- The manufacturer of a drug
- A medical society or association
- A pharmacy association
- A public interest group concerned with drug abuse
- A state or local government agency
- An individual citizen

When a petition is received by the DEA, the agency begins its own investigation of the drug. The DEA also may begin an investigation of a drug at any time based upon information received from law enforcement laboratories, state and local law enforcement and regulatory agencies, or other sources of information. Once the DEA has collected the necessary data, the DEA Administrator, by authority of the Attorney General, requests from HHS a scientific and medical evaluation and recommendation as to whether the drug or other substance should be controlled or removed from control. This request is sent to the Assistant Secretary for Health of HHS.

The Assistant Secretary, by authority of the Secretary, compiles the information and transmits back to the DEA: a medical and scientific evaluation regarding the drug or other substance, a recommendation as to whether the drug should be controlled, and in what schedule it should be placed.

The medical and scientific evaluations are binding on the DEA with respect to scientific and medical matters and form a part of the scheduling decision. Once the DEA has received the scientific and medical evaluation from HHS, the Administrator will evaluate all available data and make a final decision whether to propose that a drug or other substance should be removed or controlled and into which schedule it should be placed.

If a drug does not have a potential for abuse, it cannot be controlled. Although the term "potential for abuse" is not defined in the CSA, there is much discussion of the term in the legislative history of the Act. The following items are indicators that a drug or other substance has a potential for abuse:

- There is evidence that individuals are taking the drug or other substance in amounts sufficient to create a hazard to their health or to the safety of other individuals or to the community.

- There is significant diversion of the drug or other substance from legitimate drug channels.

- Individuals are taking the drug or other substance on their own initiative rather than on the basis of medical advice from a practitioner.

- The drug is a new drug so related in its action to a drug or other substance already listed as having a potential for abuse to make it likely that the drug will have the same potential for abuse as such drugs, thus making it reasonable to assume that there may be significant diversions from legitimate channels, significant use contrary to or without medical advice, or that it has a substantial capability of creating hazards to the health of the user or to the safety of the community. Of course, evidence of actual abuse of a substance is indicative that a drug has a potential for abuse.

In determining into which schedule a drug or other substance should be placed, or whether a substance should be decontrolled or rescheduled, certain factors are required to be considered. These factors are listed in Section 201 (c), (21 U.S.C. § 811 (c)) of the CSA as follows:

- **The drug's actual or relative potential for abuse.**

- **Scientific evidence of the drug's pharmacological effect, if known.** The state of knowledge with respect to the effects of a specific drug is, of course, a major consideration. For example, it is vital to know whether or not a drug has a hallucinogenic effect if it is to be controlled due to that effect. The best available knowledge of the pharmacological properties of a drug should be considered.

- **The state of current scientific knowledge regarding the substance.** Criteria 2 and 3 are closely related. However, 2 is primarily concerned with pharmacological effects and 3 deals with all scientific knowledge with respect to the substance.

- **Its history and current pattern of abuse.** To determine whether or not a drug should be controlled, it is important to know the pattern of abuse of that substance.

- **The scope, duration, and significance of abuse.** In evaluating existing abuse, the DEA Administrator must know not only the pattern of abuse, but also whether the abuse is widespread.

- **What, if any, risk there is to the public health.** If a drug creates dangers to the public health, in addition to or because of its abuse potential, then these dangers must also be considered by the Administrator.

- **The drug's psychic or physiological dependence liability.** There must be an assessment of the extent to which a drug is physically addictive or psychologically habit-forming.

Schedule I

- The drug or other substance has a high potential for abuse.
- The drug or other substance has no currently accepted medical use in treatment in the United States.
- There is a lack of accepted safety for use of the drug or other substance under medical supervision.
- Examples of Schedule I substances include heroin, gamma-hydroxybutyric acid (GHB), lysergic acid diethylamide (LSD), marijuana, and methaqualone.

Schedule II

- The drug or other substance has a high potential for abuse.

- The drug or other substance has a currently accepted medical use in treatment in the United States or a currently accepted medical use with severe restrictions.

- Abuse of the drug or other substance may lead to severe psychological or physical dependence.

- Examples of Schedule II substances include morphine, phencyclidine (PCP), cocaine, methadone, hydrocodone, fentanyl, and methamphetamine.

Schedule III

- The drug or other substance has less potential for abuse than the drugs or other substances in Schedules I and II.

- The drug or other substance has a currently accepted medical use in treatment in the United States.

- Abuse of the drug or other substance may lead to moderate or low physical dependence or high psychological dependence.

- Anabolic steroids, codeine products with aspirin or Tylenol, and some barbiturates are examples of Schedule III substances.

Schedule IV

- The drug or other substance has a low potential for abuse relative to the drugs or other substances in Schedule III.

- The drug or other substance has a currently accepted medical use in treatment in the United States.

- Abuse of the drug or other substance may lead to limited physical dependence or psychological dependence relative to the drugs or other substances in Schedule III.

- Examples of drugs included in Schedule IV are alprazolam, clonazepam, and diazepam.

Schedule V

- The drug or other substance has a low potential for abuse relative to the drugs or other substances in Schedule IV.

- The drug or other substance has a currently accepted medical use in treatment in the United States.

- Abuse of the drug or other substances may lead to limited physical dependence or psychological dependence relative to the drugs or other substances in Schedule IV.

- Cough medicines with codeine are examples of Schedule V drugs.

When the DEA Administrator has determined that a drug or other substance should be controlled, decontrolled, or rescheduled, a proposal to take action is published in the Federal Register. The proposal invites all interested persons to file comments with the DEA and may also request a hearing with the DEA. If no hearing is requested, the DEA will evaluate all comments received and publish a final order in the Federal Register, controlling the drug as proposed or with modifications based upon the written comments filed. This order will set the effective dates for imposing the various requirements of the CSA.

If a hearing is requested, the DEA will enter into discussions with the party or parties requesting a hearing in an attempt to narrow the issue for litigation. If necessary, a hearing will then be held before an Administrative Law Judge. The judge will take evidence on factual issues and hear arguments on legal questions regarding the control of the drug. Depending on the scope and complexity of the issues, the hearing may be brief or quite extensive. The Administrative Law Judge, at the close of the hearing, prepares findings of fact and conclusions of law and a recommended decision that is submitted to the DEA Administrator. The DEA Administrator will review these documents, as well as the underlying material, and prepare her/his own findings of fact and conclusions of law (which may or may not be the same as those drafted by the Administrative Law Judge). The DEA Administrator then publishes a final order in the Federal Register either scheduling the drug or other substance or declining to do so.

Once the final order is published in the Federal Register, interested parties have 30 days to appeal to a U.S. Court of Appeals to challenge the order. Findings of fact by the Administrator are deemed conclusive if supported by "substantial evidence." The order imposing controls is not stayed during the appeal, however, unless so ordered by the court.

Emergency or Temporary Scheduling

The CSA was amended by the Comprehensive Crime Control Act (CCCA) of 1984. This Act included a provision which allows the

DEA Administrator to place a substance, on a temporary basis, into Schedule I, when necessary, to avoid an imminent hazard to public safety.

This emergency scheduling authority permits the scheduling of a substance which is not currently controlled, is being abused, and is a risk to public health while the formal rulemaking procedures described in the CSA are being conducted. This emergency scheduling applies only to substances with no accepted medical use.

A temporary scheduling order may be issued for two years with a possible extension of up to one year if formal scheduling procedures have been initiated. The notice of intent and order are published in the Federal Register, as are the proposals and orders for formal scheduling. (21 U.S.C. § 811 (h))

Controlled Substance

Controlled substance analogues are substances that are not formally controlled substances, but may be found in illicit trafficking. They are structurally or pharmacologically similar to Schedule I or II controlled substances and have no legitimate medical use. A substance that meets the definition of a controlled substance analogue and is intended for human consumption may be treated under the CSA as if it were a controlled substance in Schedule I. (21 U.S.C. § 802(32), 21 U.S.C. § 813)

International Treaty Obligations

United States treaty obligations may require that a drug or other substance be controlled under the CSA, or rescheduled if existing controls are less stringent than those required by a treaty. The procedures for these scheduling actions are found in Section 201 (d)of the Act. (21 U.S.C. § 811 (d))

The United States is a party to the Single Convention on Narcotic Drugs of 1961, which was designed to establish effective control over international and domestic traffic in narcotics, coca leaf, cocaine, and *Cannabis*. A second treaty, the Convention on Psychotropic Substances of 1971, which entered into force in 1976 and was ratified by Congress in 1980, is designed to establish comparable control over stimulants, depressants, and hallucinogens.

Section 7.2

Combat Methamphetamine Epidemic Act

This section includes text excerpted from "CMEA (Combat
Methamphetamine Epidemic Act)," DEA Diversion Control Division,
September 27, 2006. Reviewed January 2019.

What Is the Combat Methamphetamine Epidemic Act of 2005?

The Combat Methamphetamine Epidemic Act (CMEA) of 2005 was
signed into law on March 9, 2006 to regulate, among other things,
retail over-the-counter (OTC) sales of ephedrine, pseudoephedrine, and
phenylpropanolamine products. Retail provisions of the CMEA include
daily sales limits and monthly purchase limits, placement of product
out of direct customer access, sales logbooks, customer ID, employee
training, and self-certification of regulated sellers. The CMEA is found
as Title VII of the USA PATRIOT Improvement and Reauthorization
Act of 2005 (Public Law 109–177).

Why Was the Combat Methamphetamine Epidemic Act Passed?

Ephedrine, pseudoephedrine, and phenylpropanolamine are precursor chemicals used in the illicit manufacture of methamphetamine
or amphetamine. They are also common ingredients used to make
cough, cold, and allergy products. Methamphetamine laboratories have
been found in homes, cars, hotel rooms, storage facilities—these are
generally referred to as "small toxic labs." Passage of the CMEA was
accomplished to curtail the illicit production of methamphetamine and
amphetamine. States that have enacted similar or more restrictive
retail regulations have seen a dramatic drop in small toxic labs.

What Is Methamphetamine?

Methamphetamine is a powerfully addictive drug that severely
affects users' minds and bodies, ruins lives, and endangers communities and the environment. Chronic use can lead to extremely violent behavior, the neglect of user's children, and an inability to cope
with the ordinary demands of life. Unfortunately, methamphetamine
is unique in that making it is easy but dangerous, posing the risk

of explosion, exposing families, children, and neighborhoods to toxic chemicals.

Is Methamphetamine Production and Abuse a Nationwide Problem?

Methamphetamine or "meth" has become a tremendous challenge for the entire nation. A clandestine methamphetamine laboratory has been found in every state over the past five years. A July 18, 2006, National Association of Counties (NACo) survey found that meth is the leading drug-related local law enforcement problem in the country. The survey of 500 county law enforcement officials in 44 states found that meth continues to be the number one drug problem—more counties (48%) report that meth is the primary drug problem—more than cocaine (22%), marijuana (22%) and heroin (3%) combined. In addition, according to the survey, crimes related to meth continue to grow—55 percent of law enforcement officials report an increase in robberies or burglaries in the last year and 48 percent report an increase in domestic violence.

Does Methamphetamine Production Have an Impact on the Environment?

Clandestine methamphetamine laboratories pose a significant danger in the community, as they contain highly flammable and explosive materials. Additionally, for each pound of methamphetamine produced, five to seven pounds of toxic waste remain, which is often introduced into the environment via streams, septic systems, and surface water runoff.

When Did the Combat Meth Act Go into Effect?

Some of the provisions of this law became effective on March 9, 2006, and others became effective on April 8, 2006. Other provisions became effective on September 30, 2006.

Do the Combat Meth Act and the Implementing Regulations Preempt State Laws?

State laws vary considerably. Some parts of a state law may be less stringent than the CMEA requirements; other parts may be more stringent. The CMEA does not preempt those requirements under state laws/regulations that are more stringent than the Act's requirements. Simply put, all persons subject to the CMEA must comply with the Act and the laws in the state(s) in which they sell scheduled listed chemical products at retail. Where the CMEA is less stringent than a state law (e.g., the state limits sales to licensed pharmacists or pharmacy technicians where the Act does not), the state requirements continue to be in force. If there are state requirements that are less stringent than the CMEA provisions (e.g., exemptions of some products), the Act supersedes the provisions.

Chapter 8

Drugs—Shatter the Myths

Can Marijuana Be Addictive?

Yes. The chances of becoming addicted to marijuana or any drug are different for each person. For marijuana, around 1 in 11 people who use it become addicted. Could you be that one?

Fact. If you smoke marijuana a lot in your teens, you could lose IQ (intelligent quotient) points (which measure intelligence) that you might never get back.

Why Do People Smoke When They Know It's So Bad for Them?

Maybe they smoke because they can't stop. People start smoking for different reasons, but most keep doing it because of one reason—they are addicted to nicotine.

Did you know? Research says that teens who see a lot of smoking in movies are more likely to start smoking themselves. Sometimes characters smoke to look edgy and rebellious, but sometimes it's just about "product placement"—the tobacco industry trying to get into your head and your pockets.

This chapter includes text excerpted from "Drugs: Shatter the Myths," National Institute on Drug Abuse (NIDA), September 2016.

Fact. Most people who smoke started before the age of 18.

Did you know? Almost one in five of the twelfth graders used a hookah in the past year? A hookah is a water pipe used to burn tobacco leaves. A lot of people think it's less harmful than smoking cigarettes, but many of the health risks are the same.

Did you know? E-cigarettes contain nicotine—the addictive drug in tobacco cigarettes—and other chemicals that may be harmful. More teens use e-cigarettes than tobacco cigarettes. Scientists have just started to research the health effects of e-cigarettes, but we do know one thing: users will inhale the same nicotine they get from a regular cigarette.

Drinking and Driving

Drinking and driving can add up to tragic endings. In the United States, about 4,300 people under age 21 die each year from injuries caused by underage drinking, more than 35 percent in car crashes.

Fact. About 4 in 10 people who begin drinking before age 15 eventually become alcoholics.

Medical Consequences of Drinking Alcohol

Getting human immunodeficiency virus (HIV) from unprotected sex. When you can't think straight because you're drunk or high, you may forget to play it safe.

Meth

Meth reduces the amount of protective saliva around the teeth. People who use meth also tend to drink a lot of sugary soda, neglect oral care, grind their teeth, and clench their jaws—all of which can cause what's known as "meth mouth." Meth users sometimes hallucinate that insects are creeping on top of or underneath their skin (called formication). The person will pick or scratch their skin, trying to get rid of the imaginary "crank bugs." Soon their face and arms are covered with open sores that can get infected.

Did you know? You are getting bombarded with messages about drugs in songs and movies. A study of popular music found that about:

- 1 in 3 songs said something about drug, alcohol, or tobacco use

- 3 in 4 rap songs said something about drug, alcohol, or tobacco use

- Of the top 100 movies over a 9-year period, more than 7 in 10 movies showed characters smoking and 1 in 3 movies showed people getting drunk

Get the facts, and make your own decisions.

Prescription Opioids

Prescription opioids, such as Vicodin® and OxyContin®, are medications that relieve pain. When taken as prescribed, they can be very effective in helping people with severe pain, such as a bad injury or pain after surgery. But they come from the same class of drugs like heroin and can be dangerous if used to get high.

Fact. More people die from prescription opioid overdoses than from heroin and cocaine combined.

How Can Prescription (RX) Drugs Be Harmful When They're Prescribed by Doctors?

Prescription drugs aren't bad—they help a lot of people. It really depends on the who, how, why, and what of it.

- Who were they prescribed for (you or someone else)?

- How are you taking them (as prescribed or not)?

- Why (to get well or to get high)?

- What else are you taking (mixing with alcohol or other drugs can be dangerous)?

Some teens abuse stimulants thinking it will improve their grades, but research tells us it may do just the opposite!

Fact. Anyone can overdose on prescription opioids or heroin.

Did you know? If a person overdoses, they could stop breathing and die. Naloxone is a drug that quickly reverses the effects of an overdose. If you see someone overdose, call 911 right away.

Did you know? Mixing pills with other drugs or with alcohol really increase your risk of death from accidental overdose. Abuse of prescription attention deficit hyperactivity disorder (ADHD) medications like Adderall® and Ritalin® can cause serious health problems, including panic attacks, seizures, and heart attacks.

Drugs and Your Brain

Different drugs do different things. But they all affect the brain—that's why drugs make you feel high, low, speeded up, or slowed down, or see things that aren't there.

Did you know? Repeated drug use can reset the brain's pleasure meter, so that without the drug, you feel hopeless and sad. Eventually, everyday fun stuff like spending time with friends or playing with your dog doesn't make you happy anymore.

Fact. Drugs mess with your brain's wiring and signals.

Does Treatment Really Work?

It takes time to recover from addiction—not only for the brain to re-adjust but to make lifestyle changes to avoid drugs. Think how hard it is for people trying to lose weight—they try different diets, exercise for a while, lose a few pounds only to gain them back—until they can make lasting changes to keep the weight off. Same with quitting drugs—it may take several rounds of treatment before it sticks.

Did you know? There are different types of treatments to meet your specific needs. You can get referrals to treatment programs by calling 800-662-4357 (a confidential hotline), or by visiting the Substance Abuse and Mental Health Services Administration (SAMHSA) online at findtreatment.samhsa.gov.

Fact. There is treatment and it works.

Chapter 9

Substance-Abuse Treatment Statistics

Estimates described refer to treatment received for illicit drug or alcohol use, or for medical problems associated with the use of illicit drugs or alcohol. This includes treatment received in the past year at any location, such as a hospital (inpatient), rehabilitation facility (outpatient or inpatient), mental-health center, emergency room, private doctor's office, prison or jail, or a self-help group, such as Alcoholics Anonymous or Narcotics Anonymous. Persons could report receiving treatment at more than one location. Specialty treatment includes treatment only at a hospital (inpatient), a rehabilitation facility (inpatient or outpatient), or a mental-health center.

Individuals who reported receiving substance-use treatment but were missing information on whether the treatment was specifically for alcohol use or illicit-drug use were not counted in estimates of either illicit-drug-use treatment or alcohol-use treatment; however, they were counted in estimates for "drug or alcohol use" treatment.

- In 2013, 4.1 million persons age 12 or older (1.5% of the population) received treatment for a problem related to the use of alcohol or illicit drugs. Of these, 1.3 million received

This chapter includes text excerpted from "Substance Dependence, Abuse, and Treatment," Substance Abuse and Mental Health Services Administration (SAMHSA), 2014. Reviewed January 2019.

treatment for the use of both alcohol and illicit drugs, 0.9 million received treatment for the use of illicit drugs but not alcohol, and 1.4 million received treatment for the use of alcohol but not illicit drugs. (Note that estimates by substance do not sum to the total number of persons receiving treatment because the total includes persons who reported receiving treatment but did not report for which substance the treatment was received.)

- The rate and the number of persons in the population age 12 or older receiving any substance-use treatment within the past year remained stable between 2012 (1.5% and 4.0 million) and 2013 (1.5% and 4.1 million). The rate and number of persons receiving any substance-use treatment within the past year in 2002 were 1.5 percent and 3.5 million. The rate in 2002 was similar to that in 2013, but the number of persons who received substance-use treatment in 2002 was lower than that in 2013.

- In 2013, among the 4.1 million persons age 12 or older who received treatment for alcohol or illicit-drug use in the past year, 2.3 million persons received treatment at a self-help group, and 1.8 million received treatment at a rehabilitation facility as an outpatient. The numbers of persons who received treatment at other locations were 1.2 million at a mental-health center as an outpatient, 1.0 million at a rehabilitation facility as an inpatient, 879,000 at a hospital as an inpatient, 770,000 at a private doctor's office, 603,000 at an emergency room, and 263,000 at a prison or jail. None of these estimates changed significantly between 2012 and 2013. The number of persons receiving treatment at a private doctor's office was lower in 2002 (523,000) than in 2013.

- In 2013, 2.5 million persons age 12 or older reported receiving treatment for alcohol use during their most recent treatment in the past year, 845,000 persons received treatment for marijuana use, and 746,000 persons received treatment for pain relievers. Estimates for receiving treatment for the use of other drugs were 584,000 for cocaine, 526,000 for heroin, 461,000 for stimulants, 376,000 for tranquilizers, and 303,000 for hallucinogens. None of these estimates changed significantly between 2012 and 2013.

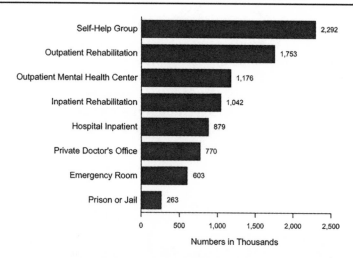

Figure 9.1. *Locations Where Substance Use Treatment Was Received among Persons Age 12 or Older: 2013.*

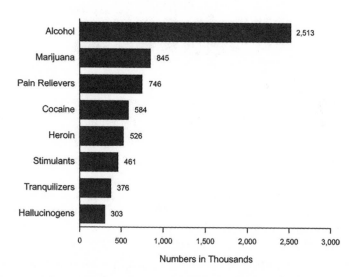

Figure 9.2. *Substances for Which Most Recent Treatment Was Received in the Past Year among Persons Age 12 or Older: 2013.*

- The numbers of persons age 12 or older who received their most recent treatment in the past year for alcohol, marijuana, cocaine, hallucinogens, inhalants, and sedatives were similar in 2002 and 2013. However, the number of persons who received treatment for tranquilizers increased from 2002 (197,000 persons) to 2013 (376,000 persons). The number who received treatment for heroin increased from 277,000 persons in 2002 to 526,000 persons in 2013. The number who received treatment for nonmedical use of prescription pain relievers increased from 2002 (360,000 persons) to 2013 (746,000 persons). The number who received treatment for stimulants increased from 268,000 persons in 2002 to 461,000 persons in 2013.

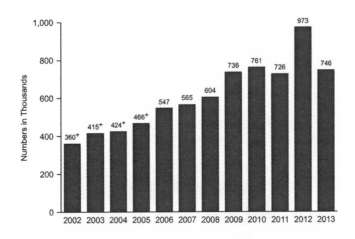

Figure 9.3. *Received Most Recent Treatment in the Past Year for the Use of Pain Relievers among Persons Age 12 or Older: 2002–2013.*

Need for and Receipt of Specialty Treatment

The following paragraphs discuss the need for and receipt of treatment for a substance-use problem at a "specialty" treatment facility. Specialty treatment is defined as treatment received at any of the following types of facilities: hospitals (inpatient only), drug or alcohol rehabilitation facilities (inpatient or outpatient), or mental-health centers. It does not include treatment at an emergency room, private doctor's office, self-help group, prison or jail, or hospital as an outpatient. An individual is defined as needing treatment for an alcohol or drug-use problem if he or she met the *Diagnostic and Statistical Manual of Mental Disorders, IV (DSM-IV)* diagnostic criteria for alcohol or illicit-drug dependence or abuse in the past 12 months or if he or she received specialty treatment for alcohol use or illicit-drug use in the past 12 months.

In the following paragraphs, an individual needing treatment for an illicit-drug-use problem is defined as receiving treatment for her or his drug-use problem only if he or she reported receiving specialty treatment for illicit-drug use in the past year. Thus, an individual who needed treatment for illicit-drug use but received specialty treatment only for alcohol use in the past year or who received treatment for illicit-drug use only at a facility not classified as a specialty facility was not counted as receiving treatment for illicit-drug use. Similarly, an individual who needed treatment for an alcohol-use problem was counted as receiving alcohol-use treatment only if the treatment was received for alcohol use at a specialty treatment facility. Individuals who reported receiving specialty substance-use treatment but were missing information on whether the treatment was specifically for alcohol use or drug use were not counted in estimates of specialty drug use treatment or in estimates of specialty alcohol-use treatment; however, they were counted in estimates for "drug or alcohol use" treatment.

In addition to questions about symptoms of substance-use problems that are used to classify respondents' need for treatment based on *DSM-IV* criteria, the National Survey on Drug Use and Health (NSDUH) includes questions asking respondents about their perceived need for treatment (i.e., whether they felt they needed treatment or counseling for illicit-drug use or alcohol use). In this report, estimates for the perceived need for treatment are discussed only for persons who were classified as needing treatment (based on *DSM-IV* criteria) but did not receive treatment at a specialty facility. Similarly, estimates for whether a person made an effort to get treatment are discussed only for persons who felt the need for treatment and did not receive it.

Illicit-Drug or Alcohol-Use Treatment and Treatment Need

- In 2013, 22.7 million persons age 12 or older needed treatment for an illicit-drug or alcohol-use problem (8.6 percent of persons age 12 or older). The number in 2013 was similar to the numbers in 2002 to 2012 (ranging from 21.6 million to 23.6 million). The rate in 2013 was similar to the rates in 2011 (8.4%) and 2012 (8.9%), but it was lower than the rates in 2002 to 2010 (ranging from 9.2 to 9.8%).

- In 2013, 2.5 million persons (0.9% of persons age 12 or older and 10.9% of those who needed treatment) received treatment at a specialty facility for an illicit-drug or alcohol problem.

The number in 2013 was similar to the numbers in 2002 (2.3 million) and in 2004 through 2012 (ranging from 2.3 million to 2.6 million), and it was higher than the number in 2003 (1.9 million). The rate in 2013 was not different from the rates in 2002 to 2012 (ranging from 0.8 to 1.0%).

- In 2013, 20.2 million persons (7.7% of the population age 12 or older) needed treatment for an illicit-drug or alcohol-use problem but did not receive treatment at a specialty facility in the past year. The number in 2013 was similar to the numbers in 2002 to 2012 (ranging from 19.3 million to 21.1 million). The rate in 2013 was similar to the rates in 2010 to 2012 (ranging from 7.5 to 8.1%), but it was lower than the rates in 2002 to 2009 (ranging from 8.3 to 8.8%).

- Of the 2.5 million persons age 12 or older who received specialty substance-use treatment in 2013, 875,000 received treatment for alcohol use only, 936,000 received treatment for illicit-drug use only, and 547,000 received treatment for both alcohol and illicit-drug use. These estimates in 2013 were similar to the estimates in 2012 and 2002.

- Among persons in 2013 who received their most recent substance-use treatment at a specialty facility in the past year, 41.7 percent reported using private health insurance as a source of payment for their most recent specialty treatment, 40.6 percent reported using their "own savings or earnings," 29.0 percent reported using Medicaid, 29.0 percent reported using public assistance other than Medicaid, 26.8 percent reported using Medicare, and 23.0 percent reported using funds from family members. None of these estimates changed significantly between 2012 and 2013.

- In 2013, among the 20.2 million persons age 12 or older who were classified as needing substance-use treatment but not receiving treatment at a specialty facility in the past year, 908,000 persons (4.5%) reported that they perceived a need for treatment for their illicit-drug or alcohol-use problem. Of these 908,000 persons who felt they needed treatment but did not receive treatment in 2013, 316,000 (34.8%) reported that they made an effort to get treatment, and 592,000 (65.2%) reported making no effort to get treatment. These estimates were stable between 2012 and 2013.

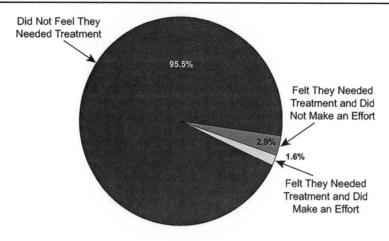

Did Not Feel They
Needed Treatment

95.5%

Felt They Needed
Treatment and Did
Not Make an Effort

2.9%

1.6%

Felt They Needed
Treatment and Did
Make an Effort

20.2 Million Needing But Not Receiving
Treatment for Illicit-Drug or Alcohol Use

Figure 9.4. *Perceived Need for and Effort Made to Receive Specialty Treatment among Persons Age 12 or Older Needing But Not Receiving Treatment for Illicit Drug or Alcohol Use: 2013.*

- The rate and the number of youth age 12 to 17 who needed treatment for an illicit-drug or alcohol-use problem in 2013 (5.4 percent and 1.3 million) were lower than those in 2012 (6.3 percent and 1.6 million), 2011 (7.0 percent and 1.7 million), 2010 (7.5 percent and 1.8 million), and 2002 (9.1 percent and 2.3 million). Of the 1.3 million youth who needed treatment in 2013, 122,000 received treatment at a specialty facility (about 9.1 percent of the youth who needed treatment), leaving about 1.2 million who needed treatment for a substance-use problem but did not receive it at a specialty facility.

- Based on 2010–2013 combined data, commonly reported reasons for not receiving illicit-drug or alcohol-use treatment among persons age 12 or older who needed and perceived a need for treatment but did not receive treatment at a specialty facility were (a) not ready to stop using (40.3 percent), (b) no health coverage and could not afford cost (31.4 percent), (c) possible negative effect on job (10.7 percent), (d) concern that receiving treatment might cause neighbors/community to have a negative opinion (10.1 percent), (e) not knowing where to go for treatment (9.2 percent), and (f) no program having type of treatment (8.0 percent).

- Based on 2010–2013 combined data, among persons age 12 or older who needed but did not receive illicit-drug or alcohol-use treatment, felt a need for treatment, and made an effort to receive treatment, commonly reported reasons for not receiving treatment were (a) no health coverage and could not afford cost (37.3 percent), (b) not ready to stop using (24.5 percent), (c) did not know where to go for treatment (9.0 percent), (d) had health coverage but did not cover treatment or did not cover cost (8.2 percent), and (e) no transportation or inconvenient (8.0 percent).

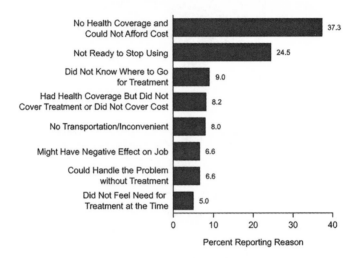

Figure 9.5. *Reasons for Not Receiving Substance Use Treatment among Persons Age 12 or Older Who Needed and Made an Effort to Get Treatment But Did Not Receive Treatment and Felt They Needed Treatment: 2010–2013 Combined.*

Illicit-Drug Use Treatment and Treatment Need

- In 2013, the number of persons age 12 or older needing treatment for an illicit-drug-use problem was 7.6 million (2.9 percent of the total population). The number in 2013 was similar to the number in each year from 2002 through 2012 (ranging from 7.2 million to 8.1 million). The rate of persons needing treatment for an illicit-drug-use problem in 2013 was lower than the rates in 2002 (3.3 percent) and 2004 (3.3 percent), but it was similar to the rates in 2012 and 2003 (3.1 percent each year) and in 2005 to 2011 (ranging from 2.8 to 3.2 percent).

- Of the 7.6 million persons age 12 or older who needed treatment for an illicit-drug-use problem in 2013, 1.5 million (0.6 percent of the total population and 19.5 percent of persons who needed treatment) received treatment at a specialty facility for an illicit-drug-use problem in the past year. The number in 2013 was similar to the numbers in 2012 (1.5 million), 2002 (1.4 million), and in 2004 to 2011 (ranging from 1.2 million to 1.6 million), but it was higher than the number in 2003 (1.1 million). The rate in 2013 was similar to the rates in 2002 to 2012 (ranging from 0.5 to 0.6 percent).

- There were 6.1 million persons (2.3 percent of the total population) who needed but did not receive treatment at a specialty facility for an illicit-drug-use problem in 2013. The number in 2013 was similar to the numbers in 2002 to 2012 (ranging from 5.8 million to 6.6 million). The rate in 2013 was similar to the rates in 2006 to 2012 (ranging from 2.3 to 2.5 percent), but it was lower than the rates in 2002 to 2005 (ranging from 2.6 to 2.8 percent).

- Of the 6.1 million persons age 12 or older who needed but did not receive specialty treatment for illicit-drug use in 2013, 395,000 (6.4 percent) reported that they perceived a need for treatment for their illicit-drug-use problem, and 5.7 million did not perceive a need for treatment. The number of persons in 2013 who needed treatment for an illicit-drug-use problem but did not perceive a need for treatment was similar to the number in 2012 (5.9 million). However, the number of persons who needed treatment and perceived a need for treatment for an illicit-drug problem in 2013 was lower than the number in 2012 (588,000 persons).

- Of the 395,000 persons age 12 or older in 2013 who felt a need for treatment for use of illicit drugs, 148,000 reported that they made an effort to get treatment, and 247,000 reported making no effort to get treatment. These estimates in 2013 for making or not making an effort to get treatment were similar to those in 2012.

- In 2013, among youth age 12 to 17, 908,000 persons (3.6 percent) needed treatment for an illicit-drug-use problem, but only 90,000 received treatment at a specialty facility (10.0 percent of youth age 12 to 17 who needed treatment), leaving 817,000 youth who needed treatment but did not receive it at a specialty facility.

These estimates in 2013 were similar to those in 2012, except that the number and the rate of youth who needed treatment for an illicit-drug-use problem in 2013 were lower than those in 2012 (1.0 million and 4.2 percent).

• Among persons age 12 or older who needed but did not receive illicit-drug use treatment and felt they needed treatment (based on 2010–2013 combined data), the commonly reported reasons for not receiving treatment were (a) no health coverage and could not afford cost (42.1 percent), (b) not ready to stop using (27.5 percent), (c) concern that receiving treatment might cause neighbors/community to have negative opinion (15.9 percent), (d) possible negative effect on job (15.2 percent), (e) not knowing where to go for treatment (12.8 percent), and (f) having health coverage that did not cover treatment or did not cover the cost (9.6 percent).

Alcohol-Use Treatment and Treatment Need

• In 2013, the number of persons age 12 or older needing treatment for an alcohol-use problem was 18.0 million (6.9 percent of the population age 12 or older). The number in 2013 was similar to the numbers in 2010 to 2012 (ranging from 17.4 million to 18.6 million) and in 2002, 2003, and 2008 (ranging from 18.2 million to 19.1 million). However, the number in 2013 was lower than the numbers in 2004 to 2007 and in 2009 (ranging from 19.4 million to 19.6 million). The rate in 2013 (6.9 percent) was similar to the rates in 2011 (6.8 percent) and 2012 (7.0 percent), but it was lower than the rates in 2002 to 2010 (ranging from 7.3 to 8.0 percent).

• Among the 18.0 million persons age 12 or older who needed treatment for an alcohol-use problem in 2013, 1.4 million (0.5 percent of the total population and 7.9 percent of the persons who needed treatment for an alcohol-use problem) received alcohol-use treatment at a specialty facility. The number and the rate of the need and receipt of treatment at a specialty facility for an alcohol-use problem in 2013 did not change significantly since 2002 (ranging from 1.3 million to 1.7 million and from 0.5 to 0.7 percent).

• The number of persons age 12 or older who needed but did not receive treatment at a specialty facility for an alcohol-use problem in 2013 (16.6 million) was similar to the numbers in

2002 (17.1 million), 2003 (16.9 million), and from 2008 to 2012 (ranging from 15.9 million to 17.7 million), but it was lower than the numbers from 2004 to 2007 (ranging from 17.8 million to 18.0 million). The rate in 2013 (6.3 percent of the population age 12 or older) was similar to the rates in 2010 to 2012 (ranging from 6.2 to 6.7 percent), but it was lower than the rates in 2002 to 2009 (ranging from 7.0 to 7.4 percent).

- Among the 16.6 million persons age 12 or older who needed but did not receive specialty treatment for an alcohol-use problem in 2013, 554,000 persons (3.3 percent) felt they needed treatment for their alcohol-use problem. The number and rate in 2013 were similar to those in 2012 (665,000 persons and 4.0 percent) and 2002 (761,000 persons and 4.5 percent). Of the 554,000 persons in 2013 who perceived a need for treatment for an alcohol-use problem but did not receive specialty treatment, 353,000 did not make an effort to get treatment, and 201,000 made an effort but were unable to get treatment.

- The number and the rate of youth age 12 to 17 who needed treatment for an alcohol-use problem in 2013 (735,000 and 3.0 percent) were lower than those in 2012 (889,000 and 3.6 percent). Of the youth in 2013 who needed treatment for an alcohol-use problem, only 73,000 received treatment at a specialty facility (0.3 percent of all youth and 10.0 percent of youth who needed treatment). These estimates were similar to those in 2012. The number and the rate of youth who needed but did not receive treatment for an alcohol-use problem in 2013 (662,000 and 2.7 percent) were lower than those in 2012 (814,000 and 3.3 percent).

- Among persons age 12 or older who needed but did not receive alcohol-use treatment and felt they needed treatment (based on 2010–2013 combined data), commonly reported reasons for not receiving treatment were (a) not ready to stop using (50.5 percent), (b) no health coverage and could not afford cost (26.4 percent), (c) not finding a program that offered the type of treatment (7.6 percent), (d) not knowing where to go for treatment (7.3 percent), (e) possible negative effect on job (7.1 percent), (f) no transportation or inconvenient (7.0 percent), (g) could handle the problem without treatment (6.8 percent), and (h) having health coverage that did not cover treatment or did not cover cost (6.7 percent).

Part Two

Drug Abuse and Specific Populations

Chapter 10

Adolescent Drug Abuse

Chapter Contents

Section 10.1

Trends in Adolescent Drug Abuse

This section contains text excerpted from the following
sources: Text in this section begins with excerpts from "Monitoring
the Future," National Institute on Drug Abuse (NIDA), December
2018; Text under the heading "2017 Monitoring the Future Survey"
is excerpted from "Monitoring the Future Survey: High School
and Youth Trends," National Institute on Drug
Abuse (NIDA), December 2018.

Since 1975 the Monitoring the Future (MTF) survey has measured
drug and alcohol use and related attitudes among adolescent students
nationwide. Survey participants report their drug use behaviors across
three time periods: lifetime, past year, and past month. Overall, 44,482
students from 392 public and private schools participated in 2017's
Monitoring the Future survey. The survey is funded by the National
Institute on Drug Abuse (NIDA), a component of the National Institutes of Health (NIH), and conducted by the University of Michigan.
Results from the survey are released each fall.

2017 Monitoring the Future Survey

The 2017 Monitoring the Future (MTF) survey of drug use and
attitudes among eighth, tenth, and twelfth graders in hundreds of
schools across the country continues to report promising trends, with
past-year use of illicit drugs other than marijuana holding steady at
the lowest levels in over two decades—5.8 percent among eighth graders, 9.4 percent among tenth graders, and 13.3 percent among twelfth
graders. This is down from peak rates of 13.1 percent for eighth graders
in 1996, 18.4 percent for tenth graders in 1996, and 21.6 percent for
twelfth graders in 2001.

In 2016, use of many substances reached the lowest levels since
the survey's inception (or since the survey began asking about them)
and held steady in 2017, or in some cases, dropped even more. Substances at historic low levels of use include alcohol and cigarettes,
heroin, prescription opioids, 3,4-methylenedioxymethamphetamine
(MDMA) (ecstasy or Molly), methamphetamine, amphetamines, and
sedatives. Other illicit drugs showed five-year declines, such as synthetic marijuana, hallucinogens other than lysergic acid diethylamide (LSD), and over-the-counter (OTC) cough and cold medications.
Five-year trends, however, did reveal an increase in LSD use among

high school seniors, although use still remains lower compared to its peak in 1996.

The survey also found a general decline in perceived risk of harm from using a number of substances and declining disapproval of people who use them. For example, the percentage of eighth graders who think that occasional use of synthetic marijuana or OTC cough and cold medications is less than it was last year and in prior years. Among tenth graders, there was a decrease in the proportion of students who perceive a risk of harm when trying inhalants, powder cocaine, or OTC cough and cold medications once or twice. High-school seniors reported reduced perception of harm in occasional cocaine, heroin, and steroid use, and reduced disapproval of trying LSD.

Opioids

Despite the continued rise in opioid and overdose deaths and high levels of opioid misuse among adults, lifetime, past-year, and past-month misuse of prescription opioids (narcotics other than heroin) dropped significantly over the last five years in twelfth graders (the only grade surveyed in this category). Vicodin use notably dropped by 51 percent in eighth graders, 67 percent in tenth graders, and 74 percent in twelfth graders. Interestingly, teens also think these drugs are not as easy to get as they used to be. Only 35.8 percent of twelfth graders said they were easily available in the 2017 survey, compared to more than 54 percent in 2010.

Marijuana

In 2016 marijuana use declined among tenth graders and remains unchanged among eighth and twelfth graders compared to five years ago, despite the changing state marijuana laws. In 2016, use of marijuana reached its lowest levels in more than two decades among eighth and tenth graders in 2016; the one slight increase in 2017 was past-month use among tenth graders, which returned to 2014–2015 levels after a decrease in 2016. Daily use of marijuana has declined among eighth graders over the past five years to 0.7 percent. Among twelfth graders, 6 percent continue to report daily use, which corresponds to about 1 in 16 high-school seniors. Among all grades, perceptions of harm and disapproval around marijuana use continue to decrease, with a smaller percentage eighth and tenth graders thinking that regular marijuana use is harmful, and fewer tenth and twelfth graders disapproving of regular marijuana use. While only 29.0 percent of twelfth graders report that regular marijuana use poses a great risk (half of what it was 20 years ago), disapproval among twelfth graders remains somewhat high, with 64.7 percent reporting they disapprove of adults smoking marijuana regularly.

In 2017, daily marijuana use exceeds daily cigarette use among eighth (0.8 versus 0.6%), tenth (2.9 versus 2.2%) and twelfth (5.9 versus 4.2%) graders. This is the first year in which daily marijuana use appeared to outpace daily cigarette use among eighth graders-this flip occurred in tenth graders in 2014 and in twelfth graders in 2015, reflecting a steep decline in daily cigarette use and fairly stable daily marijuana use.

Alcohol

Alcohol use and binge drinking continued to show a significant five-year decline among all grades. Past-month use of alcohol was reported by 8.0 percent, 19.7 percent, and 33.2 percent of eighth, tenth, and twelfth graders, respectively, compared to 11.0 percent, 27.6 percent, and 41.5 percent in 2012. Daily alcohol use and binge drinking (defined as consuming five or more drinks sometime in the past two weeks) also decreased significantly among all grades between 2012 and 2017. Unlike previous years, however, there were not significant declines in alcohol use between 2016 and 2017. Also, the perception of risk of binge drinking (BD) significantly decreased in tenth graders in 2017.

The percentage of high school teens who reported ever using alcohol dropped by as much as 60 percent compared to peak years. The 2017's survey found that 23.1 percent of eighth graders reported ever trying alcohol, which is a 60 percent drop from the peak of 55.8 percent in 1994. Among tenth graders, lifetime use fell by 40 percent from 72.0 percent in 1997 to 42.2 percent in 2017. Among twelfth graders, there was a significant 25 percent drop in lifetime alcohol use from 81.7 percent in 1997 to 61.5 percent in 2017.

Nicotine and Tobacco

Use of traditional cigarettes has continued to decline to the lowest levels in the survey's history. Significant five-year declines by more than half for daily use and for use of one-half pack or more per day were reported by all grades. Daily cigarette use was reported by 0.6 percent of eighth graders, 2.2 percent of tenth graders, and 4.2

percent of twelfth graders in 2017. This was down from peaks of 10.4 percent and 18.3 percent among eighth and tenth graders in 1996 and a peak of 24.6 percent of twelfth graders in 1997.

Use of other tobacco products including hookah and smoke-less tobacco declined among high school seniors. Among twelfth graders, tobacco use with a hookah fell from 13.0 percent to 10.1 percent in the last year; past-year hookah rates have declined by 45 percent in the past five years. Lifetime and past-month use of smokeless tobacco declined in twelfth graders from 2016 to 2017 and showed a five-year decline in all grades.

For the first time in 2017, the MTF survey asked high school students about vaping specific substances ever, in the past year, and in the past-month. Past-year vaping was reported by 13.3 percent of eighth graders, 23.9 percent of tenth graders, and 27.8 percent of twelfth graders. Vaping was the third most common form of substance use in high school seniors and tenth graders (after alcohol and marijuana) and the second most common among eighth graders (after alcohol).

Students were also asked what substances they had consumed via vaping—nicotine, marijuana, or "just flavoring." Past-year vaping of flavoring alone was most common (reported by 11.8% of eighth graders, 19.3% of tenth graders, and 20.6% of twelfth graders), followed by vaping nicotine (7.5, 15.8, and 18.8%) and marijuana (3.0, 8.1, and 9.5%).

The available survey data regarding vaping also reveal a difference in perception of harm when nicotine is specifically mentioned. While 20.3 percent of eighth graders reported thinking it is harmful to regularly use e-cigarettes, 38.2 percent reported thinking it is harmful to regularly vape an e-liquid containing nicotine. Similar differences were also seen in tenth graders (19.4% reported thinking it is harmful to use e-cigarettes regularly versus 33.3% perceiving harm in regularly vaping a liquid that contains nicotine) and twelfth graders (16.1 versus 27.0%).

Synthetic Drugs

Past-year use of synthetic cannabinoids (K2/herbal incense, sometimes called "fake weed" or "synthetic marijuana") has dropped significantly in the six years since the survey began tracking use of these substances. Since 2011, reported use among twelfth graders has dropped from 11.4 to 3.7 percent. Use has also fallen from 4.4 to 2.0 percent among eighth graders and from 8.8 to 2.7 percent among tenth graders since 2012. In recent years, use of another synthetic drug called "bath salts" (technically, synthetic cathinones) among youth has become a concern. The MTF survey began tracking past-year synthetic cathinone use in 2012, and since then, there has been a decrease among twelfth graders from 1.3 to 0.6 percent in 2017. Use among tenth graders has declined to 0.4 percent from a peak of 0.9 percent in 2013.

Section 10.2

Reasons Adolescents Try Drugs and Alcohol

This section contains text excerpted from the following sources: Text under the heading "Why Do Adolescents Take Drugs?" is excerpted from "Principles of Adolescent Substance Use Disorder Treatment: A Research-Based Guide," National Institute on Drug Abuse (NIDA), January 2014. Reviewed January 2019; Text beginning with the heading "Is Underage Drinking a Serious Health Problem?" is excerpted from "Alcohol," National Institute on Drug Abuse (NIDA) for Teens, January 2016.

Why Do Adolescents Take Drugs?

Adolescents experiment with drugs or continue taking them for several reasons, including:

- **To fit in.** Many teens use drugs "because others are doing it"—or they think others are doing it—and they fear not being accepted in a social circle that includes drug-using peers.

- **To feel good.** Abused drugs interact with the neurochemistry of the brain to produce feelings of pleasure. The intensity of this euphoria differs by the type of drug and how it is used.

- **To feel better.** Some adolescents suffer from depression, social anxiety, stress-related disorders, and physical pain. Using drugs may be an attempt to lessen these feelings of distress. Stress especially plays a significant role in starting and continuing drug use as well as returning to drug use (relapsing) for those recovering from an addiction.

- **To do better.** Ours is a very competitive society, in which the pressure to perform athletically and academically can be intense. Some adolescents may turn to certain drugs such as illegal or prescription stimulants because they think those substances will enhance or improve their performance.

- **To experiment.** Adolescents are often motivated to seek new experiences, particularly those they perceive as thrilling or daring.

Is Underage Drinking a Serious Health Problem?

Underage drinking is drinking alcohol before a person turns 21, which is the minimum legal drinking age in the United States. Underage drinking is a serious problem, as you may have seen from your friends' or your own experiences. Alcohol is the most commonly used substance of abuse among young people in America, and drinking when you're underage puts your health and safety at risk.

Why Do Teens Drink Alcohol?

Teens drink for a variety of reasons. Some teens want to experience new things. Others feel pressured into drinking by peers. And some are looking for a way to cope with stress or other problems. Unfortunately, drinking will only make any problems a person has already worse, not better.

Section 10.3

Adolescents and Prescription-Drug Misuse

This section includes text excerpted from "Prescription Drugs," National Institute on Drug Abuse (NIDA) for Teens, March 2017.

What Is Prescription-Drug Misuse?

Prescription-drug misuse has become a significant public-health problem, because misuse can lead to addiction, and even overdose deaths. Also known as:

- **Opioids.** Happy pills, hillbilly heroin, oc, oxy, oxycotton, percs, and vikes

- **Depressants.** A-minus, barbs, candy, downers, phennies, reds, red birds, sleeping pills, tooies, tranks, yellow jackets, yellows, and zombie pills

- **Stimulants.** Bennies, black beauties, hearts, roses, skippy, the smart drug, speed, and vitamin R, and uppers

For teens, it is a growing problem.

- After marijuana and alcohol, prescription drugs are the most commonly misused substances by Americans age 14 and older.

- Teens misuse prescription drugs for a number of reasons, such as to get high, to stop pain, or because they think it will help them with schoolwork.

- Many teens get the prescription drugs they misuse from friends and relatives, sometimes without the person knowing.

- Boys and girls tend to misuse some types of prescription drugs for different reasons. For example, boys are more likely to misuse prescription stimulants to get high, while girls tend to misuse them to stay alert or to lose weight.

What Makes Prescription Drugs Unsafe

Prescription drugs are often strong medications, which is why they require a prescription in the first place. Every medication has some risk for harmful effects, sometimes serious ones. Doctors consider the potential benefits and risks to each patient before prescribing medications and take into account a lot of different factors as described below. When they are misused, they can be just as dangerous as drugs that are made illegally.

- **Personal information.** Before prescribing a drug, health providers take into account a person's weight, how long they've been prescribed the medication, other medical conditions, and what other medications they are taking. Someone misusing prescription drugs may overload their system or put themselves at risk for dangerous drug interactions that can cause seizures, coma, or even death.

- **Form and dose.** Doctors know how long it takes for a pill or capsule to dissolve in the stomach, release drugs to the blood, and reach the brain. When misused, prescription drugs may be taken in larger amounts or in ways that change the way the drug works in the body and brain, putting the person at greater risk for an overdose. For example, when people who misuse OxyContin® crush and inhale the pills, a dose that normally works over the course of 12 hours hits the central nervous system (CNS) all at once. This effect increases the risk for addiction and overdose.

- **Side effects.** Prescription drugs are designed to treat a specific illness or condition, but they often affect the body in other ways, some of which can be uncomfortable and in some cases, dangerous. These are called side effects. For example, opioid pain relievers can help with pain, but they can also cause constipation and sleepiness. Stimulants, such as Adderall, increase a person's ability to pay attention, but they also raise blood pressure and heart rate, making the heart work harder. These side effects can be worse when prescription drugs are not taken as prescribed or are used in combination with other substances.

How Prescription Drugs are Misused

- **Taking someone else's prescription medication.** Even when someone takes another person's medication for its intended purposes (such as to relieve pain, to stay awake, or to fall asleep) it is considered misuse.

- **Taking a prescription medication in a way other than prescribed.** Taking your own prescription in a way that it is not meant to be taken is also misuse. This includes taking more of the medication than prescribed or changing its form—for example, breaking or crushing a pill or capsule and then snorting the powder.

- **Taking a prescription medication to get high.** Some types of prescription drugs also can produce pleasurable effects or "highs." Taking the medication only for the purpose of getting high is considered prescription-drug misuse.

- **Mixing it with other drugs.** In some cases, if you mix your prescription drug with alcohol and certain other drugs, it is considered misuse and it can be dangerous.

Commonly Misused Prescription Drugs

There are three kinds of prescription drugs that are commonly misused.

- **Opioids**—used to relieve pain, such as Vicodin, OxyContin®, or codeine

- **Depressants**—used to relieve anxiety or help a person sleep, such as Valium or Xanax

- **Stimulants**—used for treating attention deficit hyperactivity disorder (ADHD), such as Adderall and Ritalin

How Many Teens Use Prescription Drugs?

Prescription and over-the-counter (OTC) drugs are the most commonly misused substances by Americans age 14 and older, after marijuana and alcohol.

The table below shows the percentage of teens who misuse prescription drugs.

Table 10.1. Monitoring the Future Study: Trends in Prevalence of Any Prescription Drug for Twelfth Graders; 2014–2017 (In Percent)*

		12th Graders			
Drug	**Time Period**	**2014**	**2015**	**2016**	**2017**
Any Prescription Drug	Lifetime	[19.90]	18.3	18	16.5
	Past Year	[13.90]	12.9	12	10.9
	Past Month	6.4	5.9	5.4	4.9

* Data in brackets indicate statistically significant change from the previous year.

Section 10.4

Adolescent Marijuana Use

This section includes text excerpted from "Marijuana
Use in Adolescence," U.S. Department of Health and
Human Services (HHS), June 18, 2018.

Marijuana is the most commonly used substance among adolescents after alcohol. Young people who use marijuana may experience poor health outcomes. Unfortunately, fewer adolescents believe that marijuana use is a threat than in the past. This belief may undermine prevention efforts.

How Common Is Adolescent Marijuana Use?
Current Use and Trends

Marijuana use is more common among older adolescents than younger youth. In 2016, the following percentages of young people reported using marijuana at least once in the past-month:

- Five percent of students in eighth grade

- Fourteen percent of students in tenth grade

- Twenty-three percent of students in twelfth grade, and

- Twenty-two percent of college students and young adults

Unlike drinking alcohol or smoking tobacco, current marijuana use among adolescents has increased in the past 10 years for students in twelfth grade. Current substance use is defined as having used the substance (e.g., alcohol, tobacco, or marijuana) in the last 30 days. Figure 10.1 shows that both current alcohol and cigarette use among students in twelfth grade declined by at least 10 percentage points (44 to 33% and 22 to 10%, respectively) while marijuana use increased by four percentage points (19 to 23%) from 2007 to 2017.

Vaping is a popular and relatively new way to use marijuana and other substances. To vape marijuana, a person breathes in vapor, aerosol, or mist that contains hash oil or other forms of *Cannabis* through an electronic or battery-powered device. Vaping devices include e-cigarettes, including "mods," and e-pens. These devices may not be easily

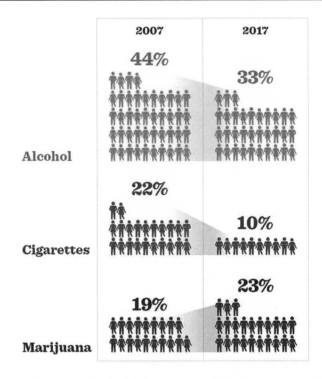

Figure 10.1. *Trends in Alcohol, Cigarette, and Marijuana Use: 30-Day Prevalence in Twelfth Graders*

identifiable as e-cigarettes and can resemble other electronic devices such as a universal serial bus (USB) flash drive.

In 2017, a national survey began asking high school students about specific substances that they vaped: nicotine, marijuana, and "just flavoring." Among students in eighth grade, two percent reported vaping marijuana in the past 30 days, compared to four percent of students in tenth grade students, and five percent of students in twelfth grade. More students across all grade levels reported vaping nicotine or flavored oil than reported vaping marijuana.

What Adolescents Think about Marijuana

Adolescents typically do not think using marijuana is as risky as using other substances. This belief has been steadily growing. When asked, "How much do you think people risk harming themselves (physically or in other ways) if they smoke marijuana regularly," less than one-third of high school seniors responded that there was a "great risk" in 2016. Ten years ago, more than half of high-school seniors (58%) believed it was a great risk.

Students' disapproval of other people using marijuana regularly has also declined. In 2006, 83 percent of high school seniors disapproved of people 18 years or older smoking marijuana regularly, but only 69 percent disapproved in 2016.

However, much variation exists among states in marijuana use and their views of the risks among youth ages 12 to 17.

Section 10.5

Adolescents and Opioids

This section includes text excerpted from "Opioids and Adolescents," U.S. Department of Health and Human Services (HHS), November 29, 2017.

The opioid crisis has received much attention in the United States. More people than ever are dying from opioid overdose; in 2016, over 42,000 people were killed by opioids. Across 52 areas in 45 states opioid overdoses increased by 30 percent from July 2016 through September 2017. In October 2017, President Trump declared the opioid crisis a public-health emergency and pledged resources to address it.

Some opioids, such as heroin, are illegal. However, many opioids are legal and are prescribed by healthcare providers to treat pain; these include oxycodone (OxyContin®), hydrocodone (Vicodin®), codeine, and morphine, among others. Use of these prescription drugs for short durations, as prescribed by a doctor, is generally safe. However, use of illegal opioids and misuse of prescription opioids can lead to addiction and even overdose or death. Misuse can include taking a drug that has been prescribed for someone else, taking a prescribed medicine differently than prescribed (for example, at a higher dose or for a longer period of time), or taking it to get high.

Fortunately, there is a concerted and multi-pronged response to this significant public-health problem. Federal and state governments are prioritizing the problem, and various government and public-health agencies are offering tools (many listed below) to help community-based organizations, healthcare providers, and parents and families deal with the problem. The scientific and medical communities are working to develop and encourage the use of safe, effective, nonaddictive treatments to manage chronic pain as well as more effective treatments for opioid-use disorders (OUDs). Parents and families of adolescents are also key to the prevention of and early intervention in opioid misuse.

Prevalence of Adolescent Opioid Misuse

Prescription-drug misuse, which can include opioids, is among the fastest growing drug problems in the United States. In 2016, 3.6 percent of adolescents age 12 to 17 reported misusing opioids over the past year. This percentage is twice as high among older adolescents and young adults age 18 to 25. The vast majority of this misuse is due to prescription opioids, not heroin.

Fortunately, opioid misuse is decreasing. For example, among high school seniors, past year misuse of pain medication, excluding heroin, decreased to 4.2 percent in 2017. The past-year misuse of Vicodin decreased from a peak of 10.5 percent in 2003 to 2.0 percent in 2017, and Oxycontin® misuse has decreased from the peak rate of 5.5 percent in 2005 to 2.7 percent in 2017. Furthermore, students in the twelfth grade believe that opioids are harder to obtain than in the past. In 2010, 54 percent of students in twelfth grade believed that these drugs were easily accessible, as compared to 35.8 percent in 2017.

Death from overdose is the most serious consequence of prescription drug misuse. And while the number of deaths from drug overdose remains quite low overall, the rate of overdose deaths among adolescents is increasing. In 2015, 4,235 youth age 15 to 24 died from a drug-related overdose; over half of these were attributable to opioids. The health consequences of opioid misuse affect a much larger number of people. For example, the Centers for Disease Control and Prevention (CDC) estimates that for every young adult overdose death, there are 119 emergency room visits and 22 treatment admissions.

Risk and Protective Factors

All adolescents are at risk for misusing opioids, though, as documented in this report, there are a wide range of factors that can either increase the risk of prescription-drug misuse or help protect against it. For example:

- Individuals at increased risk of opioid misuse include those with acute and chronic pain, physical health problems, or a history of mental illness (such as depression) or other substance use or misuse. Youth who have witnessed a family member overdose or who have a large number of friends who misuse prescription drugs also are at increased risk. National data show that nearly half of adolescents ages 12 to 17 who reported misusing pain relievers said they were given or bought them from a friend or relative. This number is over half for young adults ages 18 to 25 who reported misusing pain relievers.

- Individuals at lower risk include those who commit to doing well in school and finishing school and those who are concerned about the dangers of prescription drugs. Additionally, youth who have a strong bond with their parents and whose parents express disapproval of substance use have a lower risk of misuse.

Section 10.6

School Dropouts and Substance Abuse

This section includes text excerpted from "Substance Use among 12th Grade Age Youth, by Dropout Status," Substance Abuse and Mental Health Services Administration (SAMHSA), August 15, 2017.

High school graduation is a key milestone on the pathway to success for many Americans; however, many youth drop out of high school each year. In the United States, about 82 percent of youth who enter public high school as freshmen eventually graduate from high school in four years (calculated from the average freshman graduation rate and the adjusted cohort graduation rate). This indicates that approximately one out of five students did not graduate with a regular high school diploma within four years of the first time they started ninth grade. According to the 2012 Current Population Survey (CPS), approximately 478,000 youth age 16 to 18 were "status dropouts," meaning that they were not enrolled in high school and had not earned a high school diploma or alternative credential. Younger youth were more likely than older youth to be enrolled in school. For example, the 2012 CPS data show that high-school enrollment rates by age group were

95.4 percent for 16-year-olds and 90.1 percent for 17-year-olds. Students who fail to graduate face a wide array of negative consequences including higher rates of unemployment, earning less when employed, being more likely to receive public assistance, being more likely to suffer poor health, and being more likely to have higher rates of criminal behavior and incarceration. In addition, the failure to complete high school has intergenerational implications on socioeconomic attainment because children whose parents did not complete high school are more likely to perform poorly in school and eventually drop out themselves.

The National Survey on Drug Use and Health (NSDUH) is an annual survey of the U.S. civilian, noninstitutionalized population age 12 years or older. One of NSDUH's strengths is the stability of the survey design, which allows for multiple years of data to be combined to examine specific subgroups in the United States, such as high-school dropouts. NSDUH is a face-to-face household interview survey that is fielded continuously throughout each year. NSDUH assesses current educational attainment and school enrollment status for all respondents age 12 or older. Specifically, NSDUH asks respondents about their current age, current school enrollment status, last grade completed, and age when they last attended school. This permits NSDUH to classify each youth respondent as in school or not in school (i.e., a dropout). This measure is slightly different from alternate measures that identify whether individuals were able to attain their high school diploma or General Educational Development (GED) within four years of starting high school, a common metric for assessing high school completion.

NSDUH, which is a cross-sectional study, is unable to collect this measure. For this report, the NSDUH data were used to identify twelfth-grade-aged youth and whether they had dropped out of school. Youth age 16 to 18 were categorized into three groups:

- Twelfth-grade-aged students—youth age 16 to 18 who were in or entering the twelfth grade

- Twelfth-grade-aged dropouts—youth age 16 to 18 who had not completed high school or earned a GED, were not currently attending or were on vacation from school, and were considered twelfth-grade-aged based on the last grade they had completed and their age when they stopped attending school

- Other—youth age 16 to 18 who completed high school or earned a GED, youth age 16 to 18 in eleventh grade or lower, and youth age 16 who were not considered twelfth-grade-aged (based on criteria discussed in group 2)

This section focuses on the first two of these groups, which are collectively referred to as twelfth-grade-aged youth; comparisons of past-month (current) substance use between twelfth-grade students and twelfth-grade-aged dropouts are provided. The remaining youth (group 3) are not included in estimates in this report. All findings in this report are annual averages from the 2002 to 2014 National Survey on Drug Use and Health (NSDUH) data from about 136,200 respondents age 16 to 18, including 4,800 youth who met the high-school dropout criteria.

High-School Dropout Status

About one in nine (11.3%) twelfth-grade-aged youth had dropped out of high school, with males having been more likely than females to have dropped out (12.7 versus 9.9%; Figure 10.2). The percentage of high-school dropouts varied widely by race/ethnicity, ranging from 23.0 percent of American Indian or Alaska Native twelfth-grade-aged youth to one. One percent of Asian twelfth-grade-aged youth. When compared with the percentage of twelfth-grade-aged youth in the nation overall who have dropped out of high school (11.3%), the percentages of White (10.0%) and Asian (1.1%) youth who had dropped out of high school were lower, whereas the percentages of American Indian or Alaska Native (23.0%) and Hispanic (17.8%) youth were higher.

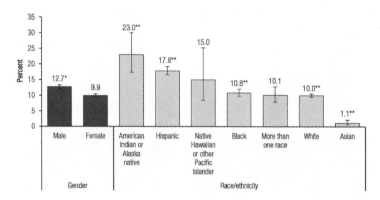

Figure 10.2. *High-School Dropout Status among Twelfth-Grade-Aged Youth, by Gender and Race/Ethnicity: 2002 to 2014.* (Source: SAMHSA, Center for Behavioral Health Statistics and Quality, National Surveys on Drug Use and Health (NSDUHs), 2002 to 2005, 2006 to 2010, and 2011 to 2014.)

* Difference between males and females is statistically significant at the .05 level.
** Difference between this estimate and the national average is statistically significant at the .05 level.

Substance Use by High-School Dropout Status

Twelfth-grade-aged dropouts were more likely than twelfth-grade-aged students to engage in current cigarette use, alcohol use, and binge alcohol use (Figure 10.3). Binge alcohol use is defined as drinking five or more drinks on the same occasion on at least 1 day in the past 30 days, and heavy alcohol use is defined as having this number of drinks on the same occasion on 5 or more days in the past 30 days. Based on combined 2002 to 2014 NSDUH data, 55.9 percent of twelfth-grade-aged dropouts were current cigarette users compared with 20.2 percent of twelfth-grade-aged students. Regarding alcohol use, 41.1 percent of twelfth-grade-aged dropouts were current alcohol drinkers compared with 33.7 percent of twelfth-grade-aged students, and 31.8 percent of twelfth-grade-aged dropouts were current binge drinkers compared with 22.1 percent of twelfth-grade-aged students.

Twelfth-grade-aged dropouts were more likely than twelfth-grade-aged students to engage in past-month illicit-drug use, with 31.4 percent of twelfth-grade-aged dropouts using any illicit drugs in the past-month compared with 18.1 percent of twelfth-grade-aged students. Illicit-drug use is defined as the use of marijuana, cocaine (including

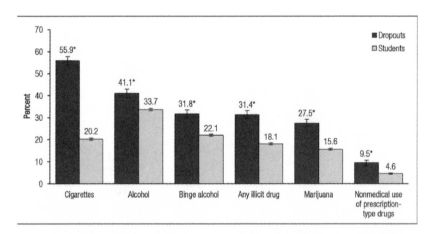

Figure 10.3. *Past-Month Substance Use among Twelfth-Grade-Aged Youth, by Dropout Status: 2002 to 2014* (Source: SAMHSA, Center for Behavioral Health Statistics and Quality, National Surveys on Drug Use and Health (NSDUHs), 2002 to 2005, 2006 to 2010, and 2011 to 2014.)

* Difference between twelfth-grade-aged students and twelfth-grade-aged dropouts is statistically significant at the .05 level.

crack), inhalants, hallucinogens, heroin, or prescription-type drugs used nonmedically. As the use of marijuana and the misuse of prescription-type psychotherapeutic drugs are the two most common forms of illicit-drug use in the United States, this report focuses on focuses on these specific substances. These forms of illicit-drug use were higher among high-school dropouts. For example, 27.5 percent of twelfth-grade-aged dropouts were current marijuana users compared with 15.6 percent of twelfth-grade-aged students. In addition, 9.5 percent of twelfth-grade-aged dropouts were misusing prescription-type drugs compared with 4.6 percent of twelfth-grade-aged students.

Male and Female Substance Use by Dropout Status

The pattern of higher past-month substance use among twelfth-grade-aged dropouts persisted for both male and female youth. Substance use was more likely among twelfth-grade-aged male dropouts than among similarly age male students (Figure 10.4). For example, twelfth-grade-aged male dropouts were much more likely than similarly age male students to be current cigarette users (59.0 versus 21.9%). There were also higher percentages of twelfth-grade-aged male dropouts than similarly age male students who were past-month alcohol

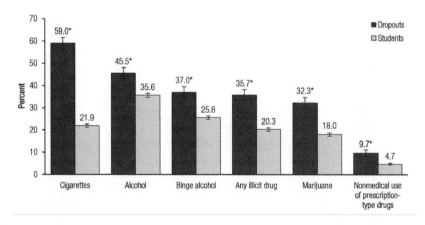

Figure 10.4. *Past-Month Substance Use among Twelfth-Grade-Aged Male Youth, by Dropout Status: 2002 to 2014.* (Source: SAMHSA, Center for Behavioral Health Statistics and Quality, National Surveys on Drug Use and Health (NSDUHs), 2002 to 2005, 2006 to 2010, and 2011 to 2014.)

* Difference between twelfth-grade-aged students and twelfth-grade-aged dropouts is statistically significant at the .05 level.

users (45.5 versus 35.6%) or who were binge alcohol users (37.0 versus 25.6%). Illicit-drug use was also more likely among twelfth-grade-aged male dropouts than among similarly age male students. Specifically, twelfth-grade-aged male dropouts were much more likely than similarly age male students to be current any illicit-drug users (35.7 versus 20.3%), to engage in marijuana use (32.3 versus 18.0%), and to engage in nonmedical use of prescription-type drugs (9.7 versus 4.7%).

As shown in (Figure 10.5), differences in past-month substance use by dropout status among females were similar to those for males. Overall, substance use was also more likely among twelfth-grade-aged female dropouts than similarly age female students (Figure 10.5). Specifically, twelfth-grade-aged female dropouts were much more likely than similarly age female students to be current cigarette users (51.7 versus 18.6%). With regards to past-month alcohol use, twelfth-grade-aged female dropouts were much more likely than similarly age female students to drink alcohol (35.1 versus 31.8%) and to engage in binge alcohol use (24.6 versus 18.5%). In addition, there were also differences in past-month illicit-drug use with twelfth-grade-aged female dropouts being more likely than similarly age female students to engage in any illicit-drug use (25.5 versus 15.9%), engage in marijuana use (21.1 versus 13.2%), and engage in nonmedical use of prescription-type drugs (9.1 versus 4.5%).

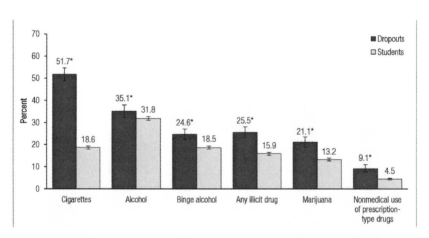

Figure 10.5. *Past-Month Substance Use among Twelfth-Grade-Aged Female Youth, by Dropout Status: 2002 to 2014.* (Source: SAMHSA, Center for Behavioral Health Statistics and Quality, National Survey on Drug Use and Health (NSDUHs), 2002 to 2005, 2006 to 2010, and 2011 to 2014.)

* Difference between twelfth-grade-aged students and twelfth-grade-aged dropouts is statistically significant at the .05 level.

Substance Use by Dropout Status and Race/Ethnicity

NSDUH asks a series of questions about race/ethnicity. First, respondents are asked about their Hispanic origin, then they are asked to identify which racial group best describes them: white, black or African American, American Indian or Alaska Native, Native Hawaiian, Other Pacific Islander, Asian, or other. Respondents may select more than one race. This analysis focuses on comparisons between twelfth-grade-aged dropouts and similarly age students for respondents who were non-Hispanic White, non-Hispanic Black, or Hispanic (Figures 9.6 to 9.8). Estimates of substance use by dropout status are not presented for youth in other racial/ethnic groups because of low precision.

Substance use varied by dropout status among racial/ethnic groups; however, the relationship between high-school dropout status and substance use was similar for those youth who were non-Hispanic White and non-Hispanic Black. For example, non-Hispanic White and Black youth who were twelfth-grade-aged dropouts were consistently more likely to engage in past-month substance use than their peers who were still in school (Figures 9.6 and 9.7). For example, current cigarette use was nearly three times higher among non-Hispanic White dropouts than among non-Hispanic White students (68.4

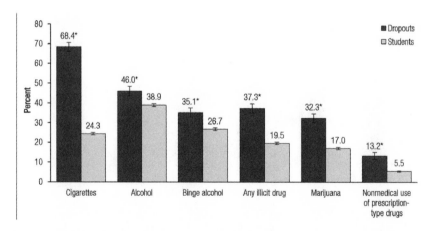

Figure 10.6. *Past-Month Substance Use among Twelfth Grade–Aged White Youth, by Dropout Status: 2002 to 2014.* (Source: SAMHSA, Center for Behavioral Health Statistics and Quality, National Surveys on Drug Use and Health (NSDUHs), 2002 to 2005, 2006 to 2010, and 2011 to 2014.)

* Difference between twelfth-grade-aged students and twelfth-grade-aged dropouts is statistically significant at the .05 level.

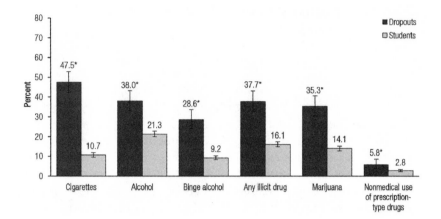

Figure 10.7. *Past-Month Substance Use among Twelfth-Grade-Aged Black Youth, by Dropout Status: 2002 to 2014.* (Source: SAMHSA, Center for Behavioral Health Statistics and Quality, National Surveys on Drug Use and Health (NSDUHs), 2002 to 2005, 2006 to 2010, and 2011 to 2014.)

* Difference between twelfth-grade-aged students and twelfth-grade-aged dropouts is statistically significant at the .05 level.

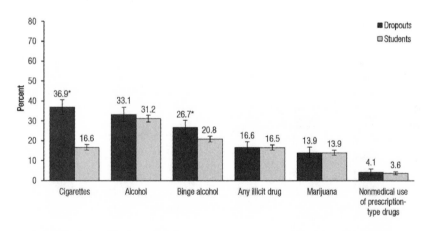

Figure 10.8. *Past-Month Substance Use among Twelfth-Grade-Aged Hispanic Youth, by Dropout Status: 2002 to 2014.* (Source: SAMHSA, Center for Behavioral Health Statistics and Quality, National Surveys on Drug Use and Health (NSDUHs), 2002 to 2005, 2006 to 2010, and 2011 to 2014.)

* Difference between twelfth-grade-aged students and twelfth-grade-aged dropouts is statistically significant at the .05 level.

versus 24.3%). Similarly, the percentage of non-Hispanic Black dropouts who were current smokers was also higher than the percentage of smokers among non-Hispanic Black students (47.5 versus 10.7%). By contrast, substance use did not differ significantly between twelfth-grade-aged Hispanic dropouts and those who were still in school, with the exception of cigarette use (36.9% among dropouts versus 16.6% among students) and binge alcohol use (26.7% among dropouts versus 20.8% among students) (Figure 10.8).

Conclusion

Dropping out of high school is related to many negative socioeconomic and health outcomes. According to combined 2002 to 2014 NSDUH data, an annual average of about one in nine twelfth-grade-aged youth dropout of high school. This report shows that twelfth-grade-aged dropouts (with a few exceptions) were more likely than similarly age youth who were still in school to have used various substances in the past-month (e.g., cigarettes, alcohol, binge alcohol use, marijuana, nonmedical use of prescription-type drugs, any illicit drugs). The NSDUH data are not suited for determining whether a youth's substance use preceded dropping out of high school or developed after dropping out. Regardless, this report indicates that youth who have dropped out of high school have an elevated risk of substance use.

Substance use is a preventable public-health issue. Prevention efforts targeted to youth and to those at risk of dropping out of high school might improve youth' future educational, employment and financial, and health outcomes. Continuing efforts are needed to educate youth, parents, teachers, physicians, service providers, and policymakers about youth substance use.

Chapter 11

Drug Use among College Students

College is a time when young people transition to adulthood, with many living independently and making behavioral-health decisions without direct parental oversight. In 2014, there were an estimated 12.4 million college students age 15 to 24 in the United States. As these youth enter adulthood, substance use appears common for many of them. More than one-third of full-time college students age 18 to 22 engaged in binge drinking in the past month; about 1 in 5 used an illicit drug in the past month. Substance use constitutes one of the most serious public-health issues for young people in the United States, creating negative health, social, and economic consequences for adolescents, their families, and communities, and for the nation as a whole.

The Center for Behavioral Health Statistics and Quality (CBHSQ) within the Substance Abuse and Mental Health Services Administration (SAMHSA) collects, analyzes, and disseminates behavioral-health data from sources such as the National Survey on Drug Use and Health (NSDUH), a national data-collection clearinghouse that offers insight into substance use and treatment among the civilian, noninstitutionalized population age 12 or older, including young adults in college. This

This chapter includes text excerpted from "A Day in the Life of College Students Age 18 to 22: Substance Use Facts," Substance Abuse and Mental Health Services Administration (SAMHSA), May 26, 2016.

issue of *The CBHSQ Report* uses NSDUH data to presents information about substance use among full-time and part-time college students age 18 to 22.

NSDUH respondents are asked about their past-year and past-month use of alcohol and illicit drugs, which includes nine categories: marijuana, cocaine (including crack), heroin, hallucinogens, and inhalants, as well as the nonmedical use of prescription-type pain relievers, tranquilizers, stimulants, and sedatives. Marijuana is categorized as an illicit drug because marijuana use remains illegal under federal law in all states (under the Controlled Substances Act: www.fda.gov/regulatoryinformation/legislation/ucm148726.htm), although the laws regarding marijuana use have changed in a number of states over the past decade.

All estimates in this report are annual averages based on combined 2011 to 2014 NSDUH data. Because NSDUH data were combined from multiple years, the estimates that are presented in this report represent annual averages. In the combined 2011 to 2014 NSDUH data, there were about 25,400 college students age 18 to 22 who participated in the survey, of whom 21,000 were full-time students and 4,300 were part-time students. These sample sizes represent an annual average of 9.0 million full-time students and 2.0 million part-time students. This report presents the estimated number of first-time substance users on an average day by college-enrollment status. Given that there are more full-time college students than part-time college students, the number of full-time college students engaging in substance use for the first time will be higher than the number of part-time college students engaging in substance use for the first time. This is because presenting the estimated number of users on an average day does not standardize the number of users across varying population sizes and, as a result, it is not useful to compare the number of users who are part-time to the number of users who are full-time. The scale used in the graphics differs for full-time and part-time college students, reflecting the difference in the overall population sizes for both groups.

First-Time Substance Use
Full-Time College Students

The combined 2011 to 2014 NSDUH data indicate there was an annual average of about 9.0 million full-time college students age 18 to 22 in the United States. According to NSDUH data, 9.9 percent of full-time college students age 18 to 22 drank alcohol for the first time in the past year. Of the 9.0 million full-time college students in the United States, 6.0 percent of used illicit drugs for the first time in the past year. On an average day during the past year, full-time college students used the following substances for the first time:

- 2,179 full-time college students drank alcohol

- 1,326 full-time college students used an illicit drug

- 1,299 full-time college students used marijuana

- 649 full-time college students used hallucinogens

- 559 full-time college students used prescription-type pain relievers nonmedically

- 447 full-time college students used cocaine

- 415 full-time college students used licit or illicit stimulants nonmedically

- 166 full-time college students used inhalants

- 39 full-time college students used methamphetamine

- 19 full-time college students used heroin

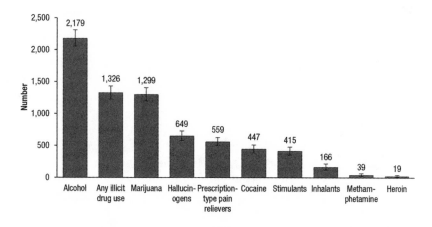

Figure 11.1. *Number of Full-Time College Students Age 18 to 22 Who Used Alcohol or Illicit Drugs for the First Time on an Average Day.* (Source: SAMHSA, Center for Behavioral Health Statistics and Quality, National Surveys on Drug Use and Health (NSDUHs), 2011 and 2014.)

Note: Annual averages based on combined 2011 to 2014 data.

Part-Time College Students

The combined 2011 to 2014 NSDUH data indicate there was an annual average of about 2.0 million part-time college students age 18 to 22 in the United States. According to NSDUH data, 8.9 percent of part-time college students age 18 to 22 drank alcohol for the first time in the past year. Of the roughly 2.0 million part-time college students in the United States, 3.8 percent used illicit drugs for the first time in the past year. On an average day during the past year, part-time college students used the following substances for the first time:

- 453 part-time college students drank alcohol

- 174 part-time college students used an illicit drug

- 153 part-time college students used marijuana

- 129 part-time college students used prescription-type pain relievers nonmedically

- 117 part-time college students used hallucinogens

- 80 part-time college students used cocaine

- 53 part-time college students used inhalants

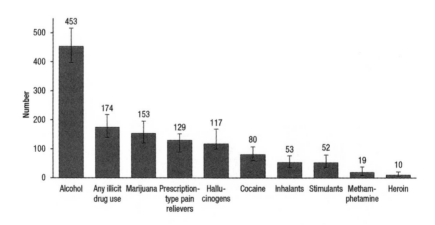

Figure 11.2. *Number of Part-Time College Students Age 18 to 22 Who Used Alcohol or Illicit Drugs for the First Time on an Average Day. (Source: SAMHSA, Center for Behavioral Health Statistics and Quality, National Surveys on Drug Use and Health (NSDUHs), 2011 and 2014.)*

Note: Annual averages based on combined 2011 to 2014 data.

- 52 part-time college students used licit or illicit stimulants nonmedically

- 19 part-time college students used methamphetamine

- 10 part-time college students used heroin

Alcohol and Drug Use
Full-Time College Students

Nearly 5.4 million full-time college students (60.1 percent of this population) drank alcohol in the past month, with 3.5 million engaging in binge drinking and 1.2 million engaging in heavy alcohol use (39.0 and 13.2 percent, respectively). Nearly 2.0 million full-time college students (22.2 percent) used an illicit drug in the past month.

On an average day during the past year, full-time college students used the following:

- 1.2 million full-time college students drank alcohol

- 703,759 full-time college students used marijuana

- 11,338 full-time college students used cocaine

- 9,808 full-time college students used hallucinogens

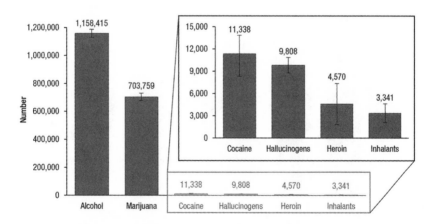

Figure 11.3. *Number of Full-Time College Students Age 18 to 22 Who Used Alcohol or Illicit Drugs on an Average Day. (Source: SAMHSA, Center for Behavioral Health Statistics and Quality, National Surveys on Drug Use and Health (NSDUHs), 2011 and 2014.)*

Note: Annual averages based on combined 2011 to 2014 data.

- 4,570 full-time college students used heroin

- 3,341 full-time college students used inhalants

Full-time college students who used alcohol in the past month drank an average of 4.1 drinks per day on the days on which they drank. Full-time college students who used alcohol in the past month drank on an average of 6.4 days per month.

Part-Time College Students

For part-time college students, 1.1 million (56.4 percent of this population) drank alcohol in the past month, with 707,000 engaging in binge drinking and 207,000 engaging in heavy alcohol use (35.5 and 10.4 percent, respectively). Nearly 448,000 part-time college students (22.5 percent) used an illicit drug in the past month.

On an average day during the past year, part-time college students used the following substances:

- 239,212 part-time college students drank alcohol

- 195,020 part-time college students used marijuana

- 3,629 part-time college students used cocaine

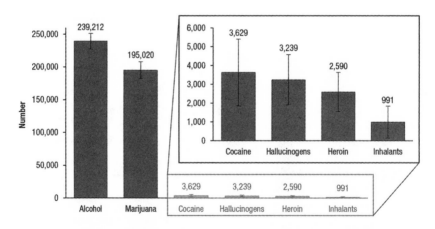

Figure 11.4. *Number of Part-Time College Students Age 18 to 22 Who Used Alcohol or Illicit Drugs on an Average Day.* (Source: SAMHSA, Center for Behavioral Health Statistics and Quality, National Surveys on Drug Use and Health (NSDUHs), 2011 and 2014.)

Note: Annual averages based on combined 2011 to 2014 data.

- 3,239 part-time college students used hallucinogens

- 2,590 part-time college students used heroin

- 991 part-time college students used inhalants

Part-time college students who used alcohol in the past month drank an average of 3.8 drinks per day on the days on which they drank. Part-time college students who used alcohol in the past month drank on an average of 6.4 days per month.

Discussion

College is often the time when young people begin to engage in substance use. Findings in this report show that, on an average day, alcohol and marijuana were the substances most frequently initiated by both full-time and part-time college students. Heroin and meth-amphetamine were the least frequently initiated substances by both populations. Because there are more full-time college students than part-time students, it is not useful to compare the number of full-time and part-time college students who are using substances because the differences between the numbers reflect the varying population sizes rather than the proportion of the populations using (i.e., differences in percentages). However, it is possible to compare the information in the report on the average number of drinks consumed by full-time and part-time students. This comparison revealed that the average number of alcoholic drinks consumed by full-time college students slightly exceeded the average number of drinks consumed by part-time college students on days on which they drank alcohol; however, the levels of binge and heavy alcohol use indicate that this is a concern in both populations. Many full-time and part-time college students engaged in binge drinking and in heavy alcohol use.

Although college affords young people numerous new experiences, neither substance-use initiation nor substance abuse are universal col-lege experiences. Providing college students with credible and accurate information about the harm associated with substance use is crucial to prevention. To learn about SAMHSA's efforts to promote behavioral health among students and prevent substance use, go to www.samhsa.gov/school-campus-health/.

Chapter 12

Substance-Abuse Issues of Concern to Women

Chapter Contents

Section 12.1

Alcohol-Use Disorder, Substance-Use Disorder, and Addiction among Women

This section includes text excerpted from "Alcohol Use Disorder, Substance Use Disorder, and Addiction," Office on Women's Health (OWH), U.S. Department of Health and Human Services (HHS), August 28, 2018.

Using drugs illegally and drinking too much alcohol can affect your mental health, physical health, and relationships. Some people, who misuse alcohol or drugs, become addicted. Addiction is a disease of the brain, but it can be treated. Women may have a harder time quitting certain substances. Women may also need help with resources for daycare or eldercare when trying to get treatment for alcohol- or substance-use disorders (SUDs).

How Common Is Alcohol-Use Disorder among Women?

No one factor can predict whether a woman will have trouble with alcohol. Women who are or have are more likely to develop an alcohol-use disorder (AUD).

- About 15 million people in the United States have an AUD, including nearly 8 million women.

- Alcohol use can start early in life. In a survey, more than 1 in 5 girls and teens ages 12 to 20 said they'd had a drink in the past month.

- Lesbians and bisexual women (especially young women) are at higher risk for drug abuse, heavy drinking, and binge drinking than other women are.

- Among women who drink, 13 percent have more than seven drinks per week. According to a survey, binge drinking is also on the rise in older women. Drinking four or more drinks on any given day or drinking more than seven drinks in a week raises a woman's risk of developing alcohol-use disorder.

How Does Alcohol Abuse or Misuse Affect Women?

Men are more likely than women to misuse alcohol and have alcohol-use disorder, but women are more likely to experience harmful health effects from alcohol. Women absorb more alcohol pound for pound than men, and it takes longer for women's bodies to digest alcohol.

Women who drink while pregnant also put their babies at risk for fetal alcohol spectrum disorder (FASD), which can cause serious problems for the baby during and after pregnancy. FASD can cause physical, mental, and behavioral disabilities. There is no amount of alcohol that has been proven safe to drink during pregnancy.

Women who misuse alcohol are more at risk of:

- **Alcoholic liver disease.** Women are more likely than men to develop liver inflammation (alcoholic hepatitis) and to die from cirrhosis (chronic liver disease).

- **Brain disease.** Alcoholism can cause diseases of the brain, such as dementia and memory loss, by changing how your cells work or by damaging brain cells.

- **Cancer.** Alcohol can cause several different types of cancer, including breast cancer. The more alcohol you drink, the higher your risk of cancer caused by alcohol. Just one drink a day can increase your risk of breast cancer by five percent before menopause and nine percent after menopause.

- **Heart disease.** Long-term, heavy drinking is a leading cause of heart disease.

- **Osteoporosis.** Long-term, heavy drinking, especially during adolescence or young adulthood, greatly weakens bones, increasing the risk of a broken bone later in life.

How Common Is Prescription-Drug Abuse among Women?

Nearly 27 million U.S. women (about 13%) have used illegal drugs or misused prescription drugs in the past year.

Women often abuse prescription drugs for different reasons than men do. Two common reasons women misuse prescription drugs are to lose weight and to fight exhaustion. Women also report higher rates of chronic pain and are more likely to be prescribed pain medicine than men are.

Prescription-drug misuse among women is on the rise. According to the Centers for Disease Control and Prevention (CDC):

- From 1999 to 2015, deaths from prescription painkiller overdoses increased more than twice as fast among women as among men.

- Each day, about 18 women die of prescription drug overdose.

- For every woman who dies of a prescription painkiller overdose, go to the emergency department for painkiller misuse or abuse.

Who Is at Risk for Alcohol-Use Disorder or Substance-Use Disorder?

A woman is more likely to misuse alcohol or drugs if she experiences:

- Parents and siblings with alcohol or drug problems

- A partner who drinks too much or misuses drugs

- Needing more and more of a drug or alcohol to get the same high

- A history of depression

- A history of childhood physical or sexual abuse

How Can You Tell If You Have a Problem with Alcohol or Drugs?

Answering the following questions can help you find out whether you or someone close to you has a problem with drinking or drugs.

- Have you ever felt that you drink too much and should cut down?

- Have you ever felt bad or guilty about your drinking?

- Have you ever had a drink as soon as you woke up to steady your nerves or to get rid of a hangover?

- Have you ever used a drug for nonmedical reasons?

- Has using drugs or alcohol created problems for you at home or at work?

- Do your family or friends complain about your drug or alcohol use?

- Have you gotten in fights or broken the law because you were on drugs or drunk?

- Do you continue to use drugs or alcohol even though you know it's harmful?

One "yes" answer suggests a possible problem. If you responded yes to more than one question, it is very likely that you have a problem.

Talk to a doctor, nurse, or mental-health professional as soon as possible. You may need to talk to a psychiatrist, psychologist, or substance-abuse counselor. Your doctor may also want to test your blood or urine to help design a treatment program for you.

How Is Treatment for Women Different from Treatment for Men?

Although women usually use drugs less often and in smaller amounts than men do, by the time women get treatment, they often have worse symptoms. This is because drugs and alcohol affect women and men differently. Women are more likely to become addicted to drugs or alcohol with smaller amounts of those substances.

Women may also have a harder time quitting certain substances, especially tobacco products. Women's bodies process the chemicals in tobacco differently from men's. Women are not as likely to be successful at quitting tobacco by using a nicotine patch or gum.

Women may also face unique barriers to getting treatment for drug and alcohol problems. Women may be pregnant or breastfeeding and unwilling to tell someone that they are addicted because they fear losing custody of their child. Women may be more likely to face additional barriers to treatment, such as needing daycare or eldercare.

Section 12.2

Substance Use While Pregnant and Breastfeeding

This section includes text excerpted from "Substance Use While Pregnant and Breastfeeding," National Institute on Drug Abuse (NIDA), July 2018.

Research shows that use of tobacco, alcohol, or illicit drugs or misuse of prescription drugs by pregnant women can have severe health consequences for infants. This is because many substances pass easily through the placenta, so substances that a pregnant woman takes also reach the fetus. Available research shows that smoking tobacco or marijuana, taking prescription pain relievers, or using illegal drugs during pregnancy is associated with double or even triple the risk of stillbirth. Estimates suggest that about five percent of pregnant women use one or more addictive substances.

Regular use of some drugs can cause neonatal abstinence syndrome (NAS), in which the baby goes through withdrawal upon birth. Most research in this area has focused on the effects of opioids (prescription pain relievers or heroin). However, data has shown that use of alcohol, barbiturates, benzodiazepines, and caffeine during pregnancy may also cause the infant to show withdrawal symptoms at birth. The type and severity of an infant's withdrawal symptoms depend on the drug(s) used, how long and how often the birth mother used, how her body breaks the drug down, and whether the infant was born full term or prematurely.

Symptoms of drug withdrawal in a newborn can develop immediately or up to 14 days after birth and can include:

- Blotchy skin coloring

- Diarrhea

- Excessive or high-pitched crying

- Abnormal sucking reflex

- Fever

- Hyperactive reflexes

- Increased muscle tone

- Irritability

- Poor feeding

- Rapid breathing

- Seizures

- Sleep problems

- Slow weight gain

- Stuffy nose and sneezing

- Sweating

- Trembling

- Vomiting

Effects of using some drugs could be long term and possibly fatal to the baby:

- Birth defects

- Low birth weight

- Premature birth

- Small head circumference

- Sudden infant death syndrome (SIDS)

Illegal Drugs
Marijuana (Cannabis)

More research needs to be done on how marijuana use during pregnancy could impact the health and development of infants, given changing policies about access to marijuana, significant increases in the number of pregnant women seeking substance-use disorder (SUD) treatment for marijuana use, and confounding effects of polysubstance use, unfortunately, given the unreliable nature of self-reported data, the number of women who use marijuana while pregnant is unknown.

There is no human research connecting marijuana use to the chance of miscarriage, although animal studies indicate that the risk for miscarriage increases if marijuana is used early in pregnancy. Some associations have been found between marijuana use during pregnancy and future developmental and hyperactivity disorders in children. There is substantial evidence of a statistical association between marijuana smoking among pregnant women and low birth weight. Researchers theorize that elevated levels of carbon dioxide might restrict fetal growth in women who use marijuana during pregnancy. Evidence is mixed related to premature birth, although some evidence suggests long-term use may elevate these risks. Given the potential of marijuana to negatively impact the developing brain, the American College of Obstetricians and Gynecologists (ACOG) recommends that obstetrician-gynecologists counsel women against using marijuana while trying to get pregnant, during pregnancy, and while they are breastfeeding.

Some women report using marijuana to treat severe nausea associated with their pregnancy; however, there is no research confirming that this is a safe practice, and it is generally not recommended. Women considering using medical marijuana while pregnant should not do so without checking with their healthcare provider. Animal studies have shown that moderate concentrations of Tetrahydrocannabinol (THC), when administered to mothers while pregnant or nursing, could have long-lasting effects on the child, including increasing stress responsivity and abnormal patterns of social interactions. Animal studies also show learning deficits in prenatally exposed individuals.

Human research has shown that some babies born to women who used marijuana during their pregnancies display altered responses to visual stimuli, increased trembling, and a high-pitched cry, which could indicate problems with neurological development. In school, marijuana-exposed children are more likely to show gaps in problem-solving skills, memory, and the ability to remain attentive. More research is needed, however, to disentangle marijuana-specific effects from those of other environmental factors that could be associated with a mother's marijuana use, such as an impoverished home environment or the mother's use of other drugs. Prenatal marijuana exposure is also associated with an increased likelihood of a person using marijuana as a young adult, even when other factors that influence drug use are considered.

The number of women who use marijuana while pregnant is unknown. One study found that about 20 percent of pregnant women 24-years-old and younger screened positive for marijuana. However, this study also found that women were about twice as likely to screen positive for marijuana use via a drug test than they state in self-reported measures. This suggests that self-reported rates of marijuana use in pregnant females is not an accurate measure of marijuana use and may be an underestimation.

Very little is known about marijuana use and breastfeeding. One study suggests that moderate amounts of THC find their way into breast milk when a nursing mother uses marijuana. Some evidence shows that exposure to THC through breast milk in the first month of life could result in decreased motor development at one year of age. There have been no studies to determine if exposure to THC during nursing is linked to effects later in the child's life. With regular use, THC can accumulate in human breast milk to high concentrations. Because a baby's brain is still forming, THC consumed in breast milk could affect brain development. Given all these uncertainties, nursing mothers are discouraged from using marijuana. New mothers using medical marijuana should be vigilant about coordinating care between the doctor recommending their marijuana use and the pediatrician caring for their baby.

Stimulants (Cocaine and Methamphetamine)

It is not completely known how a pregnant woman's cocaine use affects her child since cocaine-using women are more likely to also use other drugs such as alcohol, to have poor nutrition, or to not seek prenatal care. All of these factors can affect a developing fetus, making it difficult to isolate the effects of cocaine.

Research does show, however, that pregnant women who use cocaine are at higher risk for maternal migraines and seizures, premature membrane rupture, and placental abruption (separation of the placental lining from the uterus). Pregnancy is accompanied by normal cardiovascular changes, and cocaine use exacerbates these changes—sometimes leading to serious problems with high blood pressure (hypertensive crisis), spontaneous miscarriage, preterm labor, and difficult delivery. Babies born to mothers who use cocaine during pregnancy may also have low birth weight and smaller head circumferences and are shorter in length than babies born to mothers who do not use cocaine. They also show symptoms of irritability, hyperactivity, tremors, high-pitched cry, and excessive sucking at birth. These symptoms may be due to the effects of cocaine itself, rather than withdrawal since cocaine and its metabolites are still present in the baby's body up to five to seven days after delivery. Estimates suggest that there are about 750,000 cocaine-exposed pregnancies every year.

Pregnant women who use methamphetamine have a greater risk of preeclampsia (high blood pressure and possible organ damage), premature delivery, and placental abruption. Their babies are more likely to be smaller and to have low birth weight. In a large, longitudinal study of children prenatally exposed to methamphetamine, exposed children had increased emotional reactivity and anxiety/depression, were more withdrawn, had problems with attention, and showed cognitive problems that could lead to poorer academic outcomes.

MDMA (Ecstasy, Molly)

More research is needed on the effects of 3,4-methylenedioxymethamphetamine (MDMA) use during pregnancy. What research exists suggests that prenatal MDMA exposure may cause learning, memory, and motor problems in the baby.

Heroin

Heroin use during pregnancy can result in neonatal abstinence syndrome (NAS) specifically associated with opioid use. NAS occurs when heroin passes through the placenta to the fetus during pregnancy, causing the baby to become dependent on opioids. Symptoms include excessive crying, high-pitched cry, irritability, seizures, and gastrointestinal (GI) problems, among others.

Other Substances
Alcohol

Alcohol use while pregnant can result in fetal alcohol spectrum disorders (FASDs), a general term that includes fetal alcohol syndrome (FAS), partial fetal alcohol syndrome (pFAS), alcohol-related disorders of brain development, and alcohol-related birth defects. These effects can last throughout life, causing difficulties with motor coordination, emotional control, schoolwork, socialization, and holding a job.

Fetal alcohol exposure occurs when a woman drinks while pregnant. Alcohol can disrupt fetal development at any stage during pregnancy—including at the earliest stages before a woman even knows she is pregnant.

There is little research into how a nursing mother's alcohol use might affect her breastfed baby. What science suggests is that, contrary to folklore, alcohol does not increase a nursing mother's milk production, and it may disrupt the breastfed child's sleep cycle. The American Academy of Pediatrics (AAP) recommends that alcohol drinking should be minimized during the months a woman nurses and daily intake limited to no more than two ounces of liquor, 8 ounces of wine, or 2 average beers for a 130-pound woman. In this case, nursing should take place at least two hours after drinking to allow the alcohol to be reduced or eliminated from the mother's body and milk. This will minimize the amount of alcohol passed to the baby.

Nicotine (Tobacco Products and E-Cigarettes)

Almost ten percent of pregnant women in the United States have smoked cigarettes in the past month. Carbon monoxide and nicotine from tobacco smoke may interfere with the oxygen supply to the fetus. Nicotine also readily crosses the placenta, and concentrations of this drug in the blood of the fetus can be as much as 15 percent higher than in the mother. Smoking during pregnancy increases the risk for certain birth defects, premature birth, miscarriage, and low birth weight and is estimated to have caused more than 1,000 infant deaths each year. Newborns of smoking mothers also show signs of stress and drug withdrawal consistent with what has been reported in infants exposed to other drugs. In some cases, smoking during pregnancy may be associated with SIDS, as well as learning and behavioral problems and an increased risk of obesity in children. In addition, smoking more than one pack a day during pregnancy nearly doubles the risk that the affected child will become addicted to tobacco if that child starts smoking. Even a mother's secondhand exposure to cigarette smoke can cause problems; such exposure is associated with premature birth and low birth weight, for example.

Research provides strong support that nicotine is a gateway drug, making the brain more sensitive to the effects of other drugs such as cocaine. This shows that pregnant women who use nicotine may be affecting their fetus's brain in ways they may not anticipate. Additionally, e-cigarettes (or e-vaporizers) sometimes contain nicotine. Therefore, those products may also pose a risk to the fetus's health.

Similar to pregnant women, nursing mothers are also advised against using tobacco. New mothers who smoke should be aware that nicotine is passed through breast milk, so tobacco use can impact the infant's brain and body development—even if the mother never smokes near the baby. There is also evidence that the milk of mothers who smoke smells and may taste like cigarettes. It is unclear whether this will make it more likely that exposed children may find tobacco flavors/smells more appealing later in life.

Secondhand Smoke

Newborns exposed to secondhand smoke are at greater risk for SIDS, respiratory illnesses (asthma, respiratory infections, and bronchitis), ear infections, cavities, and increased medical visits and hospitalizations. If a woman smokes and is planning a pregnancy, the ideal time to seek smoking cessation help is before she becomes pregnant.

Section 12.3

Negative Consequences of Prenatal Exposure to Drugs

This section contains text excerpted from the following sources:
Text under the heading "Prenatal Exposure to Substance Use:
A Growing Concern" is excerpted from "Infants with Prenatal
Substance Exposure," Substance Abuse and Mental Health Services
Administration (SAMHSA), June 25, 2018; Text beginning with the
heading "Effects of Prenatal Exposure to Substance Use" is excerpted
from "Health Consequences of Drug Misuse," National Institute on
Drug Abuse (NIDA), March 2017; Text under the heading "What You
Need to Do" is excerpted from "Pregnancy and Substance Abuse,"
MedlinePlus, National Institutes of Health (NIH), January 3, 2017.

Prenatal Exposure to Substance Use: A Growing Concern

Each year, an estimated 15 percent of infants are affected by prenatal alcohol or illicit drug exposure. Prenatal exposure to alcohol,
tobacco, and illicit drugs has the potential to cause a wide spectrum
of physical and developmental challenges for these infants. Coordinated services and early intervention for pregnant women with substance-use disorders (SUDs) and their infants are critical in preparing
families for optimal bonding, health, and well-being.

Effects of Prenatal Exposure to Substance Use

Studies show that various drugs may result in miscarriage, premature birth, low birth weight, and a variety of behavioral and cognitive
problems in the child. A baby can also be born dependent on the drug
if the mother uses it regularly—a condition called neonatal abstinence
syndrome (NAS).

Drugs That May Have Adverse Prenatal Effects

Drugs that may have adverse prenatal effects include:

- Cocaine
- Heroin
- Inhalants
- Marijuana

- 3,4-methylenedioxymethamphetamine (MDMA)

- Methamphetamine

- Nicotine

- Prescription and over-the-counter (OTC) drugs

What You Need to Do

When you are pregnant, you are not just "eating for two." You also breathe and drink for two. If you smoke, use alcohol or take illegal drugs, so does your unborn baby.

To protect your baby, you should avoid:

- **Tobacco.** Smoking during pregnancy passes nicotine, carbon monoxide, and other harmful chemicals to your baby. This could cause many problems for your unborn baby's development. It raises the risk of your baby being born too small, too early, or with birth defects. Smoking can also affect babies after they are born. Your baby would be more likely to develop diseases such as asthma and obesity. There is also a higher risk of dying from sudden infant death syndrome (SIDS).

- **Drinking alcohol.** There is no known amount of alcohol that is safe for a woman to drink during pregnancy. If you drink alcohol when you are pregnant, your child could be born with lifelong fetal alcohol syndrome disorders (FASDs). Children with FASD can have a mix of physical, behavioral, and learning problems.

- **Illegal drugs.** Using illegal drugs such as cocaine and methamphetamines may cause underweight babies, birth defects, or withdrawal symptoms after birth.

- **Misusing prescription drugs.** If you are taking prescription medicines, carefully follow your healthcare provider's instructions. It can be dangerous to take more medicines than you are supposed to, use them to get high or take someone else's medicines. For example, misusing opioids can cause birth defects, withdrawal in the baby, or even loss of the baby.

If you are pregnant and you are doing any of these things, get help. Your healthcare provider can recommend programs to help you quit. You and your baby's health depend on it.

Section 12.4

What Women Need to Know about Date Rape Drugs

This section includes text excerpted from "Date Rape
Drugs," Office on Women's Health (OWH), U.S. Department of
Health and Human Services (HHS), May 22, 2018.

Date rape drugs are illegal and are sometimes used to assist a
sexual assault. Sexual assault is any type of sexual activity that a
person does not agree to. Date rape drugs often have no color, smell,
or taste, so you can't tell if you are being drugged. The drugs can make
you weak and confused—or even cause you to pass out—so that you
cannot consent to sex. Both men and women can be drugged with date
rape drugs.

What Are Date Rape Drugs?

These are drugs that are sometimes used during sexual assault.
Sexual assault is any type of sexual activity that a person does not
agree to. It can include touching that is not okay; putting something
into the vagina; rape; and attempted rape.

Date rape drugs are powerful and dangerous. They can be slipped
into your drink when you are not looking. The drugs often have no
color, smell, or taste, so you can't tell if you are being drugged. The
drugs can make you become weak and confused—or even pass out—
so that you cannot consent to sex. If you are drugged, you might not
remember what happened while you were drugged. Date rape drugs
may be used on both females and males.

These drugs also are known as "club drugs" because they tend to
be used at dance clubs, concerts, and raves.

The term "date rape" is widely used. But most experts prefer the
term "drug-facilitated sexual assault." These drugs also are used to
help people commit other crimes, like robbery and physical assault.
They are used on both men and women. The term "date rape" also can
be misleading because the person who commits the crime might not
be dating the victim. Rather, it could be an acquaintance or stranger.

What Are the Most Common Date Rape Drugs?

The three most common date rape drugs are:

- **Rohypnol.** Rohypnol is the trade name for flunitrazepam. Abuse of two similar drugs appears to have replaced Rohypnol abuse in some parts of the United States. These are: clonazepam (marketed as Klonopin in the United States and Rivotril in Mexico) and alprazolam (marketed as Xanax). Rohypnol is also known as:

  - Circles
  - Forget Pill
  - LA Rochas
  - Lunch Money
  - Mexican Valium
  - Mind Erasers
  - Poor Man's Quaalude
  - R-2
  - Rib
  - Roach
  - Roach-2
  - Roches
  - Roofies
  - Roopies
  - Rope
  - Rophies
  - Ruffies
  - Trip-and-Fall
  - Whiteys

- **GHB**, which is short for gamma-hydroxybutyric acid. GHB is also known as:

  - Bedtime scoop
  - Cherry meth
  - Easy lay
  - Energy drink
  - G
  - Gamma 10
  - Georgia home boy
  - G-Juice
  - Gook
  - Goop
  - Great hormones
  - Grievous bodily harm (GBH)
  - Liquid E
  - Liquid ecstasy
  - Liquid X
  - PM
  - Saltwater
  - Soap
  - Somatomax
  - Vita-G

- **Ketamine**, also known as:

  - Black hole
  - Bump

- Cat Valium
- Green
- Jet
- K
- K-Hole

- Kit kat
- Psychedelic heroin
- Purple
- Special K
- Superacid

What Do the Drugs Look Like?

- Rohypnol comes as a pill that dissolves in liquids. Some are small, round, and white. Newer pills are oval and green-gray in color. When slipped into a drink, a dye in these new pills makes clear liquids turn bright blue and makes dark liquids turn cloudy. But this color change might be hard to see in a dark drink, like cola or dark beer, or in a dark room. Also, the pills with no dye are still available. The pills may be ground up into a powder.

- GHB has a few forms: a liquid with no odor or color, white powder, and a pill. It might give your drink a slightly salty taste. Mixing it with a sweet drink, such as fruit juice, can mask the salty taste.

- Ketamine comes as a liquid and a white powder.

What Effects Do These Drugs Have on the Body?

These drugs are very powerful. They can affect you very quickly and without your knowing. The length of time that the effects last varies. It depends on how much of the drug is taken and if the drug is mixed with other drugs or alcohol. Alcohol makes the drugs even stronger and can cause serious health problems—even death.

Rohypnol

The effects of Rohypnol can be felt within 30 minutes of being drugged and can last for several hours. If you are drugged, you might look and act like someone who is drunk. You might have trouble standing. Your speech might be slurred. Or you might pass out. Rohypnol can cause these problems:

- Muscle relaxation or loss of muscle control
- Difficulty with motor movements

132

- Drunk feeling
- Problems talking
- Nausea
- Can't remember what happened while drugged
- Loss of consciousness
- Confusion
- Problems seeing
- Dizziness
- Sleepiness
- Lower blood pressure
- Stomach problems
- Death

Gamma-Hydroxybutyric Acid

GHB takes effect in about 15 minutes and can last three or four hours. It is very potent: A very small amount can have a big effect. So it's easy to overdose on GHB. Most GHB is made by people in home or street "labs." So, you don't know what's in it or how it will affect you. GHB can cause these problems:

- Relaxation
- Drowsiness
- Dizziness
- Nausea
- Problems seeing
- Loss of consciousness
- Seizures
- Can't remember what happened while drugged
- Problems breathing
- Tremors
- Sweating
- Vomiting

- Slow heart rate
- Dream-like feeling
- Coma
- Death

Ketamine

Ketamine is very fast-acting. You might be aware of what is happening to you, but unable to move. It also causes memory problems. Later, you might not be able to remember what happened while you were drugged. Ketamine can cause these problems:

- Distorted perceptions of sight and sound
- Lost sense of time and identity
- Out of body experiences
- Dream-like feeling
- Feeling out of control
- Impaired motor function
- Problems breathing
- Convulsions
- Vomiting
- Memory problems
- Numbness
- Loss of coordination
- Aggressive or violent behavior
- Depression
- High blood pressure
- Slurred speech

Are These Drugs Legal in the United States?

Some of these drugs are legal when lawfully used for medical purposes. But that doesn't mean they are safe. These drugs are powerful and can hurt you. They should only be used under a doctor's care and order.

- Rohypnol is not legal in the United States. It is legal in Europe and Mexico, where it is prescribed for sleep problems and to assist anesthesia before surgery. It is brought into the United States illegally.

- Ketamine is legal in the United States for use as an anesthetic for humans and animals. It is mostly used on animals. Veterinary clinics are robbed for their ketamine supplies.

- GHB was made legal in the United States to treat problems from narcolepsy (a sleep disorder). Distribution of GHB for this purpose is tightly restricted.

Is Alcohol a Date Rape Drug? What about Other Drugs?

Any drug that can affect judgment and behavior can put a person at risk for unwanted or risky sexual activity. Alcohol is one such drug. In fact, alcohol is the drug most commonly used to help commit sexual assault. When a person drinks too much alcohol:

- It's harder to think clearly.

- It's harder to set limits and make good choices.

- It's harder to tell when a situation could be dangerous.

- It's harder to say "no" to sexual advances.

- It's harder to fight back if a sexual assault occurs.

- It's possible to blackout and to have memory loss.

The club drug "ecstasy" 3,4-methylenedioxymethamphetamine (MDMA) has been used to commit sexual assault. It can be slipped into someone's drink without the person's knowledge. Also, a person who willingly takes ecstasy is at greater risk of sexual assault. Ecstasy can make a person feel "lovey-dovey" towards others. It also can lower a person's ability to give reasoned consent. Once under the drug's influence, a person is less able to sense danger or to resist a sexual assault.

Even if a victim of sexual assault drank alcohol or willingly took drugs, the victim is not at fault for being assaulted. It is never okay to have sexual contact with someone without their consent. Sexual assault is always the responsibility of the person who commits the assault. Sexual assault is never the victim's fault, regardless of the circumstances.

How Can You Protect Yourself from Being a Victim?

Consider the following tips to protect yourself from being a victim:

- Don't accept drinks from other people.
- Open containers yourself.
- Keep your drink with you at all times, even when you go to the bathroom.
- Don't share drinks.
- Don't drink from punch bowls or other common, open containers. They may already have drugs in them.
- If someone offers to get you a drink from a bar or at a party, go with the person to order your drink. Watch the drink being poured and carry it yourself.
- Don't drink anything that tastes or smells strange. Sometimes, GHB tastes salty.
- Have a nondrinking friend with you to make sure nothing happens.
- If you realize you left your drink unattended, pour it out.
- If you feel drunk and haven't drunk any alcohol—or, if you feel like the effects of drinking alcohol are stronger than usual—get help right away.

Are There Ways to Tell If You Might Have Been Drugged and Raped?

It is often hard to tell. Most victims don't remember being drugged or assaulted. The victim might not be aware of the attack until 8 or 12 hours after it occurred. These drugs also leave the body very quickly. Once a victim gets help, there might be no proof that drugs were involved in the attack. But there are some signs that you might have been drugged:

- You feel drunk and haven't drunk any alcohol—or, you feel like the effects of drinking alcohol are stronger than usual.
- You wake up feeling very hungover and disoriented or having no memory of a period of time.
- You remember having a drink but cannot recall anything after that.

- You find that your clothes are torn or not on right.

- You feel like you had sex, but you cannot remember it.

What Should You Do If You Think You've Been Drugged and Raped?

If you think that you might have been drugged and raped, then:

- **Get medical care right away.** Call 911 or have a trusted friend take you to a hospital emergency room. Don't urinate, douche, bathe, brush your teeth, wash your hands, change clothes, or eat or drink before you go. These things may give evidence of the rape. The hospital will use a "rape kit" to collect evidence.

- **Call the police from the hospital.** Tell the police exactly what you remember. Be honest about all your activities. Remember, nothing you did—including drinking alcohol or doing drugs—can justify rape.

- **Ask the hospital to take a urine (pee) sample that can be used to test for date rape drugs.** The drugs leave your system quickly. Rohypnol stays in the body for several hours, and can be detected in the urine up to 72 hours after taking it. GHB leaves the body in 12 hours. Don't urinate before going to the hospital.

- **Don't pick up or clean up where you think the assault might have occurred.** There could be evidence left behind— such as on a drinking glass or bed sheets.

- **Get counseling and treatment.** Feelings of shame, guilt, fear, and shock are normal. A counselor can help you work through these emotions and begin the healing process. Calling a crisis center or a hotline is a good place to start. One national hotline is the National Sexual Assault hotline at 800-656-4673.

Chapter 13

Cigarette Smoking and Tobacco Use among People of Low Socioeconomic Status

Adults who have lower levels of educational attainment, who are unemployed, or who live at, near, or below the U.S. federal poverty level are considered to have low socioeconomic status (SES).

According to the U.S. Census Bureau, the poverty rate in 2016 was 12.7 percent. In 2017, the percentage of people age 18 and older who had completed only high school was 28.9 percent, and the percentage who had completed high school up to grade 11 but had no diploma was 4.2 percent.

In the United States, people living below the poverty level and people having lower levels of educational attainment have higher rates of cigarette smoking than the general population.

This chapter includes text excerpted from "Cigarette Smoking and Tobacco Use among People of Low Socioeconomic Status," Center for Disease Control and Prevention (CDC), March 7, 2018.

Tobacco Use Prevalence

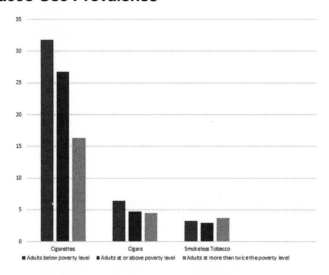

Figure 13.1. *Current Use* of Cigarettes, Cigars, and Smokeless Tobacco among Adults Living Below Poverty Level Compared with Adults Living at or above Poverty Level.*

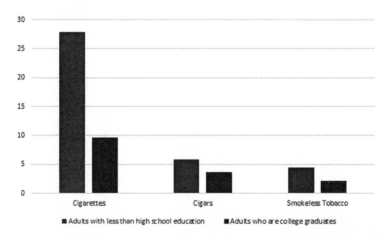

Figure 13.2. *Current Use* of Cigarettes, Cigars, and Smokeless Tobacco among Adults with Less Than High School Education Compared With Adults Who Are College Graduates.*

* "Current Use" is defined as self-reported consumption of cigarettes, cigars, or smokeless tobacco in the past 30 days (at the time of survey).
† Data taken from the National Survey on Drug Use and Health, 2016, and refer to adults age 18 years and older.

Health Effects

Cigarette smoking disproportionately affects the health of people with low SES. Lower income cigarette smokers suffer more from diseases caused by smoking than do smokers with higher incomes.

- Populations in the most socioeconomically deprived groups have higher lung cancer risk than those in the most affluent groups.

- People with less than a high-school education have higher lung cancer incidence than those with a college education.

- People with family incomes of less than $12,500 have higher lung cancer incidence than those with family incomes of $50,000 or more.

- People living in rural, deprived areas have 18 to 20 percent higher rates of lung cancer than people living in urban areas.

- Lower-income populations have less access to healthcare, making it more likely that they are diagnosed at later stages of diseases and conditions.

Patterns of Cigarette Smoking

People with low SES tend to smoke cigarettes more heavily.

- People living in poverty smoke cigarettes for a duration of nearly twice as many years as people with a family income of three times the poverty rate.

- People with a high-school education smoke cigarettes for a duration of more than twice as many years as people with at least a bachelor's degree.

- Blue-collar workers are more likely to start smoking cigarettes at a younger age and to smoke more heavily than white-collar workers.

Secondhand Smoke Exposure

Secondhand smoke exposure is higher among people living below the poverty level and those with less education.

- Low SES populations are more likely to suffer the harmful health consequences of exposure to secondhand smoke.

- Blue-collar workers are more likely to be exposed to secondhand smoke at work than white-collar workers.

- Service workers, especially bartenders and wait staff, report the lowest rates of workplace smoke-free policies than other occupation categories.

Quitting Behavior

People of low SES are just as likely to make quit attempts but are less likely to quit smoking cigarettes than those who are not.

- An estimated 66.6 percent of adult current daily cigarette smokers living below the poverty level attempt to quit smoking cigarettes compared with 69.9 percent of those living at or above the poverty level.

- An estimated 39.0 percent of adult current daily cigarette smokers with no high school diploma attempt to quit smoking compared with 44.0 percent of those with some college education.

- Adults who live below the poverty level have less success in quitting (34.5%) than those who live at or above the poverty level (57.5%).

- Adults with less than a high-school education (9 to 12 years, but no diploma) have less success in quitting (43.5%) than those with a college education or greater (73.9%).

- Blue-collar and service workers are less likely to quit smoking than white-collar workers.

Tobacco Industry Marketing and Targeting

Tobacco companies often target their advertising campaigns toward low-income neighborhoods and communities.

- Researchers have found a higher density of tobacco retailers in low-income neighborhoods.

- Tobacco companies have historically targeted women of low SES through distribution of discount coupons, point-of-sale discounts, direct-mail coupons, and development of brands that appeal to these women.

Culturally appropriate anti-smoking health marketing strategies and mass media campaigns such as the CDC's Tips From Former Smokers national tobacco education campaign, as well as CDC-recommended tobacco prevention and control programs and policies, can help reduce the burden of disease among people of low SES status.

Chapter 14

Substance Abuse in the Workplace

Substance use negatively affects U.S. industry through lost productivity, workplace accidents and injuries, employee absenteeism, low morale, and increased illness. U.S. companies lose billions of dollars a year because of employees' alcohol and drug use and related problems. Research shows that the rate of substance use varies by occupation and industry.

The National Survey on Drug Use and Health (NSDUH) gathers information about substance use and dependence or abuse. NSDUH defines illicit drugs as marijuana/hashish, cocaine (including crack), inhalants, hallucinogens, heroin, or prescription-type drugs used nonmedically. Heavy alcohol use is defined as drinking five or more drinks on the same occasion (i.e., at the same time or within a couple of hours of each other) on 5 or more days in the past 30 days. NSDUH also includes a series of questions to assess symptoms of dependence on or abuse of alcohol or illicit drugs during the past year. These questions are used to classify persons as dependent on or abusing substances based on criteria in the fourth edition of the *Diagnostic and Statistical Manual of Mental Disorders (DSM-IV)*. In this chapter, dependence on or abuse of alcohol or illicit drugs is referred to as a "substance-use disorder."

This chapter includes text excerpted from "Substance Use and Substance Use Disorder by Industry," Substance Abuse and Mental Health Services Administration (SAMHSA), April 16, 2015. Reviewed January 2019.

This chapter contains one of the several reports designed to update SAMHSA's Analytic Series A-29, Worker Substance Use and Workplace Policies and Programs, published in 2007. To enhance the statistical power and analytic capability and ensure consistency in time frames across all of the updated reports, 5-year time periods were chosen. This issue of The Center for Behavioral Health Statistics and Quality (CBHSQ) Report uses combined data from the 2008 to 2012 surveys to present estimates of substance-use behaviors (past-month illicit-drug use and past-month heavy alcohol use) and past-year substance-use disorder among persons age 18 to 64 who are employed full time by industry category. Full-time employment is defined as working 35 or more hours per week and working in the past week or having a job despite not working in the past week. NSDUH includes questions to assess the type of business or industry in which these respondents worked. Using the North American Industry Classification System (NAICS) developed by the U.S. Census Bureau, 19 major industry groupings were identified.

The analyses presented in this report includes comparisons of the 2008 to 2012 rates of illicit-drug use and heavy alcohol use across industries and comparisons of the 2008 to 2012 rates with the 2003 to 2007 rates within each industry. For this report, testing for differences across industry groupings included two phases. First, differences across industries were assessed by making pair-wise comparisons between industries (e.g., the rates for each industry were compared with those of every other industry) to identify whether any industry had significantly higher rates than all other industries. A second test was conducted to assess whether significant differences between industries were the result of differences in the age and gender composition of the industry. Previous research has shown that males have higher substance-use rates than females and adults age 18 to 25 have higher substance-use rates than older adults. As a result, male-dominated or youth-dominated industries could have higher substance-use rates at the overall level, but when the industry's age and gender distribution was taken into account, the industry might not differ from other industries. The final part of this chapter presents comparisons of combined 2008 to 2012 data with combined 2003 to 2007 data.

Substance Use by Industry Category

Rates of substance-use behaviors and substance-use disorder varied across industry groupings. The overall rate of past-month heavy alcohol use among full-time workers age 18 to 64 was 8.7 percent. Rates of past-month heavy alcohol use ranged from 17.5 percent among workers in the mining industry to 4.4 percent among workers in the healthcare and social-assistance industry.

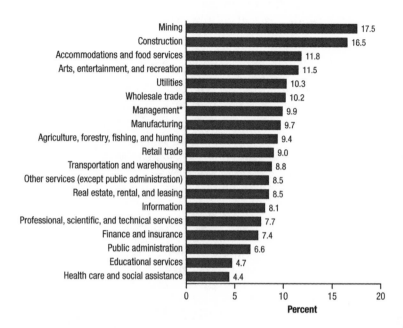

Figure 14.1. *Past-Month Heavy Alcohol Use among Adults Age 18 to 64 Employed Full Time, by Industry Category: Combined 2008 to 2012.* (Source: SAMHSA, Center for Behavioral Health Statistics and Quality, National Surveys on Drug Use and Health (NSDUHs) 2008 to 2010 (Revised March 2012) and 2011 to 2012.)

Workers in the mining (17.5%) and construction (16.5%) industries had the highest rates of past-month heavy alcohol use. For the workers in the construction industry, this finding remained true even when controlling for gender and age differences across industries. This indicates that there is something unique about past-month heavy alcohol use for the construction industry that would remain even if the construction industry had the same gender and age distribution of any other industry. However, for the mining industry, this higher rate did not remain when controlling for age or gender differences. This indicates that the high heavy alcohol use rate in the mining industry can be attributed to the demographic composition of the mining industry.

The overall rate of past month illicit-drug use among full-time workers age 18 to 64 was 8.6 percent. Rates of past-month illicit-drug use ranged from 19.1 percent among workers in the accommodations and food services industry to 4.3 percent among workers in the public-administration industry. These findings remained true even when controlling for gender and age differences across industries.

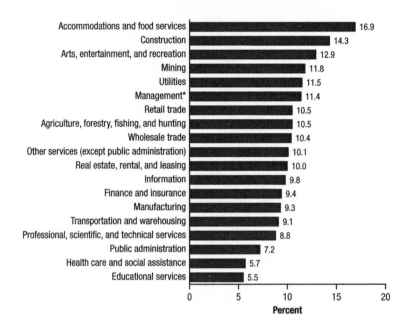

Figure 14.2. *Past-Month Illicit-Drug Use among Adults Age 18 to 64 Employed Full Time, by Industry Category: Combined 2008 to 2012.* (Source: SAMHSA, Center for Behavioral Health Statistics and Quality, National Surveys on Drug Use and Health (NSDUHs) 2008 to 2010 (Revised March 2012) and 2011 to 2012.)

The overall rate of past-year substance-use disorder among full-time workers age 18 to 64 was 9.5 percent. Rates of past-year substance-use disorder ranged from 16.9 percent among workers in the accommodations and food-services industry to 5.5 percent among workers in the educational-services industry. Although the accommodations and food-services industry group had the highest rate of past-year substance-use disorder, this finding did not remain true after controlling for age and gender distributions. This indicates that the high rate can be attributed to the demographic composition of the accommodation and food-services industry.

146

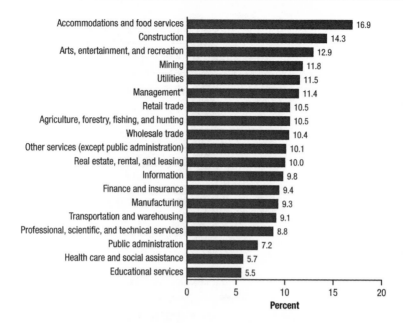

Figure 14.3. *Past-Year Substance-Use Disorder among Adults Age 18 to 64 Employed Full Time, by Industry Category: Combined 2008 to 2012.* (Source: SAMHSA, Center for Behavioral Health Statistics and Quality, National Surveys on Drug Use and Health (NSDUHs) 2008 to 2010 (Revised March 2012) and 2011 to 2012.)

Trends

Comparisons between combined 2003 to 2007 data and combined 2008 to 2012 data show some changes in rates of substance-use behaviors or disorders by industry category. Between the two time periods, rates of past month illicit-drug use increased among workers in the accommodations and food-services industry (from 16.9 to 19.1 percent) and in the educational-services industry (from 3.7 to 4.8 percent), and decreased among workers in the construction-services industry (from 13.9 to 11.6 percent). Additionally, decreases were seen in the rates of past-year substance-use disorder in four industry categories: construction (from 17.3 to 14.3 percent), management (from 13.8 to 11.4 percent), wholesale trade (from 13.4 to 10.4 percent), and manufacturing (from 10.4 to 9.3 percent). The changes within each industry between the two time periods do not account for any changes in the demographic composition (e.g., age distribution) that may have occurred within the industries.

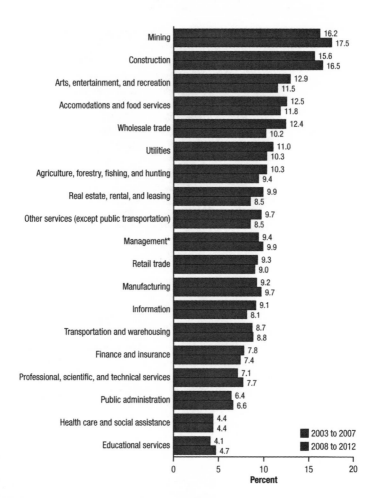

Figure 14.4. *Past-Month Heavy Alcohol Use among Adults Age 18 to 64 Employed Full Time, by Industry Category: Combined 2003 to 2007 and Combined 2008 to 2012.* (Source: SAMHSA, Center for Behavioral Health Statistics and Quality, National Surveys on Drug Use and Health (NSDUHs) 2003 to 2005, 2006 to 2010 (Revised March 2012) and 2011 to 2012.)

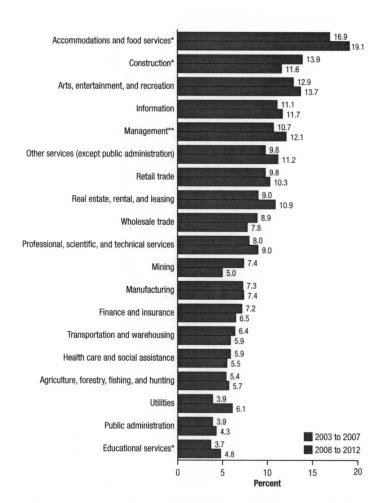

Figure 14.5. *Past-Month Illicit-Drug Use among Adults Age 18 to 64 Employed Full Time, by Industry Category: Combined 2003 to 2007 and Combined 2008 to 2012.* (Source: SAMHSA, Center for Behavioral Health Statistics and Quality, National Surveys on Drug Use and Health (NSDUHs) 2003 to 2005, 2006 to 2010 (Revised March 2012) and 2011 to 2012.)

* Difference between estimates for 2003 to 2007 and for 2008 to 2012 are statistically significant at .05 level.
** The full title of this category is "Management of companies and enterprises, administration, support, waste management, and remediation services."

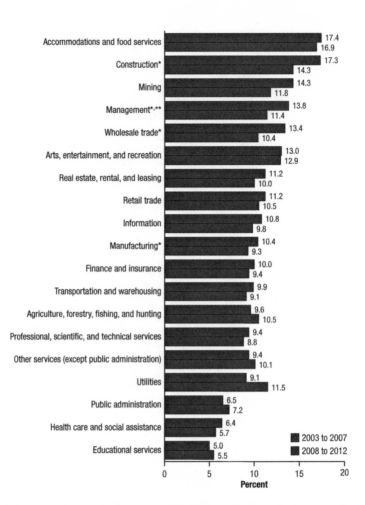

Figure 14.6. *Past-Year Substance-Use Disorder among Adults Age 18 to 64 Employed Full Time, by Industry Category: Combined 2003 to 2007 and Combined 2008 to 2012.* (Source: SAMHSA, Center for Behavioral Health Statistics and Quality, National Surveys on Drug Use and Health (NSDUHs) 2003 to 2005, 2006 to 2010 (Revised March 2012) and 2011 to 2012.)

* Difference between estimates for 2003 to 2007 and for 2008 to 2012 are statistically significant at .05 level.
** The full title of this category is "Management of companies and enterprises, administration, support, waste management, and remediation services."

Discussion

Employee heavy alcohol use, use of illicit drugs, and substance-use disorders are associated with negative work behaviors, such as absenteeism and frequent job changes. This chapter indicates that the prevalence of substance-use and substance-use disorders is not consistent across industries. For example, the lowest rates of heavy alcohol use, illicit-drug use, and substance-use disorder were generally seen in education, healthcare and social assistance, and public administration. In contrast, higher rates were generally seen in mining, construction, and accommodations, and food-services industries. There are demographic differences in the age and gender composition across industries, and some of the differences in substance-use rates across industries were statistically significant even when controlling for age or gender. Differences across industries that did not remain significant when controlling for age and gender are still important to identify. Employers in industries that have higher or lower rates of heavy alcohol use, use of illicit drugs, and substance-use disorder that can be attributed to the demographic composition of their industry can use this information when developing prevention/education programs.

When heavy alcohol use, use of illicit drugs, and substance-use disorder rates are examined over time, it appears that some industries have had a reduction in rates; however, there were increases as well. An extension of this research could examine whether the changes in use rates correspond to either change in climate in the industries (e.g., attitudes toward substance use, distribution of prevention messages) or shifts in the demographic compositions of the industries across these time periods.

Studies also have indicated that employers vary in their treatment of substance-use issues and that workplace-based Employee Assistance Programs (EAPs) can be a valuable resource for obtaining help for substance-using workers. Given the lifetime health and economic burdens from alcohol-use, illicit-drug, and substance-use disorders, this chapter illustrates the need to monitor industries individually.

Chapter 15

Seniors and Drug Abuse

Illicit-drug use generally declines as individuals move through young adulthood and into middle adulthood. Although the percentage of people with substance-use disorder (SUD) reflects the decline in use as people age, more than one million individuals age 65 or older ("older adults") had an SUD in 2014, including 978,000 older adults with an alcohol use disorder and 161,000 with an illicit-drug use disorder. Research suggests that substance use is an emerging public health issue among the nation's older adults. Illicit-drug use among adults age 50 or older is projected to increase from 2.2 to 3.1 percent between 2001 and 2020. For example, the number of older Americans with SUD is expected to rise from 2.8 million in 2002–2006 to 5.7 million by 2020. The emergence of SUD as a public health concern among older adults reflects, in part, the relatively higher drug use rates of the baby boom generation (people born between 1946 and 1964) compared with previous generations. Thus, there is a cohort of older adults who may experience the negative consequences of substance use, including physical and mental health issues, social and family problems, involvement with the criminal-justice system, and death from drug overdose. Older adults are more likely than people in other age groups to have chronic health conditions and to take prescription medication, which may further complicate adverse effects of substance use.

This chapter includes text excerpted from "A Day in the Life of Older Adults: Substance Use Facts," Substance Abuse and Mental Health Services Administration (SAMHSA), May 11, 2017.

This chapter presents information about substance use in older adults from several data sources, including information on the use of substances, admissions to treatment, and emergency department (ED) visits for substance use on a typical or average day. Data in this chapter are for adults age 65 or older and are drawn from three national data sources collected by the Center for Behavioral Health Statistics and Quality (CBHSQ) in the Substance Abuse and Mental Health Services Administration (SAMHSA). These data sources include the National Survey on Drug Use and Health (NSDUH), the Treatment Episode Data Set (TEDS), and the Drug Abuse Warning Network (DAWN).

Different years of NSDUH, TEDS, and DAWN data were used in this analysis based on the availability. All NSDUH estimates in this chapter are annual averages based on combined 2007 to 2014 NSDUH data. Combining multiple years of NSDUH data allows substance use among older adults to be examined in greater detail by improving the precision of estimates for making statistical comparisons. TEDS data provide information on admissions to substance-abuse treatment in 2012, and DAWN data provide information on drug-related ED visits in 2011.

The NSDUH collects data from a nationally representative sample of the U.S. civilian, noninstitutionalized population age 12 or older. NSDUH data are collected through face-to-face, computer-assisted interviews at the respondent's place of residence. TEDS is a nationwide compilation of data on the demographic and substance-use characteristics of admissions to substance-abuse treatment. TEDS data are reported to SAMHSA by state substance-abuse agencies and include information on admissions age 12 and older to facilities that receive some public funding. DAWN was a public-health surveillance system that monitored drug-related morbidity and mortality. DAWN used a probability sample of hospitals to produce annual estimates of drug-related ED visits for the United States and selected metropolitan areas.

Alcohol Use and Illicit-Drug Use among Older Adults

According to combined 2007 to 2014 NSDUH data, nearly 16.2 million adults age 65 or older drank alcohol in the past month, with 3.4 million reporting binge alcohol use and 772,000 reporting heavy alcohol use (data not shown). In the 2007 to 2014 NSDUHs, "binge alcohol use" was defined as drinking five or more drinks on the same occasion (i.e., at the same time or within a couple of hours of each other), and "heavy alcohol use" was defined as binge drinking on five or more days in the past 30 days. This threshold for binge drinking is higher than the threshold that is sometimes used for older adults— having more than two drinks for women and three drinks for men on a single occasion.

Combined 2007 to 2014 NSDUH data indicate that, on an average day, 6.0 million older adults used alcohol (Figure 15.1). Older adults who used alcohol in the past month drank an average of 1.8 drinks per day on the days they drank. NSDUH data indicate that older adults who used alcohol in the past month drank on an average of 11.1 days per month.

The combined 2007 to 2014 NSDUH data indicate that nearly 469,000 older adults used an illicit drug in the past month (data not shown). NSDUH includes nine of them: marijuana, cocaine (including crack), heroin, hallucinogens, and inhalants, as well as the nonmedical use of prescription-type pain relievers, tranquilizers, stimulants, and sedatives. Although the laws regarding marijuana use have changed in several states over the past decade, marijuana is categorized as an illicit drug because marijuana use remains illegal under federal laws in all states.

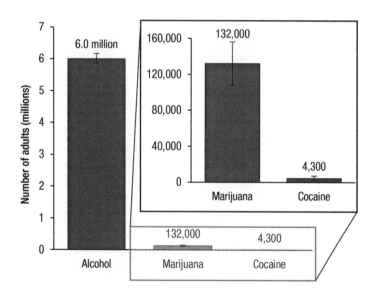

Figure 15.1. *Number of Adults Age 65 or Older Who Used Alcohol, Marijuana, or Cocaine on an Average Day: Annual Averages, 2007 to 2014 NSDUHs.* (Source: SAMHSA, Center for Behavioral Health Statistics and Quality, National Surveys on Drug Use and Health (NSDUHs), 2007 to 2014.)

On an average day during the past month, 132,000 older adults used marijuana and 4,300 used cocaine (Figure 15.1). In this report, the "average day" estimates are presented for only marijuana and cocaine. Because of small sample sizes, "average day" estimates of crack, heroin, hallucinogens, and inhalants could not be produced. The data used in the "average day" estimates are not collected for the nonmedical use of prescription-type pain relievers, tranquilizers, stimulants, and sedatives; therefore, those estimates are also not presented.

Emergency Department Visits

In 2011, DAWN estimates showed 750,529 drug-related ED visits by adults age 65 or older, where 105,982 visits involved illicit-drug use, use of alcohol in combination with other substances, or nonmedical use of pharmaceuticals (e.g., prescription medications, over-the-counter (OTC) remedies, dietary supplements) (data not shown). The remaining 644,547 ED visits by older adults primarily involved adverse reactions to and accidental ingestion of drugs. DAWN does not collect information on alcohol-only ED visits among adults.

On an average day in 2011, there were 2,056 drug-related ED visits by older adults, of which 290 involved illegal drug use, alcohol in combination with other drugs, or nonmedical use of pharmaceuticals. Nonmedical use includes ED visits where the patient misused a medication, took more than the prescribed dose of a medication, took a medication prescribed for another individual, or was poisoned by another person. On an average day in 2011, these substances were involved in the following numbers of visits (Figure 15.2):

- 118 involved prescription or nonprescription pain relievers, 80 of which involved narcotic pain relievers specified by name (e.g., hydrocodone, oxycodone)

- 48 involved benzodiazepines

- 25 involved alcohol in combination with other drugs

- 23 involved antidepressants or antipsychotics

- 13 involved cocaine

- 7 involved heroin

- 5 involved marijuana and

- 2 involved illicit amphetamines or methamphetamine

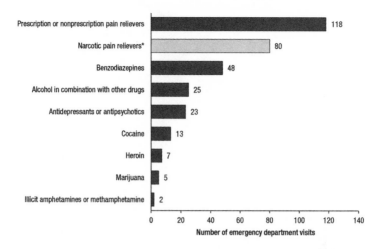

Figure 15.2. *Number of emergency-department visits for drug misuse on an average day for patients age 65 or older, by selected types of drugs: 2011 DAWN.* (Source: SAMHSA, Center for Behavioral Health Statistics and Quality, Drug Abuse Warning Network (DAWN), 2011.)

* Narcotic pain relievers are a subset of prescription or nonprescription pain relievers.

Despite the fact that illicit-drug use generally declines after young adulthood, more than one million older adults had an SUD in 2014. Emerging data suggest that substance use among older adults is a public-health issue. Findings in this report show that on an average day in the past month, older adults were using alcohol more frequently than they were using illicit drugs such as marijuana and cocaine. For example, on an average day in the past month for older adults, there were 29 admissions to treatment for alcohol use and 6 admissions to treatment for heroin or opiate use. Policymakers can use this information to help inform their assessments of substance-use problems. Increasing demands for substance-abuse treatment may require the development of new facilities and programs to address drug use among older adults.

Signs of possible substance misuse among older adults may include physical symptoms such as injuries, increased tolerance to medication, blackouts, and cognitive impairment. Psychiatric symptoms that may suggest a problem with substance misuse include sleep disturbances, anxiety, depression, and mood swings. Finally, problematic substance use may be signaled by social symptoms such as legal, financial, and family problems; loss of a spouse; and needing extra supplies of medication.

Chapter 16

Substance Abuse in the LGBT Community

People who identify as lesbian, gay, bisexual, or transgender (LGBT) often face social stigma, discrimination, and other challenges not encountered by people who identify as heterosexual. They also face a greater risk of harassment and violence. As a result of these and other stressors, sexual minorities are at increased risk for various behavioral health issues.

Many federally funded surveys have only recently started to ask about sexual orientation and gender identification in their data collections. Surveys thus far have found that sexual minorities have higher rates of substance misuse and substance-use disorders (SUDs) than people who identify as heterosexual. Therefore, it is not yet possible to establish long-term trends about substance use and SUD prevalence in LGBT populations.

Substance Use and Misuse

According to 2015 data from the National Survey on Drug Use and Health (NSDUH), adults defined as a "sexual minority" (in this chapter, meaning lesbian, gay, or bisexual) were more than twice as likely as heterosexual adults (39.1 versus 17.1%) to have used any illicit drug

This chapter includes text excerpted from "Substance Use and SUDs in LGBT Populations," National Institute on Drug Abuse (NIDA), September 2017.

in the past year. Nearly a third of sexual minority adults (30.7%) used marijuana in the past year, compared to 12.9 percent of heterosexual adults, and about 1 in 10 (10.4%) misused prescription pain relievers, compared to 4.5 percent of heterosexual adults.

A 2013 survey conducted by the U.S. Census Bureau found that a higher percentage of LGBT adults between 18 and 64 reported past-year binge drinking (five or more drinks on a single occasion) than heterosexual adults. LGBT people in treatment for SUDs initiated alcohol consumption earlier than their heterosexual counterparts.

Lesbian, gay, and bisexual (LGB) adolescents also reported higher rates of substance use compared to heterosexual adolescents. In one meta-analysis, LGB adolescents were 90 percent more likely to use substances than heterosexual adolescents, and the difference was particularly pronounced in some subpopulations; bisexual adolescents used substances at 3.4 times the rate of heterosexual adolescents, and lesbian and bisexual females used at 4 times the rate of their heterosexual counterparts.

Substance-Use Disorders and Comorbidities

LGBT people also have a greater likelihood than non-LGBT persons of experiencing a substance-use disorder (SUD) in their lifetime, and they often enter treatment with more severe SUDs.

Some common SUD treatment modalities have been shown to be effective for gay or bisexual men including motivational interviewing, social-support therapy, contingency management, and cognitive-behavioral therapy (CBT).

Addiction-treatment programs offering specialized groups for gay and bisexual men showed better outcomes for those clients compared to gay and bisexual men in nonspecialized programs; but in one study, only 7.4 percent of programs offered specialized services for LGBT patients. Available research is limited on rates of SUD among transgender populations, although research shows that transgender individuals are more likely to seek SUD treatment than the nontransgender population. Available research also suggests that treatment should address unique factors in these patients' lives that may include homophobia/transphobia, family problems, violence, and social isolation.

Sexual minorities with SUDs are more likely to have additional (comorbid or co-occurring) psychiatric disorders. For example, gay and bisexual men and lesbian and bisexual women report greater odds of frequent mental distress and depression than their heterosexual counterparts. Transgender children and adolescents have higher

160

levels of depression, suicidality, self-harm, and eating disorders than their nontransgender counterparts. Thus, it is particularly important that LGBT people in SUD treatment be screened for other psychiatric problems (as well as vice versa) and that all identifiable conditions are treated concurrently.

LGBT people are also at increased risks for human immunodeficiency virus (HIV) due to both intravenous drug use and risky sexual behaviors. HIV infection is particularly prevalent among gay and bisexual men (men who have sex with men, or MSM) and transgender women who have sex with men. SUD treatment can also help prevent HIV transmission among those at high risk. For example, addiction treatment is associated not only with reduced drug use but also with less risky sexual behavior among MSM, and those with HIV report improvements in viral load.

Chapter 17

Substance Abuse in the Racial and Ethnic Minority Populations

Racial and ethnic minorities make up about one-third of the population of the nation and are expected to become a majority by 2050. These diverse communities have unique behavioral-health needs and experience different rates of mental and/or substance-use disorders (SUDs) and treatment access.

Communities of color tend to experience a greater burden of mental and substance-use disorders often due to poorer access to care; inappropriate care; and higher social, environmental, and economic risk factors.

Substance Abuse among African Americans

There are about 44.5 million African Americans in the United States (about 14.2% of the total population). According to data from the National Survey on Drug Use and Health (NSDUH)—2014:

- The rate of illegal drug use in the last month among African Americans ages 12 and up in 2014 was 12.4 percent, compared to the national average of 10.2 percent.

This chapter includes text excerpted from "Racial and Ethnic Minority Populations," Substance Abuse and Mental Health Services Administration (SAMHSA), August 16, 2018.

- The rate of binge drinking (drinking five or more drinks on a single occasion for men) among African Americans ages 12 and up was 21.6 percent—compared with the national average of 23 percent.

- African Americans ages 12 to 20 in 2014 reported past-month alcohol use at a rate of 17.3 percent, compared with the national average of 22.8 percent. Past-month underage binge drinking was 8.5 percent for African American youth, while the national average was 13.8 percent.

Rates of mental disorders are generally low among African Americans. In 2014, 3.8 percent of African American adults ages 18 and older had a past-year mental illness and a SUD, while the national average was 3.3 percent. The 2014 national average for any mental illness in the past year for adults was 18.1 percent, compared to 16.3 percent for African American adults.

African Americans face higher rates of death from major diseases and higher rates of human immunodeficiency virus (HIV) infection than their Caucasian counterparts. African Americans in 2010 accounted for 44 percent of HIV infection cases in the country.

Substance Abuse among American Indians and Alaska Natives

There are about 5.2 million American Indians and Alaska Natives in the United States (about 1.7% of the total population). American Indians and Alaska Natives experience some of the highest rates of substance-use and mental disorders compared to other U.S. racial or ethnic groups. For instance:

- The rate of illegal drug use in the last month among American Indians and Alaska Natives ages 12 and up in 2014 was 14.9 percent.

- American Indians and Alaska Natives ages 12 to 20 in 2014 reported past-month alcohol use at a rate of 21.9 percent, compared with the national average of 22.8 percent.

- Past-month underage binge drinking was 14.3 percent for American Indian and Alaska Native youth, while the national average was 13.8 percent.

- In 2010, Native Americans had the highest rate of drug-induced death (17.1%).

Rates of mental disorders in American Indians and Alaska Natives in 2014:

- The percentage of American Indians and Alaska Natives ages 18 and up who reported a past-year mental illness was 21.2 percent.

- The rate of serious mental illness among American Indians and Alaska Natives ages 18 and up in this population was 4 percent.

- In 2014, 8.8 percent of American Indians and Alaska Natives ages 18 and up had co-occurring, past-year mental and SUDs, while the national average was 3.3 percent.

In addition, according to a 2015 fact sheet published by the Centers for Disease Control and Prevention (CDC), the suicide rate among American Indian and Alaska Native adolescents and young adults between the ages of 15 and 34 (19.5 per 100,000) is 1.5 times higher than the national average for that age group (12.2 per 100,000). The 2015 NSDUH rate of serious thoughts of suicide among those ages 18 and up was 4.8 percent for American Indians and Alaska Natives, compared with the national average of 3.9 percent.

Substance Abuse among Asian Americans, Native Hawaiians, and Other Pacific Islanders

There are about 18.2 million people who identify themselves as Asian American. There are also 1.4 million Native Hawaiians or Other Pacific Islanders in the United States. According to the 2010 U.S. Census, Asians are the fastest growing racial group in the nation.

In 2014:

- Among people, ages 12 and up, the rate of illegal drug use in the last month was 4.1 percent among Asian Americans and 15.6 percent among Native Hawaiians or other Pacific Islanders.

- The rate of binge alcohol use was lowest among Asian Americans ages 12 and up (14.5%). The binge alcohol-use rate was 18.3 percent among Native Hawaiian or other Pacific Islanders.

- The past-month binge alcohol use rate for youth ages 12 to 20 was 6.7 percent for Asian Americans, compared with the national average of 13.8 percent.

- The rate of substance dependence or abuse was 4.5 percent for Asian Americans and 10 percent for Native Hawaiians or other Pacific Islanders.

In 2014, the percentage of Asian Americans ages 18 and up reporting a past-year mental illness was 13.1 percent, and 3.1 percent of Asian Americans and 1.2 percent of Native Hawaiian or other Pacific Islanders ages 18 and older had serious thoughts of suicide, compared to the national average of 3.9 percent.

However, examination of disaggregated data unmasks disparities experienced by groups within the Asian American, Native Hawaiian, and Pacific Islander population. For instance, older Asian American women have the highest suicide rate of all U.S. women over the age of 65. Southeast Asian refugees are also at risk for posttraumatic stress disorder (PTSD) associated with trauma experienced before and after emigration to the United States.

Substance Abuse among Hispanics or Latinos

There are about 52 million Hispanics or Latinos in the United States (about 16.7% of the total population). By 2050, the number of people in this population group is expected to double to about 132.8 million, making up approximately 30 percent of the total U.S. population.

Regarding substance abuse among Hispanics or Latinos, data from the 2015 NSDUH indicate:

- The rate of illicit-drug use in the past month among Hispanic individuals ages 12 and up was 8.9 percent, while the national average was 10.2 percent.

- The rate of binge alcohol use among Hispanics or Latinos within this age group was 24.7 percent. Alcohol use in the last year among people ages 12 to 17 was 23.9 percent for Hispanic youth.

Rates of mental disorders for Hispanics or Latinos in 2014 include:

- The percentage of people ages 18 and up reporting a past-year mental illness was 15.6 percent.

- About 3.5 percent of adult Hispanics or Latinos had a serious mental illness.

- The percentage of people who reported a major depressive episode was 5.6 percent.

- About 3.3 percent of this population had a co-occurring mental-health and substance-use disorder.

Chapter 18

Drug Abuse in Other Populations

Chapter Contents

Section 18.1

Veterans and Drug Abuse

This section includes text excerpted from "Substance Abuse in the Military," National Institute on Drug Abuse (NIDA), March 2013. Reviewed January 2019.

Members of the armed forces are not immune to the substance-use problems that affect the rest of society. Although illicit-drug use is lower among U.S. military personnel than among civilians, heavy alcohol and tobacco use, and especially prescription-drug abuse, are much more prevalent and are on the rise.

The stresses of deployment during wartime and the unique culture of the military account for some of these differences. Zero-tolerance policies and stigma pose difficulties in identifying and treating substance-use problems in military personnel, as does lack of confidentiality that deters many who need treatment from seeking it.

Those with multiple deployments and combat exposure are at greatest risk of developing substance-use problems. They are more apt to engage in new-onset heavy weekly drinking and binge drinking, to suffer alcohol- and other drug-related problems, and to have greater prescribed use of behavioral-health medications. They are also more likely to start smoking or relapse to smoking.

Mental-Health Problems in Returning Veterans

Service members may carry the psychological and physical wounds of their military experience with them into subsequent civilian life. In one study, one in four veterans returning from Iraq and Afghanistan reported symptoms of a mental or cognitive disorder; one in six PTSD. These disorders are strongly associated with substance abuse and dependence, as are other problems experienced by returning military personnel, including sleep disturbances, TBI, and violence in relationships.

Young adult veterans are particularly likely to have substance-use or other mental-health problems. According to a report of veterans in 2004 to 2006, a quarter of 18- to 25-year-old veterans met the criteria for a past-year SUD, which is more than double the rate of veterans age 26 to 54 and five times the rate of veterans 55 or older.

Illicit and Prescription Drugs

According to the 2008 U.S. Department of Defense (DoD) Survey of Health-Related Behaviors (HRB) among Active Duty Military Personnel, just 2.3 percent of military personnel were past-month users of an illicit drug, compared with 12 percent of civilians. Among those age 18 to 25 (who are most likely to use drugs), the rate among military personnel was 3.9 percent, compared with 17.2 percent among civilians.

A policy of zero tolerance for drug use among DoD personnel is likely one reason why illicit-drug use has remained at a low level in the military for two decades. The policy was instituted in 1982 and is currently enforced by frequent random drug testing; service members face dishonorable discharge and even criminal prosecution for a positive drug test.

However, in spite of the low level of illicit-drug use, abuse of prescription drugs is higher among service members than among civilians and is on the increase. In 2008, 11 percent of service members reported misusing prescription drugs, up from 2 percent in 2002 and 4 percent in 2005. Most of the prescription drugs misused by service members are opioid pain medications.

The greater availability of these medications and increases in prescriptions for them may contribute to their growing misuse by service members. Pain reliever prescriptions written by military physicians quadrupled between 2001 and 2009—to almost 3.8 million. Combat-related injuries and the strains from carrying heavy equipment during multiple deployments likely play a role in this trend.

Drinking and Smoking

Alcohol use is also higher among men and women in military service than among civilians. Almost half of active-duty service members (47%) reported binge drinking in 2008—up from 35 percent in 1998. In 2008, 20 percent of military personnel reported binge drinking every week in the past month; the rate was considerably higher—27 percent—among those with high combat exposure.

In 2008, 30 percent of all service members were current cigarette smokers—comparable to the rate for civilians (29%). However, as with alcohol use, smoking rates are significantly higher among personnel who have been exposed to combat.

Suicides and Substance Use

Suicide rates in the military were traditionally lower than among civilians in the same age range, but in 2004 the suicide rate in the U.S.

Army began to climb, surpassing the civilian rate in 2008. Substance use is involved in many of these suicides. The 2010 report of the Army Suicide Prevention Task Force found that 29 percent of active-duty Army suicides from FY2005 to FY2009 involved alcohol or drug use; and in 2009, prescription drugs were involved in almost one-third of them.

Addressing the Problem

A 2012 report prepared for the DoD by the Institute of Medicine (IOM) recommended ways of addressing the problem of substance use in the military, including increasing the use of evidence-based prevention and treatment interventions and expanding access to care. The report recommends broadening insurance coverage to include effective outpatient treatments and better-equipping healthcare providers to recognize and screen for substance-use problems so that they can refer patients to appropriate, evidence-based treatment when needed. It also recommends measures such as limiting access to alcohol on bases.

The IOM Report also notes that addressing substance use in the military will require increasing confidentiality and shifting a cultural climate in which drug problems are stigmatized and evoke fear in people suffering from them.

Branches of the military have already taken steps to curb prescription-drug abuse. The Army, for example, has implemented changes that include limiting the duration of prescriptions for opioid pain relievers to six months and having a pharmacist monitor a soldier's medications when multiple prescriptions are being used.

Section 18.2

Criminal Justice Populations and Substance Abuse

This section includes text excerpted from "Principles of Drug Abuse Treatment for Criminal Justice Populations— A Research-Based Guide," National Institute on Drug Abuse (NIDA), April 2014. Reviewed January 2019.

Drug abuse is implicated in at least three types of drug-related offenses:

- Offenses defined by drug possession or sales

- Offenses directly related to drug abuse (e.g., stealing to get money for drugs)

- Offenses related to a lifestyle that predisposes the drug abuser to engage in illegal activity, for example, through association with other offenders or with illicit markets

Individuals who use illicit drugs are more likely to commit crimes, and it is common for many offenses, including violent crimes, to be committed by individuals who had used drugs or alcohol prior to committing the crime, or who were using them at the time of the offense.

According to 2012 statistics from the U.S. Department of Justice's (DOJ) Bureau of Justice Statistics (BJS), the total correctional population is estimated to be 6,937,600, with 4,794,000 individuals on probation or under parole supervision, and drug-law violations accounting for the most common type of criminal offense. In a survey of state and federal prisoners, BJS estimated that about half of the prisoners met *Diagnostic and Statistical Manual for Mental Disorders (DSM)* criteria for drug abuse or dependence, and yet fewer than 20 percent who needed treatment received it. Of those surveyed, 14.8 percent of state and 17.4 percent of federal prisoners reported having received drug treatment since admission.

Juvenile justice systems also report high levels of drug abuse. In 2008, approximately 10 percent of the estimated 2.1 million juvenile arrests were for drug-abuse or underage-drinking violations. As many as two-thirds of detained juveniles may have a substance-use disorder (SUD); female juveniles who enter the system generally have higher SUD rates than males.

Although the past several decades have witnessed an increased interest in providing substance-abuse treatment services for criminal-justice offenders, only a small percentage of offenders has access to adequate services, especially in jails and community correctional facilities. Not only is there a gap in the availability of these services for offenders, but often there are few choices in the types of services provided. Treatment that is of insufficient quality and intensity or that is not well suited to the needs of offenders may not yield meaningful reductions in drug use and recidivism. Untreated substance-abusing offenders are more likely than treated offenders to relapse to drug abuse and return to criminal behavior. This can lead to re-arrest and re-incarceration, jeopardizing public health and public safety and taxing criminal-justice system resources. Treatment is the most effective course for interrupting drug abuse/criminal justice cycle for offenders with drug abuse problems.

Drug-abuse treatment can be incorporated into criminal-justice settings in a variety of ways. Examples include treatment in prison followed by community-based treatment after release; drug courts that blend judicial monitoring and sanctions with treatment by imposing treatment as a condition of probation; and treatment under parole or probation supervision. Drug-abuse treatment can benefit from the cross-agency coordination and collaboration of criminal-justice professionals, substance-abuse treatment providers, and other social service agencies. By working together, the criminal-justice and treatment systems can optimize resources to benefit the health, safety, and well-being of the individuals and communities they serve.

Why Do People Involved in the Criminal-Justice System Continue Abusing Drugs?

The answer to this perplexing question spans basic neurobiological, psychological, social, and environmental factors. The repeated use of addictive drugs eventually changes how the brain functions. Resulting brain changes, which accompany the transition from voluntary to compulsive drug use, affect the brain's natural inhibition and reward centers, causing the addicted person to use drugs in spite of the adverse health, social, and legal consequences. Craving for drugs may be triggered by contact with the people, places, and things associated with prior drug use, as well as by stress. Forced abstinence (when it occurs) is not treatment, and it does not cure addiction. Abstinent individuals must still learn how to avoid relapse, including those who may have been abstinent for a long period of time while incarcerated.

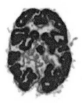 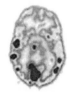 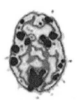

Normal   **Cocaine Abuser**   **Cocaine Abuser**
(10 days of   (100 days of
abstinence)   abstinence)

Source: Volkow et al. 1992, 1993

Figure 18.1. *Impact of Cocaine on the Human Brain*

Potential risk factors for released offenders include pressures from peers and family members to return to drug use and a criminal lifestyle. Tensions of daily life—violent associates, few opportunities for legitimate employment, lack of safe housing, and even the need to comply with correctional supervision conditions—can also create stressful situations that can precipitate relapse to drug use.

Research on how the brain is affected by drug abuse promises to teach us much more about the mechanics of drug-induced brain changes and their relationship to addiction. Research also reveals that with effective drug-abuse treatment, individuals can overcome persistent drug effects and lead healthy, productive lives.

Section 18.3

Substance-Use Disorders in People with Disabilities

This section includes text excerpted from "Substance Use Disorders in People with Physical and Sensory Disabilities," Substance Abuse and Mental Health Services Administration (SAMHSA), August 2011. Reviewed January 2019.

Approximately 23 million people in the United States, including people with disabilities, need treatment for substance-use disorders

(SUDs), a major behavioral-health disorder. In addition, more than 24 million adults in the United States experienced serious psychological distress in 2006. People with and without disabilities may face many of the same barriers to substance-abuse treatment, such as lacking insurance or sufficient funds for treatment services, or feeling that they do not need treatment.

In addition, people with disabilities may face other barriers to SUD treatment, particularly finding treatment facilities that are fully accessible. Vocational rehabilitation (VR) counselors, vocational-education providers, and others who work with people with disabilities report that their clients with SUDs have less successful vocational outcomes than clients without SUDs.

To improve outcomes, it is important that clients with disabilities and SUDs receive services for both conditions and that the disabilities do not prevent clients from receiving treatment for SUDs. This, in brief, is intended to help people who work with people with physical and sensory disabilities—hearing loss, deafness, blindness, and low vision—to better understand SUDs and assist their clients in finding accessible SUD treatment services.

What Substance-Use Disorder Is

"Substance-use disorder" is a broad term that encompasses abuse of and dependence on drugs or alcohol. It includes using illegal substances, such as heroin, marijuana, or methamphetamines, and using legal substances, such as prescription or over-the-counter (OTC) medications, in ways not prescribed or recommended.

Substance-Use Disorders Harm People with Disabilities

It is difficult to estimate the number of people with physical disabilities who have SUDs. Some studies suggest that people with disabilities have higher rates of legal and illegal substance use than the general population, whereas other studies show lower rates. Although debate exists among researchers about the prevalence of SUDs among people with disabilities, there is agreement that active SUDs can seriously harm the health and quality of life of individuals with disabilities. An active SUD can:

- Interfere with successful engagement in rehabilitation services

- Interact with prescribed medications; alcohol, for example, can interfere with antiseizure medications

- Impede coordination and muscle control

- Impair cognition

- Reduce the ability to follow self-care regimens

- Contribute to social isolation, poor communication, and domestic strife

- Contribute to poor health, secondary disabling conditions, or the hastening of disabling diseases (e.g., cirrhosis, depression, and bladder infections)

- Inhibit educational advancement

- Lead to job loss, underemployment, and housing instability

Women with Disabilities and Substance-Use Disorders

Across all age groups, more women than men are disabled. Women with co-occurring disabilities and SUDs are at high risk of experiencing physical abuse and domestic violence.

One study of people with disabilities and SUDs found that 47 percent of women reported histories of physical, sexual, or domestic violence, compared with 20 percent of men with disabilities reporting abuse experiences. In the same study, 37 percent of women reported sexual abuse, compared with 7 percent of men.

Another study found that 56 percent of women with disabilities reported abuse, with 89 percent of these reporting multiple abusive incidents. What is more, being a victim of physical or sexual abuse is a risk factor for SUD.

Substance-Use Disorder Risk Factors and Warning Signs

For some people, drug or alcohol abuse is a direct or indirect cause of their disability, for example, by their becoming intoxicated and then falling or causing a car crash. Without SUD treatment, people who had SUDs before sustaining a disability will likely continue to use substances afterward. Other people may have developed SUDs after using substances such as pain medications or alcohol to cope with aspects of their disability or to cope with social isolation or depression.

Numerous signs may suggest the presence of an active SUD. These include, but are not limited to:

- Dilated or constricted pupils
- Slurred speech
- Inability to focus, visually or cognitively
- Unsteady gait
- Blackouts
- Insomnia
- Irritability or agitation
- Depression, anxiety, low self-esteem, resentment
- Odor of alcohol on the breath
- Excessive use of aftershave or mouthwash (to mask the odor of alcohol)
- Mild tremor
- Nasal irritation (suggestive of cocaine insufflation)
- Eye irritation (suggestive of exposure to marijuana smoke)
- Odor of marijuana on clothing
- Abuse of drugs or alcohol by family members
- Many missed appointments with vocational rehabilitation (VR), job interviews, and the like
- Difficulty learning new tasks
- Attention deficits
- Lack of initiative

Some manifestations of certain disabilities may be difficult to distinguish from the signs of SUDs mentioned above. For example, people with multiple sclerosis may have an unsteady gait, slurred speech, and memory impairment. Other signs, such as depression or anxiety, may indicate a different, distinct behavioral-health condition.

Substance-Use Disorder Risk Factors for People with Disabilities

The following are some of the SUD risk factors for people with disabilities:

- Pain
- Access to prescription pain medications
- Chronic medical problems
- Depression
- Social isolation
- Enabling by caregivers
- Unemployment
- Limited education
- Low socioeconomic level
- Little exposure to SUD prevention education
- History of physical or sexual abuse

Part Three

Drugs of Abuse

Chapter 19

Introduction to Drug Classes

The Controlled Substances Act (CSA) regulates five classes of drugs:

1. **Narcotics.** Also known as "opioids," the term "narcotic" comes from the Greek word for "stupor" and originally referred to a variety of substances that dulled the senses and relieved pain. Though some people still refer to all drugs as "narcotics," today "narcotic" refers to opium, opium derivatives, and their semi-synthetic substitutes. A more current term for these drugs, with less uncertainty regarding its meaning, is "opioid." Examples include the illicit drug heroin and pharmaceutical drugs such as OxyContin®, Vicodin, codeine, morphine, methadone, and fentanyl.

2. **Depressants.** Depressants will put you to sleep, relieve anxiety and muscle spasms, and prevent seizures. Barbiturates are older drugs and include butalbital (Fiorina), phenobarbital, Pentothal, Seconal, and Nembutal. A person can rapidly develop dependence on and tolerance to barbiturates, meaning a person needs more and more of them to feel and function normally. This makes them unsafe, increasing the likelihood of coma or death. Benzodiazepines were developed to replace barbiturates, though they still share many of the undesirable side effects including tolerance and dependence. Some examples are Valium, Xanax, Halcion, Ativan, Klonopin, and Restoril.

This chapter includes text excerpted from "Drugs of Abuse," U.S. Drug Enforcement Administration (DEA), June 15, 2017.

Rohypnol is a benzodiazepine that is not manufactured or legally marketed in the United States, but it is used illegally. Lunesta, Ambien, and Sonata are sedative-hypnotic medications approved for the short-term treatment of insomnia that shares many of the properties of benzodiazepines. Other central nervous system (CNS) depressants include meprobamate, methaqualone (Quaalude), and the illicit drug GHB.

3. **Stimulants.** Stimulants speed up the body's systems. This class of drugs includes prescription drugs such as amphetamines (Adderall and Dexedrine), methylphenidate (Concerta and Ritalin), diet aids (such as Didrex, Bontril, Preludin, Fastin, Adipex P, Ionamin, and Meridia), and illicitly produced drugs such as methamphetamine, cocaine, and methcathinone.

4. **Hallucinogens.** Hallucinogens are found in plants and fungi or are synthetically produced and are among the oldest known group of drugs used for their ability to alter human perception and mood.

5. **Anabolic steroids.** Anabolic steroids are synthetically produced variants of the naturally occurring male hormone testosterone that are abused in an attempt to promote muscle growth, enhance athletic or other physical performance, and improve physical appearance. Testosterone, nandrolone, stanozolol, methandienone, and boldenone are some of the most frequently abused anabolic steroids.

Each class has distinguishing properties, and drugs within each class often produce similar effects. However, all controlled substances, regardless of class, share a number of common features. This introduction will familiarize you with these shared features and define the terms frequently associated with these drugs.

All controlled substances have abuse potential or are immediate precursors to substances with abuse potential. With the exception of anabolic steroids, controlled substances are abused to alter mood, thought, and feeling through their actions on the central nervous system (brain and spinal cord).

Some of these drugs alleviate pain, anxiety, or depression. Some induce sleep and others energize. Though some controlled substances are therapeutically useful, the "feel good" effects of these drugs contribute to their abuse. The extent to which a substance is reliably capable of producing intensely pleasurable feelings (euphoria) increases the likelihood of that substance being abused.

Chapter 20

Anabolic Steroids and Related Drugs Used as Performance Enhancers

Chapter Contents

Section 20.1

Anabolic Steroids

This section includes text excerpted from "Anabolic Steroids,"
National Institute on Drug Abuse (NIDA), August 2018.

What Are Anabolic Steroids?

Anabolic steroids are synthetic, or human-made, variations of the
male sex hormone testosterone. The proper term for these compounds
is "anabolic-androgenic steroids" (AAS). "Anabolic" refers to muscle
building, and "androgenic" refers to increased male sex characteristics.
Some common names for anabolic steroids are gear, juice, roids, and
stackers.

Healthcare providers can prescribe steroids to treat hormonal
issues, such as delayed puberty. Steroids can also treat diseases that
cause muscle loss, such as cancer and acquired immune deficiency
syndrome (AIDS). But some athletes and bodybuilders misuse these
drugs in an attempt to boost performance or improve their physical
appearance.

The majority of people who misuse steroids are male weightlifters
in their twenties or thirties. Anabolic steroid misuse is much less common in women. It is difficult to measure steroid misuse in the United
States because many national surveys do not measure it. However,
use among teens is generally minimal. The 2016 National Institute on
Drug Abuse (NIDA)-funded Monitoring the Future study has shown
that past-year misuse of steroids has declined among eighth and tenth
graders, while holding steady for twelfth graders.

How Do People Misuse Anabolic Steroids?

People who misuse anabolic steroids usually take them orally, inject
them into muscles, or apply them to the skin as a gel or cream. These
doses may be 10 to 100 times higher than doses prescribed to treat
medical conditions.

Commons patterns for misusing steroids include:

- **Cycling**—taking multiple doses for a period of time, stopping for
  a time, and then restarting

- **Stacking**—combining two or more different steroids and mixing
  oral and/or injectable types

- **Pyramiding**—slowly increasing the dose or frequency of steroid misuse, reaching a peak amount, and then gradually tapering off to zero

- **Plateauing**—alternating, overlapping, or substituting with another steroid to avoid developing a tolerance

There is no scientific evidence that any of these practices reduce the harmful medical consequences of these drugs.

How Do Anabolic Steroids Affect the Brain?

Anabolic steroids work differently from other drugs of abuse; they do not have the same short-term effects on the brain. The most important difference is that steroids do not directly activate the reward system to cause a "high"; they also do not trigger rapid increases in the brain chemical dopamine, which reinforces most other types of drug-taking behavior.

Misuse of anabolic steroids might lead to negative mental effects, such as:

- Paranoid (extreme, unreasonable) jealousy

- Extreme irritability and aggression ("roid rage")

- Delusions—false beliefs or ideas

- Impaired judgment

- Mania

What Are Other Health Effects of Anabolic Steroids?

Aside from mental effects, steroid use commonly causes severe acne. It also causes the body to swell, especially in the hands and feet.

Long-Term Effects

Anabolic steroid misuse might lead to serious, even permanent, health problems such as:

- Kidney problems or failure

- Liver damage and tumors

- Enlarged heart, high blood pressure, and changes in blood cholesterol, all of which increase the risk of stroke and heart attack, even in young people

- Increased risk of blood clots

Several other effects are gender- and age-specific effects:
In men:

- Shrinking testicles
- Decreased sperm count
- Baldness
- Development of breasts
- Increased risk for prostate cancer

In women:

- Growth of facial hair or excess body hair
- Decreased breast size
- Male-pattern baldness
- Changes in or stopping of the menstrual cycle
- Enlarged clitoris
- Deepened voice

In teens:

- Stunted growth (when high hormone levels from steroids signal to the body to stop bone growth too early)
- Stunted height (if teens use steroids before their growth spurt)

Some of these physical changes, such as shrinking sex organs in men, can add to mental side effects such as mood disorders.

Are Anabolic Steroids Addictive?

Even though anabolic steroids do not cause the same high as other drugs, they can lead to a substance-use disorder (SUD). A SUD occurs when a person continues to misuse steroids, even though there are serious consequences for doing so. The most severe form of a SUD is addiction. People might continue to misuse steroids despite physical problems, high costs to buy the drugs, and negative effects on their relationships. These behaviors reflect steroids' addictive potential. Research has further found that some steroid users turn to other drugs, such as opioids, to reduce sleep problems and irritability caused by steroids.

People who misuse steroids might experience withdrawal symptoms when they stop use, including:

- Fatigue

- Restlessness

- Loss of appetite

- Sleep problems

- Decreased sex drive

- Steroid cravings

One of the more serious withdrawal symptoms is depression, which can sometimes lead to suicide attempts.

How Can People Get Treatment for Anabolic Steroid Addiction?

Some people seeking treatment for anabolic steroid addiction have found a combination of behavioral therapy and medications to be helpful.

In certain cases of addiction, patients have taken medicines to help treat symptoms of withdrawal. For example, healthcare providers have prescribed antidepressants to treat depression and pain medicines for headaches and muscle and joint pain. Other medicines have been used to help restore the patient's hormonal system.

Section 20.2

Clenbuterol

This section includes text excerpted from "Clenbuterol," DEA Diversion Control Division, November 2013. Reviewed January 2019.

Clenbuterol is a potent, long-lasting bronchodilator that is prescribed for human use outside of the United States. It is abused generally by bodybuilders and athletes for its ability to increase lean muscle mass and reduce body fat (i.e., repartitioning effects). However, clenbuterol is also associated with significant adverse cardiovascular and neurological effects.

Licit Uses of Clenbuterol

In the United States, clenbuterol is not approved for human use; it is only approved for use in horses. In 1998, the U.S. Food and Drug Administration (FDA) approved the clenbuterol-based Ventipulmin Syrup, manufactured by Boehringer Ingelheim Vetmedica, Inc., as a prescription-only drug for the treatment of airway obstruction in horses (0.8 to 3.2 μg/kg twice daily). This product is not intended for human use or drug-taking use in food-producing animals.

Outside the U.S., clenbuterol is available by prescription for the treatment of bronchial asthma in humans. It is available in tablets (0.01 or 0.02 mg per tablet) and liquid preparations. The recommended dosage is 0.02 to 0.03 mg twice daily.

Chemistry and Pharmacology of Clenbuterol

Clenbuterol is a beta2 (β2)-adrenergic agonist. Stimulation of the beta2-adrenergic receptors on bronchial smooth muscle produces bronchodilation. However, clenbuterol, like other beta-adrenergic agonists, can produce adverse cardiovascular and neurological effects, such as heart palpitations, muscle tremors, and nervousness. Activation of beta-adrenergic receptors also accounts for clenbuterol's ability to increase lean muscle mass and reduce body fat, although the downstream mechanisms by which it does so have yet to be clearly defined.

After ingestion, clenbuterol is readily absorbed (70 to 80%) and remains in the body for a while (25 to 39 hours). As a result of its long half-life, the adverse effects of clenbuterol are often prolonged.

Illicit Uses of Clenbuterol

Clenbuterol is abused for its ability to alter body composition by reducing body fat and increasing skeletal muscle mass. It is typically abused by athletes and bodybuilders at a dose of 60 to 120 μg per day. It is often used in combination with other performance-enhancing drugs, such as anabolic steroids and growth hormone. It is also illicitly administered to livestock for its repartitioning effects. This has resulted in several outbreaks of acute illness in Spain, France, Italy, China, and Portugal 0.5 to 3 hours after individuals ingested liver and meat containing clenbuterol residues. The symptoms, which included increased heart rate, nervousness, headache, muscular tremor, dizziness, nausea, vomiting, fever, and chills, typically resolved within 2 to 6 days. Consequently, the U.S. and Europe actively monitor urine and tissue samples from livestock for the presence of clenbuterol.

There have also been reports of clenbuterol-tainted heroin and cocaine. Although no deaths were attributed to the clenbuterol exposures, the individuals were hospitalized for up to several days due to clenbuterol intoxication.

Clenbuterol: User Population

Clenbuterol is typically abused by athletes. It is thought to be more popular among female athletes as the repartitioning effects are not associated with the typical androgenic side effects (i.e., facial hair, deepening of the voice, and thickening of the skin) of anabolic steroids. Professional athletes in several different sports have tested positive for clenbuterol. Clenbuterol is also marketed and abused for weight-loss purposes.

Illicit Distribution of Clenbuterol

Clenbuterol is readily available on the Internet as tablets, syrup, and an injectable formulation. The drug is purportedly obtained by illegal importation from other countries where it food-producing for human use. According to the National Forensic Laboratory Information System (NFLIS) and the System to Retrieve Information from Drug Evidence (STRIDE), 16 exhibits were identified as clenbuterol in 2011, 13 exhibits were identified in 2012 and 2 exhibits were identified in the first quarter of 2013. The relatively small numbers of drug seizures are likely a result of low enforcement priority due to the noncontrolled status of clenbuterol in the United States.

Control Status of Clenbuterol

Clenbuterol is currently not controlled under the Controlled Substances Act (CSA). However, clenbuterol is listed by the World Anti-Doping Agency (WADA) and the International Olympic Committee (IOC) as a performance-enhancing drug. Therefore, athletes are barred from its use.

Section 20.3

Human Growth Hormone (hGH)

This section includes text excerpted from "Human
Growth Hormone," DEA Diversion Control Division, October 2018.

Human growth hormone (hGH) is a naturally occurring polypeptide hormone secreted by the pituitary gland and is essential for body growth. Daily secretion of hGH increases throughout childhood, peaking during adolescence, and steadily declining thereafter. In 1985, synthetic hGH was developed and approved by the U.S. Food and Drug Administration (FDA) for specific uses. However, it is commonly abused by athletes, bodybuilders, and aging adults for its ability increase muscle mass and decrease body fat, as well as its purported potential to improve athletic performance and reverse the effects of aging.

Licit Uses of Human Growth Hormone

Several FDA-approved injectable hGH preparations are available by prescription from a supervising physician for clearly and narrowly defined indications. In children, hGH is approved for the treatment of poor growth due to Turner syndrome, Prader-Willi syndrome, and chronic renal insufficiency, hGH insufficiency/deficiency, for children born small for gestational age, and for idiopathic short stature. Accepted medical uses in adults include the treatment of the wasting syndrome of acquired immunodeficiency syndrome (AIDS) and hGH deficiency. The recommended dosage is 40g/kg/day for children and 25g/kg/day for adults. The FDA-approved injectable formulations are available as liquid preparations, or as powder with a diluent for reconstitution.

Chemistry and Pharmacology of Human Growth Hormone

Using recombinant deoxyribonucleic acid (DNA) technology, two forms of synthetic hGH were developed, somatropin and somatrem. Somatropin is identical to the endogenous pituitary-derived hGH, whereas somatrem has an extra amino acid on the N-terminus. Both synthetic forms have similar biological actions and potencies as the endogenous hGH polypeptide. Synthetic hGH also is chemically indistinguishable from the naturally occurring hormone in blood and urine tests. hGH binds to growth hormone receptors present on cells throughout the body. hGH functions to regulate body composition, fluid homeostasis, glucose and lipid metabolism, skeletal muscle and bone growth, and possibly cardiac functioning. Sleep, exercise, and stress all increase the secretion of hGH.

The use of hGH is associated with several adverse effects, including edema, carpal tunnel syndrome (CTS), joint pain, muscle pain, and abnormal skin sensations (e.g., numbness and tingling). It may also increase the growth of preexisting malignant cells, and increase the possibility of developing diabetes.

hGH is administered by subcutaneous or intramuscular injection. The circulating half-life of hGH is relatively short half-life (20 to 30 minutes), while its biological half-life is much longer (9 to 17 hours) due to its indirect effects.

Illicit Uses of Human Growth Hormone

Human growth hormone is illicitly used as an antiaging agent, to improve athletic performance, and for bodybuilding purposes. It is marketed, distributed, and illegally prescribed off-label to aging adults to replenish declining hGH levels and reverse age-related bodily deterioration. It is also abused for its ability to alter body composition by reducing body fat and increasing skeletal muscle mass. It is often used in combination with other performance-enhancing drugs, such as anabolic steroids. Athletes also use it to improve their athletic performance, although the ability of hGH to increase athletic performance is debatable.

Human Growth Hormone: Abuser Population

Athletes, bodybuilders, and aging adults are the primary abusers of hGH. Because the illicit use of synthetic hGH is difficult to detect, its use in sports is believed to be widespread. Over the past few years, numerous professional athletes have admitted to using hGH. Bodybuilders, and celebrities also purportedly use it for its ability to alter body composition. Aging adults looking to reverse the effects of aging are increasingly using synthetic hGH.

Illicit Distribution of Human Growth Hormone

The illicit distribution of hGH occurs as the result of physicians illegally prescribing it for off-label uses, and for the treatment of

FDA-approved medical conditions without examination and supervision. Illicit distribution also involves diverted hGH obtained through theft, smuggled hGH illegally imported from other countries, and counterfeit hGH.

The illicit distribution of injectable synthetic hGH formulations is thought to be primarily through Internet pharmacies, as well as wellness and anti-aging clinics and websites. Internet pharmacies are often partnered with a physician willing to write prescriptions for a fee without a physical examination. Individuals may also obtain hGH and other performance-enhancing drugs (e.g., anabolic steroids) without a prescription through the black market.

According to Drug Enforcement Administration's (DEA) National Forensic Laboratory Information System (NFLIS), law enforcement officials submitted five hGH exhibits to federal, state, and local forensic laboratories in 2011 and 2012, that has remained relatively stable with the exception of 2014 in which 15 exhibits were identified as hGH. In more recent years, the number of hGH exhibits have decreased to five in 2015, one in 2016, and nine in 2017. Various oral preparations (e.g., sprays and pills) purported to contain hGH are also marketed and distributed. However, hGH is only available in the injectable form. The hGH molecule is too large for absorption across the lining of the oral mucosa and the hormone is digested by the stomach before absorption can occur.

Control Status of Human Growth Hormone

Human growth hormone is not controlled under the Controlled Substances Act (CSA). However, as part of the 1990 Anabolic Steroids Control Act (ASCA), the distribution and possession, with the intent to distribute, of hGH "for any use other than the treatment of a disease or other recognized medical condition, where such use has been authorized by the Secretary of U.S. Health and Human Services (HHS) and pursuant to the order of a physician" was criminalized as a five-year felony under the penalties chapter of the Food, Drug, and Cosmetics Act (FDCA) of the FDA.

hGH is listed by the World Anti-Doping Agency and the International Olympic Committee (IOC) as a performance-enhancing drug barring athletes from using it.

Chapter 21

Cannabinoids

Chapter Contents

Section 21.1

Cannabis *and Cannabinoids*

This section includes text excerpted from "Cannabis and
Cannabinoids (PDQ®)—Patient Version," National
Cancer Institute (NCI), December 20, 2017.

What Is Cannabis*?*

Cannabis, also known as marijuana, is a plant from Central Asia
that is grown in many parts of the world. The *Cannabis* plant produces
a resin containing compounds called cannabinoids. Some cannabinoids
are psychoactive (acting on the brain and changing mood or consciousness). In the United States, *Cannabis* is a controlled substance and
has been classified as a Schedule I agent (a drug with high potential
for abuse and no currently accepted medical use).

Clinical trials that study medicinal *Cannabis* in cancer are limited.
To do research with *Cannabis* in the United States, researchers must
file an investigational new drug (IND) application with the U. S. Food
and Drug Administration (FDA), receive a Schedule I license from the
U.S. Drug Enforcement Administration (DEA), and gain approval from
the National Institute on Drug Abuse (NIDA).

By federal law, the possession of *Cannabis* is illegal in the United
States outside of approved research settings. However, a growing number of states, territories, and the District of Columbia have enacted
laws to legalize medical marijuana.

What Are Cannabinoids?

Cannabinoids are active chemicals in *Cannabis* that cause druglike effects throughout the body, including the central nervous system
(CNS) and the immune system. They are also known as phytocannabinoids. The main active cannabinoid in *Cannabis* is delta-9-tetrahydrocannabinol (THC). Another active cannabinoid is cannabidiol (CBD),
which may relieve pain and lower inflammation without causing the
"high" of delta-9-THC.

Cannabinoids are used for treating the side effects of cancer, but
other possible effects of cannabinoids include:

- Antiinflammatory activity

- Blocking cell growth

- Preventing the growth of blood vessels that supply tumors

- Antiviral activity

- Relieving muscle spasms caused by multiple sclerosis (MS)

What Is the History of the Medical Use of Cannabis?

The use of *Cannabis* for medicinal purposes dates back at least 3,000 years. It came into use in Western medicine in the nineteenth century and was said to relieve pain, inflammation, spasms, and convulsions.

In 1937, the U.S. Treasury began taxing *Cannabis* under the Marijuana Tax Act at one dollar per ounce for medicinal use and one hundred dollars per ounce for nonmedical use. The American Medical Association (AMA) opposed this regulation of *Cannabis* and did not want studies of its potential medicinal benefits to be limited. In 1942, *Cannabis* was removed from the U.S. Pharmacopoeia because of continuing concerns about its safety. In 1951, Congress passed the Boggs Act, which included *Cannabis* with narcotic drugs for the first time.

Under the Controlled Substances Act passed by Congress in 1970, marijuana was classified as a Schedule I drug. Other Schedule I drugs include heroin, Lysergic acid diethylamide (LSD), mescaline, methaqualone, and gamma-hydroxybutyrate (GHB).

Although *Cannabis* was not believed to have any medicinal use, the U.S. government distributed it to patients on a case-by-case basis under the compassionate use of investigational new drug program (IND) started in 1978. This program was closed to all the patients in 1992 as recommended by the Secretary of U.S. Department of Health and Human Services (HHS).

Researchers have studied how cannabinoids act on the brain and other parts of the body. Cannabinoid receptors (molecules that bind cannabinoids) have been discovered in brain cells and nerve cells in other parts of the body. The presence of cannabinoid receptors on immune system cells suggests that cannabinoids may have a role in immunity.

Nabiximols (Sativex) is a *Cannabis* extract that contains delta-9-THC and cannabidiol (CBD). Nabiximols is approved in Canada (under the notice of compliance with conditions) for the relief of pain in patients with advanced cancer or multiple sclerosis (MS).

How Is Cannabis Administered?

Cannabis may be taken by mouth or may be inhaled. When taken by mouth (in baked products or as an herbal tea), the main psychoactive ingredient in *Cannabis* (delta-9-THC) is processed by the liver, making an additional psychoactive chemical.

When *Cannabis* is smoked and inhaled, cannabinoids quickly enter the bloodstream. The additional psychoactive chemical is produced in smaller amounts than when taken by mouth.

A growing number of clinical trials are studying a medicine made from an extract of *Cannabis* that contains specific amounts of cannabinoids. This medicine is sprayed under the tongue.

Have Any Side Effects or Risks Been Reported from Cannabis *and Cannabinoids?*

Adverse side effects of cannabinoids may include:

* Rapid beating of the heart
* Low blood pressure
* Muscle relaxation
* Bloodshot eyes
* Slowed digestion and movement of food by the stomach and intestines.
* Dizziness
* Depression
* Hallucinations
* Paranoia

Because *Cannabis* smoke contains many of the same substances as tobacco smoke, there are concerns about how inhaled *Cannabis* affects the lungs. A study of over 5,000 men and women without cancer over a period of 20 years found that smoking tobacco was linked with some loss of lung function but that occasional and low use of *Cannabis* was not linked with loss of lung function.

As the use of *Cannabis* over a long time may have harmful effects on the endocrine and reproductive systems, rates of testicular germ cell tumors (TGCTs) in *Cannabis* users have been studied. Larger studies that follow patients over time and laboratory studies of cannabinoid receptors in TGCTs are needed to find if there is a link between *Cannabis* use and a higher risk of TGCTs.

A review of bladder cancer rates in *Cannabis* users and nonusers was done in over 84,000 men who took part in the California Men's

Health Study (CMHS). Over 16 years of follow up and adjusting for age, race/ethnic group and body mass index (BMI), rates of bladder cancer were found to be 45 percent lower in *Cannabis* users than in men who did not report *Cannabis* use.

Both *Cannabis* and cannabinoids may be addictive. Symptoms of withdrawal from cannabinoids may include:

- Irritability

- Trouble sleeping

- Restlessness

- Hot flashes

- Nausea and cramping (rarely occur)

These symptoms are mild compared to withdrawal from opiates and usually lessen after a few days.

Section 21.2

Synthetic Cannabinoids (K2/Spice)

This section includes text excerpted from "Synthetic Cannabinoids (K2/Spice)," National Institute on Drug Abuse (NIDA), February 2018.

What Are Synthetic Cannabinoids?

Synthetic cannabinoids are human-made mind-altering chemicals that are either sprayed on dried, shredded plant material so they can be smoked or sold as liquids to be vaporized and inhaled in e-cigarettes and other devices. These products are also known as herbal or liquid incense.

These chemicals are called cannabinoids because they are similar to chemicals found in the marijuana plant. Because of this similarity, synthetic cannabinoids are sometimes misleadingly called "synthetic marijuana" (or "fake weed"), and they are often marketed as safe, legal alternatives to that drug. In fact, they are not safe and may affect the brain much more powerfully than marijuana; their actual effects can be unpredictable and, in some cases, more dangerous or even life-threatening.

Synthetic cannabinoids are part of a group of drugs called new psychoactive substances (NPS). NPS are unregulated mind-altering substances that have become newly available on the market and are intended to produce the same effects as illegal drugs. Some of these substances may have been around for years but have reentered the market in altered chemical forms, or due to renewed popularity.

Manufacturers sell these products in colorful foil packages and plastic bottles to attract consumers. They market these products under a wide variety of specific brand names. Hundreds of brands now exist, including K2, Spice, Joker, Black Mamba, Kush, and Kronic.

For several years, synthetic cannabinoid mixtures have been easy to buy in drug paraphernalia shops, novelty stores, gas stations, and over the Internet. Because the chemicals used in them have no medical benefit and a high potential for abuse, authorities have made it illegal to sell, buy, or possess some of these chemicals. However, manufacturers try to sidestep these laws by changing the chemical formulas in their mixtures.

Easy access and the belief that synthetic cannabinoid products are "natural" and, therefore, harmless have likely contributed to their use among young people. Another reason for their continued use is that standard drug tests cannot easily detect many of the chemicals used in these products.

False Advertising

Synthetic cannabinoid products are often labeled "not for human consumption." Labels also often claim that they contain "natural" material taken from a variety of plants. However, the only parts of these products that are natural are the dried plant materials. Chemical tests show that the active, mind-altering ingredients are cannabinoid compounds made in laboratories.

How Do People Use Synthetic Cannabinoids?

The most common way to use synthetic cannabinoids is to smoke the dried plant material. Users also mix the sprayed plant material with marijuana or brew it as tea. Other users buy synthetic cannabinoid products as liquids to vaporize in e-cigarettes.

How Do Synthetic Cannabinoids Affect the Brain?

Synthetic cannabinoids act on the same brain cell receptors as delta-9-THC, the mind-altering ingredient in marijuana. So far, there have been few scientific studies of the effects of synthetic cannabinoids on the human brain, but researchers do know that some of them bind more strongly than marijuana to the cell receptors affected by THC, and can produce much stronger effects. The resulting health effects can be unpredictable and dangerous. Because the chemical composition of many synthetic cannabinoid products is unknown and may change from batch to batch, these products are likely to contain substances that cause dramatically different effects than the user might expect.

Synthetic cannabinoid users report some effects similar to those produced by marijuana:

- Elevated mood

- Relaxation

- Altered perception—awareness of surrounding objects and conditions

- Symptoms of psychosis—delusional or disordered thinking detached from reality

Psychotic effects include:

- Extreme anxiety

- Confusion

- Paranoia—extreme and unreasonable distrust of others

- Hallucinations—sensations and images that seem real, although they are not

What Are Some Other Health Effects of Synthetic Cannabinoids?

People who have used synthetic cannabinoids and have been taken to emergency rooms have shown severe effects including:

- Rapid heart rate

- Vomiting

- Violent behavior

- Suicidal thoughts

Synthetic cannabinoids can also raise blood pressure and cause a reduction in blood supply to the heart, as well as kidney damage and seizures. Use of these drugs is associated with a rising number of deaths.

Are Synthetic Cannabinoids Addictive?

Yes, synthetic cannabinoids can be addictive. Regular users trying to quit may have the following withdrawal symptoms:

- Headaches
- Anxiety
- Depression
- Irritability

Behavioral therapies and medications have not specifically been tested for treatment of addiction to these products. Healthcare providers should screen patients for possible co-occurring mental-health conditions.

Chapter 22

Club Drugs

Chapter Contents

Section 22.1

What Are Club Drugs?

This section contains text excerpted from the following sources:
Text in this section begins with excerpts from "Club Drugs,"
MedlinePlus, National Institutes of Health (NIH), December 28,
2016; Text beginning with the heading "How Are Club Drugs
Abused?" is excerpted from "Club Drugs," National Institute on
Drug Abuse (NIDA), December 2014. Reviewed January 2019.

Club drugs are a group of psychoactive drugs. They act on the central nervous system (CNS) and can cause changes in mood, awareness, and how you act. These drugs are often abused by young adults at all-night dance parties, dance clubs, and bars. They include

- Methylenedioxymethamphetamine (MDMA), also known as ecstasy XTC, X, E, Adam, Molly, Hug Beans, and Love Drug

- Gamma-hydroxybutyrate (GHB), also known as G, liquid ecstasy, and Soap

- Ketamine, also known as Special K, K, Vitamin K, and Jet

- Rohypnol, also known as Roofies

- Methamphetamine, also known as Speed, Ice, Chalk, Meth, Crystal, Crank, and Glass

- Lysergic acid diethylamide (LSD), also known as Acid, Blotter, and Dots

How Are Club Drugs Abused?

GHB and Rohypnol are available in odorless, colorless, and tasteless forms that are frequently combined with alcohol and other beverages. Both drugs have been used to commit sexual assaults (also known as "date rape," "drug rape," "acquaintance rape," or "drug-assisted" assault) due to their ability to sedate and incapacitate unsuspecting victims, preventing them from resisting sexual assault.

GHB is usually ingested orally, either in liquid or powder form, while Rohypnol is typically taken orally in pill form. Recent reports, however, have shown that Rohypnol is being ground up and snorted.

Both GHB and Rohypnol are also abused for their intoxicating effects, similar to other CNS depressants.

GHB also has anabolic effects (it stimulates protein synthesis) and has been used by bodybuilders to aid in fat reduction and muscle building.

Ketamine is usually snorted or injected intramuscularly.

How Do Club Drugs Affect the Brain?

GHB acts on at least two sites in the brain: the GABAB receptor and a specific GHB binding site. At high doses, GHB's sedative effects may result in sleep, coma, or death.

Rohypnol, like other benzodiazepines, acts at the GABAA receptor. It can produce anterograde amnesia, in which individuals may not remember events they experienced while under the influence of the drug.

Ketamine is a dissociative anesthetic, so called because it distorts perceptions of sight and sound and produces feelings of detachment from the environment and self. Ketamine acts on a type of glutamate receptor (NMDA receptor) to produce its effects, which are similar to those of the drug Phencyclidine (PCP). Low-dose intoxication results in impaired attention, learning ability, and memory. At higher doses, ketamine can cause dreamlike states and hallucinations; and at higher doses still, ketamine can cause delirium and amnesia.

Addictive Potential

Repeated use of GHB may lead to withdrawal effects, including insomnia, anxiety, tremors, and sweating. Severe withdrawal reactions have been reported among patients presenting from an overdose of GHB or related compounds, especially if other drugs or alcohol are involved.

Like other benzodiazepines, chronic use of Rohypnol can produce tolerance, physical dependence, and addiction.

There have been reports of people binging on ketamine, a behavior that is similar to that seen in some cocaine or amphetamine-dependent individuals. Ketamine users can develop signs of tolerance and cravings for the drug.

What Other Adverse Effects Do Club Drugs Have on Health?

Uncertainties about the sources, chemicals, and possible contaminants used to manufacture many club drugs make it extremely difficult to determine toxicity and associated medical consequences.

Nonetheless, it is known that:

- Coma and seizures can occur following the use of GHB. Combined use with other drugs such as alcohol can result in nausea and breathing difficulties. GHB and two of its precursors, gamma-butyrolactone (GBL) and 1,4 butanediol (BD), have been involved in poisonings, overdoses, date rapes, and deaths.

- Rohypnol may be lethal when mixed with alcohol and/or other CNS depressants.

- Ketamine, in high doses, can cause impaired motor function, high blood pressure, and potentially fatal respiratory problems.

What Treatment Options Exist for Persons Who Are Dependent on Club Drugs?

There is very little information available in the scientific literature about treatment for persons who abuse or are dependent on club drugs.

- There are no GHB detection tests for use in emergency rooms, and as many clinicians are unfamiliar with the drug, many GHB incidents likely go undetected. According to case reports, however, patients who abuse GHB appear to present both a mixed picture of severe problems upon admission and a good response to treatment, which often involves residential services.

- Treatment for Rohypnol follows accepted protocols for any benzodiazepine, which may consist of a 3- to 5-days inpatient detoxification program with a 24-hour intensive

- medical monitoring and management of withdrawal symptoms, since withdrawal from benzodiazepines can be life-threatening.

- Patients with a ketamine overdose are managed through supportive care for acute symptoms, with special attention to cardiac and respiratory functions.

Section 22.2

Gamma-Hydroxybutyrate (GHB)

This section includes text excerpted from "Gamma Hydroxybutyric Acid," DEA Diversion Control Division, October 2018.

Gamma-hydroxybutyric acid (GHB) is a Schedule I depressant. The GHB-containing pharmaceutical product, Xyrem®, is controlled as a Schedule III drug. GHB abuse became popular among teens and young adults at dance clubs and raves in the 1990s and gained notoriety as a date rape drug.

Licit Uses of Gamma-Hydroxybutyrate

In 2002, the U.S. Food and Drug Administration (FDA) approved Xyrem® (sodium oxybate) with orphan drug status and limited distribution through a central pharmacy. Xyrem® is approved as a treatment to reduce the incidence of cataplexy and to improve daytime sleepiness in patients with narcolepsy. The aggregate production quota for GHB in 2012 was 47,000 kilograms.

Chemistry and Pharmacology of Gamma-Hydroxybutyrate

GHB has the molecular formula $C_4H_8O_3$ and the molecular weight 104.10 g/mol. It is a powdered substance and is generally dissolved in a liquid. In liquid form, GHB is clear and colorless, and slightly salty in taste.

GHB is present in the central nervous system (CNS) in the concentrations; it is a metabolite of the neurotransmitter gamma-aminobutyric acid (GABA). Scientific data suggest that GHB can function as a neurotransmitter or neuromodulator in the brain. It produces dose-dependent depressant effects similar to those of the barbiturates and methaqualone. Low doses of GHB produce drowsiness, nausea, and visual distortion. At high doses, GHB overdose can result in unconsciousness, seizures, slowed heart rate, severe respiratory depression, decreased body temperature, vomiting, nausea, coma, or death. Sustained use of GHB can lead to addiction. Chronic abuse of GHB produces a withdrawal syndrome characterized by insomnia, anxiety, tremors, marked autonomic activation (i.e., increased heart rate and blood pressure) and occasional psychotic thoughts. Currently, there is no antidote available for GHB overdose.

Illicit Uses of Gamma-Hydroxybutyrate

GHB the for its euphoric and sedative effects. GHB is mainly self-ingested orally in a liquid mixture. It is sometimes mixed with alcohol to intensify its effects resulting in respiratory depression and coma. The average oral dose ranges from one to five grams (depending on the purity of the compound this can be 1 to 2 teaspoons mixed in a beverage). The concentration of GHB in these "home-brews" is variable, and the user is not usually aware of the actual dose they are drinking. The onset of action after oral ingestion is 15 to 30 minutes and the effects last 3 to 6 hours. The 2016 American Association of Poison Control Centers (AAPCC) report indicates that GHB accounted for 541 case mentions, 351 single exposures, 130 moderate medical outcomes, and 51 major medical outcomes. According to New DAWN ED, emergency room visits associated with GHB use increased from 1,084 in 2006 to 2,406 in 2011. GHB analogues gamma-butyrolactone (GBL) and 1,4-butanediol (BD) are often abused in place of GHB. Upon ingestion these analogues metabolize to GHB and thus produce physiological effects similar to GHB.

User Population of Gamma-Hydroxybutyrate

GHB by teens and young adults at all-night parties and raves. Peak levels of annual use were recorded in 2000 by the Monitoring the Future (MTF) survey that indicated that 1.4 percent of eighth, tenth and twelfth graders combined, reported past year GHB use. In the 2017 National Survey on Drug Use and Health (NSDUH), it was reported the lifetime use of GHB, among persons age 12 and older, slightly increased from 1,191 in 2015 to 1,401 in 2016.

Illicit Distribution

GHB is produced illegally in both domestic and foreign clandestine laboratories. The major source of GHB is through clandestine synthesis by local operators. GHB is sold usually as a white powder or as a clear liquid. GHB is packaged in vials or small bottles. At bars or "rave" parties, GHB is sold in liquid form by the capful or "swig" for 5 to $25 per cap.

National Forensic Laboratory Information System (NFLIS) data indicate that there were 223 laboratory report submissions identified as GHB by federal, state and local forensic laboratories in 2016 and 209 in 2017; that has remained fairly stable over the years.

Control Status

GHB is controlled in Schedule I of the Controlled Substances Act (CSA). Though Xyrem® is a Schedule III controlled substance, trafficking of Xyrem® is subject to Schedule I penalties.

Gamma-Butyrolactone (GBL) and 1,4-butanediol (BD) are structurally similar to GHB and there is a large body of evidence to confirm that GBL and BD has to GHB after oral administration. GBL and BD have been sold and substituted for GHB in an effort to circumvent state and federal laws. If intended for human consumption, both GBL and BD may be treated as a "controlled substance analogue" under the CSA pursuant to 21 U.S.C §§802(32) (A) and 813.

Section 22.3

Ketamine

This section includes text excerpted from "Drugs of Abuse," Get Smart About Drugs, U.S. Drug Enforcement Administration (DEA), June 15, 2017.

Ketamine is a dissociative anesthetic that has some hallucinogenic effects. It distorts perceptions of sight and sound and makes the user feel disconnected and not in control. It is an injectable, short-acting anesthetic for use in humans and animals. It is referred to as a "dissociative anesthetic" because it makes patients feel detached from their pain and environment.

Ketamine can induce a state of sedation (feeling calm and relaxed), immobility, relief from pain, and amnesia (no memory of events while under the influence of the drug). It is known for its ability to produce dissociative sensations and hallucinations. Ketamine has also been used to facilitate sexual assault.

Ketamine is produced commercially in a number of countries, including the United States. Most of the ketamine illegally distributed in the United States is diverted or stolen from legitimate sources, particularly veterinary clinics, or smuggled into the United States from Mexico.

Distribution of ketamine typically occurs among friends and acquaintances, most often at raves, nightclubs, and at private parties; street sales of ketamine are rare.

Facts about Ketamine
What Are Common Street Names?

Common street names include:

- Cat Tranquilizer, Cat Valium, Jet K, Kit Kat, Purple, Special K, Special La Coke, Super Acid, Super K, and Vitamin K

What Does It Look Like?

Ketamine comes in a clear liquid and a white or off-white powder. Powdered ketamine (100 milligrams to 200 milligrams) typically is packaged in small glass vials, small plastic bags, and capsules as well as paper, glassine, or aluminum foil folds.

How Is It Abused?

Ketamine, along with the other club drugs, has become popular among teens and young adults at dance clubs and raves. Ketamine is manufactured commercially as a powder or liquid. Powdered ketamine is also formed from pharmaceutical ketamine by evaporating the liquid using hot plates, warming trays, or microwave ovens, a process that results in the formation of crystals, which are then ground into powder.

Powdered ketamine is cut into lines known as bumps and snorted, or it is smoked, typically in marijuana or tobacco cigarettes. Liquid ketamine is injected or mixed into drinks. Ketamine is found by itself or often in combination with 3,4-Methylenedioxymethamphetamine (MDMA), amphetamine, methamphetamine, or cocaine.

What Is Its Effect on the Mind?

Ketamine produces hallucinations. It distorts perceptions of sight and sound and makes the user feel disconnected and not in control. A "Special K" trip is touted as better than that of lysergic acid diethylamide (LSD) or phencyclidine (PCP) because its hallucinatory effects are relatively short in duration, lasting approximately 30 to 60 minutes as opposed to several hours.

Slang for experiences related to Ketamine or effects of ketamine include:

- "K-land" (refers to a mellow and colorful experience)
- "K-hole" (refers to the out-of-body, near-death experience)
- "Baby food" (users sink into blissful, infantile inertia)
- "God" (users are convinced that they have met their maker)

The onset of effects is rapid and often occurs within a few minutes of taking the drug, though taking it orally results in a slightly slower onset of effects. Flashbacks have been reported several weeks after ketamine is used. Ketamine may also cause agitation, depression, cognitive difficulties, unconsciousness, and amnesia.

What Is Its Effect on the Body?

A couple of minutes after taking the drug, the user may experience an increase in heart rate and blood pressure that gradually decreases over the next 10 to 20 minutes. Ketamine can make users unresponsive to stimuli. When in this state, users experience:

- Involuntarily rapid eye movement, dilated pupils, salivation, tear secretions, and stiffening of the muscles

This drug can also cause nausea.

What Are Its Overdose Effects?

An overdose can cause unconsciousness and dangerously slowed breathing.

Which Drugs Cause Similar Effects

Other hallucinogenic drugs such as LSD, PCP, and mescaline can cause hallucinations. There are also several drugs such as gamma-hydroxybutyrate (GHB), Rohypnol, and other depressants that are misused for their amnesiac or sedative properties to facilitate sexual assault.

What Is Its Legal Status in the United States?

Since the 1970s, ketamine has been marketed in the United States as an injectable, short-acting anesthetic for use in humans and animals. In 1999, ketamine including its salts, isomers, and salts of isomers, became a Schedule III nonnarcotic substance under the Controlled Substances Act (CSA). It has a currently accepted medical use but some potential for abuse, which may lead to moderate or low physical dependence or high psychological dependence.

Section 22.4

Rohypnol

This section includes text excerpted from "Drugs of Abuse," Get Smart About Drugs, U.S. Drug Enforcement Administration (DEA), June 15, 2017.

Rohypnol is a trade name for flunitrazepam, a central nervous system (CNS) depressant that belongs to a class of drugs known as benzodiazepines. Flunitrazepam is also marketed as generic preparations and other trade name products outside of the United States.

Like other benzodiazepines, Rohypnol produces sedative-hypnotic, antianxiety, and muscle relaxant effects. This drug has never been approved for medical use in the United States by the U.S. Food and Drug Administration (FDA). Outside the United States, Rohypnol is commonly prescribed to treat insomnia. Rohypnol gamma-butyrolactone to as a "date rape" drug.

Rohypnol is smuggled into the United States from other countries, such as Mexico.

Facts about Rohypnol
What Are Common Street Names?

Common street names include:

- Circles, Forget Pill, Forget-Me-Pill, La Rocha, Lunch Money Drug, Mexican Valium, Pingus, R2, Reynolds, Roach, Roach 2, Roaches, Roachies, Roapies, Robutal, Rochas Dos, Rohypnol, Roofies, Rophies, Ropies, Roples, Row-Shay, Ruffies, and Wolfies

What Does It Look Like?

Prior to 1997, Rohypnol was manufactured as a white tablet (0.5 to 2 milligrams per tablet), and when mixed in drinks, was colorless, tasteless, and odorless. In 1997, the manufacturer responded to concerns about the drug's role in sexual assaults by reformulating the drug.

Rohypnol is now manufactured as an oblong olive green tablet with a speckled blue core that when dissolved in light-colored drinks will dye the liquid blue. However, generic versions of the drug may not contain the blue dye.

How Is It Abused?

The tablet can be swallowed whole, crushed and snorted, or dissolved in liquid. Adolescents may abuse Rohypnol to produce a euphoric effect often described as a "high." While high, they experience reduced inhibitions and impaired judgment.

Rohypnol is also used in combination with alcohol to produce an exaggerated intoxication.

In addition, abuse of Rohypnol may be associated with multiple-substance abuse. For example, cocaine users may use benzodiazepines such as Rohypnol to relieve the side effects (e.g., irritability and agitation) associated with cocaine binges.

Rohypnol is also misused to physically and psychologically incapacitate victims targeted for sexual assault. The drug is usually placed in the alcoholic drink of an unsuspecting victim to incapacitate them and prevent resistance to sexual assault. The drug leaves the victim unaware of what happened to them.

What Is Its Effect on the Mind?

Like other benzodiazepines, Rohypnol slows down the functioning of the CNS producing:

- Drowsiness (sedation), sleep (pharmacological hypnosis), decreased anxiety, and amnesia (no memory of events while under the influence of the substance)

Rohypnol can also cause:

- Increased or decreased reaction time, impaired mental functioning and judgment, confusion, aggression, and excitability

What Is Its Effect on the Body?

Rohypnol causes muscle relaxation. Adverse physical effects include:

- Slurred speech, loss of motor coordination, weakness, headache, and respiratory depression

Rohypnol also can produce physical dependence when taken regularly over a period of time.

What Are Its Overdose Effects?

High doses of Rohypnol, particularly when combined with CNS depressant drugs such as alcohol and heroin, can cause severe sedation, unconsciousness, slow heart rate, and suppression of respiration that may be sufficient to result in death.

Which Drugs Cause Similar Effects

Drugs that cause similar effects include GHB (gamma-hydroxybutyrate) and other benzodiazepines such as alprazolam (e.g., Xanax), clonazepam (e.g., Klonopin), and diazepam (e.g., Valium).

What Is Its Legal Status in the United States?

Rohypnol is a Schedule IV substance under the Controlled Substances Act (CSA). Rohypnol is not approved for manufacture, sale, use, or importation to the United States. It is legally manufactured and marketed in many countries. Penalties for possession, trafficking, and distribution involving one gram or more are the same as those of a Schedule I drug.

Chapter 23

Dissociative Drugs

Chapter Contents

Section 23.1

Dextromethorphan (DXM)

This section includes text excerpted from "Drugs of Abuse," U.S.
Drug Enforcement Administration (DEA), September 5, 2018.

Dextromethorphan (DXM) is a cough suppressor found in more than 120 over-the-counter (OTC) cold medications, either alone or in combination with other drugs such as analgesics (e.g., acetaminophen), antihistamines (e.g., chlorpheniramine), decongestants (e.g., pseudoephedrine), and/ or expectorants (e.g., guaifenesin). The typical adult dose for a cough is 15 or 30 mg taken three to four times daily. The cough-suppressing effects of DXM persist for five to six hours after ingestion. When taken as directed, side effects are rarely observed.

DXM users can obtain the drug at almost any pharmacy or supermarket, seeking out the products with the highest concentration of the drug from among all the OTC cough and cold remedies that contain it. DXM products and powder can also be purchased on the Internet.

Facts on Dextromethorphan
What Are Common Street Names?

Common street names include:

- CCC, Dex, DXM, Poor Man's PCP, Robo, Rojo, Skittles, Triple C, and Velvet

What Does It Look Like?

DXM can come in the form of:

- Cough syrup, tablets, capsules, or powder

How Is It Abused?

DXM is abused in high doses to experience euphoria and visual and auditory hallucinations. Users take various amounts depending on their body weight and the effect they are attempting to achieve. Some users ingest 250 to 1,500 milligrams in a single dosage, far more than the recommended therapeutic dosages described above.

Illicit use of DXM is referred to on the street as "Robo-tripping," "skittling," or "dexing." The first two terms are derived from the products that are most commonly abused, Robitussin and Coricidin HBP. DXM abuse has traditionally involved drinking large volumes of the OTC liquid cough preparations. More recently, however, abuse of tablet and gel-capsule preparations has increased.

These newer, high-dose DXM products have particular appeal for users. They are much easier to consume, eliminate the need to drink large volumes of unpleasant-tasting syrup, and are easily portable and concealed, allowing an abuser to continue to abuse DXM throughout the day, whether at school or work.

DXM powder, sold over the Internet, is also a source of DXM for abuse. (The powdered form of DXM poses additional risks to the user due to the uncertainty of composition and dose.)

DXM is also distributed in illicitly manufactured tablets containing only DXM or mixed with other drugs such as pseudoephedrine and/or methamphetamine.

DXM is abused by individuals of all ages, but its abuse by teenagers and young adults is of particular concern. This abuse is fueled by DXM's OTC availability and extensive "how to" abuse information on various websites.

What Is Its Effect on the Mind?

Some of the many psychoactive effects associated with high-dose DXM include:

- Confusion, inappropriate laughter, agitation, paranoia, and hallucinations

- Other sensory changes, including the feeling of floating and changes in hearing and touch

Long-term abuse of DXM is associated with severe psychological dependence. Abusers of DXM describe the following four dose-dependent "plateaus":

Table 23.1. Dose-Dependent "Plateaus"

Plateau	Dose (Mg)	Behavioral Effects
1st	100–200	Mild stimulation
2nd	200–400	Euphoria and hallucinations
3rd	300–600	Distorted visual perceptions Loss of motor coordination
4th	500–1500	Out-of-body sensations

What Is Its Effect on the Body?

DXM intoxication involves:

- Over-excitability, lethargy, loss of coordination, slurred speech, sweating, hypertension, and involuntary spasmodic movement of the eyeballs

The use of high doses of DXM in combination with alcohol or other drugs is particularly dangerous, and deaths have been reported. Approximately 5 to 10 percent of Caucasians are poor DXM metabolizers and at increased risk for overdoses and deaths. DXM taken with antidepressants can be life-threatening.

OTC products that contain DXM often contain other ingredients such as acetaminophen, chlorpheniramine, and guaifenesin that have their own effects, such as liver damage, rapid heart rate, lack of coordination, vomiting, seizures, and coma.

What Are Its Overdose Effects?

DXM overdose can be treated in an emergency room setting and generally does not result in severe medical consequences or death. Most DXM-related deaths are caused by ingesting the drug in combination with other drugs. DXM-related deaths also occur from impairment of the senses, which can lead to accidents.

A 14-year-old boy in Colorado who abused DXM died when he was hit by two cars as he attempted to cross a highway. State law enforcement investigators suspect that the drug affected the boy's depth perception and caused him to misjudge the distance and speed of the oncoming vehicles.

Which Drugs Cause Similar Effects

Depending on the dose, DXM can have effects similar to marijuana or ecstasy. In high doses, its out-of-body effects are similar to those of ketamine or Phencyclidine (PCP).

What Is Its Legal Status in the United States?

DXM is a legally marketed cough suppressant that is neither a controlled substance nor a regulated chemical under the Controlled Substances Act (CSA).

Section 23.2

Phencyclidine (PCP)

This section includes text excerpted from "Phencyclidine," DEA
Diversion Control Division, January 2013. Reviewed January 2019.

After a decline in abuse during the late 1980s and 1990s, the abuse
of phencyclidine (PCP) has increased slightly in recent years. Street
names include Angel Dust, Hog, Ozone, Rocket Fuel, Shermans, Wack,
Crystal, and Embalming Fluid. Street names for PCP combined with
marijuana include Killer Joints, Super Grass, Fry, Lovelies, Wets,
and Waters.

Licit Uses of Phencyclidine

PCP was developed in the 1950s to be used as an intravenous anesthetic in the United States, but its use was discontinued due to the
high incidence of patients experiencing postoperative delirium (POD)
with hallucinations. PCP is no longer produced or used for medical
purposes in the United States.

Chemistry and Pharmacology of Phencyclidine

Phencyclidine, 1-(1-phenylcyclohexyl) piperidine, is a white crystalline powder which is readily soluble in water or alcohol. PCP is
classified as a hallucinogen. PCP is a "dissociative" drug; it induces
distortion of sight and sound and produces feelings of detachment.

PCP's effects include sedation, immobility, amnesia, and marked
analgesia. The effects of PCP vary by the route of administration
and dose. The intoxicating effects can be produced within two to five
minutes after smoking and 30 to 60 minutes after swallowing. PCP
intoxication may last from four to eight hours; some users report experiencing subjective effects from 24 to 48 hours after using PCP. Low
to moderate doses (1 to 5 mg) induce feelings of detachment from surroundings and self, numbness, slurred speech and loss of coordination
accompanied by a sense of strength and invulnerability. A blank stare,
rapid and involuntary eye movements are the more observable effects.
Catatonic posturing, resembling that observed with schizophrenia,
is also produced. Higher doses of PCP produce hallucinations. Physiological effects include increased blood pressure, rapid and shallow
breathing, elevated heart rate and elevated temperature.

Chronic use of PCP can result in dependency with a withdrawal syndrome upon cessation of the drug. Chronic abuse of PCP can impair memory and thinking. Other effects of long-term use include persistent speech difficulties, suicidal thoughts, anxiety, depression, and social withdrawal.

Illicit Uses of Phencyclidine

PCP is abused for its mind-altering effects. It can be abused by snorting, smoking or swallowing. Smoking is the most common method of abusing PCP. Leafy material such as mint, parsley, oregano, tobacco, or marijuana is saturated with PCP, and subsequently rolled into a cigarette and smoked. A marijuana joint or cigarette dipped in liquid PCP is known as a "dipper." PCP is typically used in small quantities; 5 to 10 mg is an average dose.

User Population of Phencyclidine

PCP is predominantly abused by young adults and high-school students. In 2010, there was an estimated 53,542 emergency department visits associated with PCP use, according to the Drug Abuse Warning Network (New DAWN ED). This is a significant increase from an estimated 37,266 PCP-associated visits in 2008. The American Association of Poison Control Centers (AAPCC) National Poison Data System (NPDS) reports 747 PCP exposure case mentions and 350 single exposures in 2010. According to the 2011 National Survey on Drug Use and Health (NSDUH), 6.1 million (2.4%) individuals in the United States, age 12 and older, reported using PCP in their lifetime. The Monitoring the Future (MTF) survey indicates that PCP use among twelfth graders in the past year increased from 1.0 percent in 2010 to 1.3 percent in 2011 and then decreased to 0.9 percent in 2012.

Illicit Distribution of Phencyclidine

PCP is available in powder, crystal, tablet, capsule, and liquid forms. It is most commonly sold in powder and liquid forms. Tablets sold as 3,4-methylenedioxymethamphetamine (Ecstasy) occasionally are found to contain PCP. Prices for PCP range from $5–$15 per tablet, $20–$30 for a gram of powder PCP, and $200–$300 for an ounce of liquid PCP. The "dipper" sells for $10–$20 each.

According to the system to retrieve information from drug evidence (STRIDE) and the National Forensic Laboratory Information System

(NFLIS), 5,374 PCP reports were from federal, state, and local forensic laboratories in 2011. In the first six months of 2012, there were 2,748 PCP reports from forensic laboratories.

Control Status of Phencyclidine

On January 25, 1978, PCP was transferred from Schedule III to Schedule II under the Controlled Substances Act (CSA).

Section 23.3

Salvia divinorum

This section includes text excerpted from "Drugs of Abuse,"
U.S. Drug Enforcement Administration (DEA), September 5, 2018.

Salvia divinorum is a perennial herb in the mint family that is abused for its hallucinogenic effects. Salvia is native to certain areas of the Sierra Mazateca region of Oaxaca, Mexico. It is one of several plants that are used by Mazatec Indians for ritual divination. *Salvia divinorum* plants can be grown successfully outside of this region. They can be grown indoors and outdoors, especially in humid semi-tropical climates.

Facts about Salvia divinorum
What Are Common Street Names?

Common street names include:

• Maria Pastora, Sally-D, and Salvia

What Does It Look Like?

The plant has spade-shaped variegated green leaves that look similar to mint. The plants themselves grow to more than three feet high, have large green leaves, hollow square stems, and white flowers with purple calyces.

How Is It Abused?

Salvia can be chewed, smoked, or vaporized.

What Is Its Effect on the Mind?

Psychic effects include perceptions of bright lights, vivid colors, shapes, and body movement, as well as body or object distortions. *Salvia divinorum* may also cause fear and panic, uncontrollable laughter, a sense of overlapping realities, and hallucinations.

Salvinorin A is believed to be the ingredient responsible for the psychoactive effects of *Salvia divinorum*.

What Is Its Effect on the Body?

Adverse physical effects may include:

• Loss of coordination, dizziness, and slurred speech

Which Drugs Cause Similar Effects

When *Salvia divinorum* is chewed or smoked, the hallucinogenic effects elicited are similar to those induced by other Scheduled hallucinogenic substances.

What Is Its Legal Status in the United States?

Neither *Salvia divinorum* nor its active constituent Salvinorin A has an approved medical use in the United States. Salvia is not controlled under the Controlled Substances Act (CSA). *Salvia divinorum* is, however, controlled by a number of states. Since Salvia is not controlled by the CSA, some online botanical companies and drug promotional sites have advertised Salvia as a legal alternative to other plant hallucinogens such as mescaline.

Chapter 24

Hallucinogenic Drugs

Chapter Contents

Section 24.1

Introduction to Hallucinogens

This section includes text excerpted from "Hallucinogens,"
National Institute on Drug Abuse (NIDA), January 2016.

What Are Hallucinogens?

Hallucinogens are a diverse group of drugs that alter perception (awareness of surrounding objects and conditions), thoughts, and feelings. They cause hallucinations or sensations and images that seem real though they are not. Hallucinogens can be found in some plants and mushrooms (or their extracts) or can be human-made. People have used hallucinogens for centuries, mostly for religious rituals. Common hallucinogens include the following:

- **Ayahuasca** is a tea made from one of several Amazonian plants containing dimethyltryptamine (DMT), the primary mind-altering ingredient. Ayahuasca is also known as Hoasca, Aya, and Yagé.

- **Dimethyltryptamine (DMT)** is a powerful chemical found in some Amazonian plants. Manufacturers can also make DMT in a lab. The drug is usually a white crystalline powder. A popular name for DMT is Dimitri.

- **D-lysergic acid diethylamide (LSD)** is one of the most powerful mood-changing chemicals. It is a clear or white odorless material made from lysergic acid, which is found in a fungus that grows on rye and other grains. LSD has many other names, including Acid, Blotter, Dots, and Yellow Sunshine.

- **Peyote (mescaline)** is a small, spineless cactus with mescaline as its main ingredient. Peyote can also be synthetic. Buttons, Cactus, and Mesc are common names for peyote.

- **4-phosphoryloxy-N,N-dimethyltryptamine** (psilocybin) comes from certain types of mushrooms found in tropical and subtropical regions of South America, Mexico, and the United States. Other names for psilocybin include Little Smoke, Magic Mushrooms, Purple Passion, and Shrooms.

Some hallucinogens also cause users to feel out of control or disconnected from their body and environment. Common examples include the following:

- **Dextromethorphan (DXM)** is a cough suppressant and mucus-clearing ingredient in some over-the-counter (OTC) cold and cough medicines (syrups, tablets, and gel capsules). Robo is another popular name for DXM.

- **Ketamine** is used as a surgical anesthetic for humans and animals. Much of the ketamine sold on the streets comes from veterinary offices. While available as an injectable liquid, manufacturers mostly sell it as a powder or as pills. Other names for ketamine include K, Special K, or Cat Valium.

- **Phencyclidine (PCP)** was developed in the 1950s as a general anesthetic for surgery. It's no longer used for this purpose due to serious side effects. While PCP can be found in a variety of forms, including tablets or capsules, liquid and white crystal powder are the most common forms. PCP has various other names, such as Angel Dust, Hog, Love Boat, and Peace Pill.

- *Salvia divinorum* (**salvia**) is a plant common to southern Mexico and Central and South America. Other names for salvia are Diviner's Sage, Maria Pastora, Sally-D, and Magic Mint.

How Do People Use Hallucinogens?

People use hallucinogens in a wide variety of ways, as shown in Table 24.1.

How Do Hallucinogens Affect the Brain?

Research suggests that hallucinogens work at least partially by temporarily disrupting communication between brain chemical systems throughout the brain and spinal cord. Some hallucinogens interfere with the action of the brain chemical serotonin, which regulates:

- Mood
- Sensory perception
- Sleep
- Hunger
- Body temperature
- Sexual behavior
- Muscle control

Table 24.1. Hallucinogens

	Ayahuasca	DMT	LSD	Peyote	Psilocybin	DXM	Ketamine	PCP	Salvia
Swallowing as tablets or pills		✓	✓				✓	✓	
Swallowing as liquid		✓	✓	✓					
Consuming raw or dried	✓			✓	✓				✓
Brewing into tea	✓			✓	✓				✓
Snorting							✓	✓	
Injecting							✓	✓	
Inhaling, vaporizing, or smoking		✓						✓	✓
Absorbing through the lining in the mouth using drug-soaked paper pieces			✓						

Other hallucinogens interfere with the action of the brain chemical glutamate, which regulates:

- Pain perception

- Responses to the environment

- Emotion

- Learning and memory

Short-Term Effects

The effects of hallucinogens can begin within 20 to 90 minutes and can last as long as 6 to 12 hours. Salvia's effects are more short-lived, appearing in less than one minute and lasting less than 30 minutes. Hallucinogen users refer to the experiences brought on by these drugs as "trips," calling the unpleasant experiences "bad trips."

Along with hallucinations, other short-term general effects include:

- Increased heart rate

- Nausea

- Intensified feelings and sensory experiences

- Changes in sense of time (for example, time passing by slowly)

Specific short-term effects of some hallucinogens include:

- Increased blood pressure, breathing rate, or body temperature

- Loss of appetite

- Dry mouth

- Sleep problems

- Mixed senses (such as "seeing" sounds or "hearing" colors)

- Spiritual experiences

- Feelings of relaxation or detachment from self/environment

- Uncoordinated movements

- Excessive sweating

- Panic

- Paranoia—extreme and unreasonable distrust of others

- Psychosis—disordered thinking detached from reality

Long-Term Effects

Little is known about the long-term effects of hallucinogens. Researchers do know that ketamine users may develop symptoms that include ulcers in the bladder, kidney problems, and poor memory. Repeated use of PCP can result in long-term effects that may continue for a year or more after use stops, such as:

- Speech problems

- Memory loss

- Weight loss

- Anxiety

- Depression and suicidal thoughts

Though rare, long-term effects of some hallucinogens include the following:

- **Persistent psychosis**—a series of continuing mental problems, including:

- Visual disturbances

- Disorganized thinking

- Paranoia

- Mood changes

- **Flashbacks**—recurrences of certain drug experiences. They often happen without warning and may occur within a few days or more than a year after drug use. In some users, flashbacks can persist and affect daily functioning, a condition known as hallucinogen persisting perceptual disorder (HPPD). These people continue to have hallucinations and other visual disturbances, such as seeing trails attached to moving objects.

- Symptoms that are sometimes mistaken for other disorders, such as stroke or a brain tumor

What Are Other Risks of Hallucinogens?

Other risks or health effects of many hallucinogens remain unclear and need more research. Known risks include the following:

- Some psilocybin users risk poisoning and possibly death from using a poisonous mushroom by mistake.

- High doses of PCP can cause seizures, coma, and death, though death more often results from accidental injury or suicide during PCP intoxication. Interactions between PCP and depressants such as alcohol and benzodiazepines (prescribed to relieve anxiety or promote sleep—alprazolam (Xanax®), for instance) can also lead to coma.

- Some bizarre behaviors resulting from hallucinogens that users display in public places may prompt public-health or law-enforcement personnel intervention.

- While hallucinogens' effects on the developing fetus are unknown, researchers do know that mescaline in peyote may affect the fetus of a pregnant woman using the drug.

Are Hallucinogens Addictive?

Evidence indicates that certain hallucinogens can be addictive or that people can develop a tolerance to them. Use of some hallucinogens also produces tolerance to other similar drugs.

For example, LSD is not considered an addictive drug because it doesn't cause uncontrollable drug-seeking behavior. However, LSD does produce tolerance, so some users who take the drug repeatedly must take higher doses to achieve the same effect. This is an extremely dangerous practice, given the unpredictability of the drug. In addition, LSD produces tolerance to other hallucinogens, including psilocybin.

On the other hand, PCP is a hallucinogen that can be addictive. People who stop repeated use of PCP experience drug cravings, head-aches, and sweating as common withdrawal symptoms.

How Can People Get Treatment for Addiction to Hallucinogens?

There are no government-approved medications to treat addiction to hallucinogens. While inpatient behavioral treatments can be helpful for patients with a variety of addictions, scientists need more research to find out if behavioral therapies are effective for addiction to hallucinogens.

Section 24.2

4-Iodo-2,5-Dimethoxyphenethylamine

This section includes text excerpted from
"4-Iodo-2,5-Dimethoxyphenethylamine," DEA
Diversion Control Division, October 2018.

Street names: 2C-I, Infinity, Isabel

4-Iodo-2,5-dimethoxyphenethylamine (2C-I, 4-iodo 2,5-DMPEA) is a synthetic drug abused for its hallucinogenic effects. It has been encountered in a number of states by federal, state, and local law enforcement agencies. 2C-I has no approved medical uses in the United States.

Chemistry and Pharmacology of 4-Iodo-2,5-Dimethoxyphenethylamine

4-Iodo-2,5-dimethoxyphenethylamine is closely related to the phenethylamine hallucinogens, 1-(4-bromo 2, 5-dimethoxyphenyl)-2-aminopropane (DOB) and 2,5- dimethoxy-4-methylamphetamine (DOM). Like DOM and DOB, 2C-I displays high affinity for central serotonin receptors. 2C-I selectively binds to the 5-HT receptor system.

Drug discrimination studies in animals indicate that 2C-I produces discriminative stimulus effects that are similar to those of several Schedule I hallucinogens such as lysergic acid diethylamide (LSD), N,N-dimethyltryptamine (DMT) and methylenedioxymethamphetamine (MDMA). In rats trained to discriminate LSD, DMT or MDMA from saline, 2C-I fully substituted for these Schedule I hallucinogens.

In humans, 2C-I produces dose-dependent psychoactive effects. User reports have mentioned oral doses between 3 and 25 mg, producing LSD-like hallucinations and visual distortions, and MDMA-like empathy. Onset of subjective effects following 2C-I ingestion is around 40 minutes with peak effects occurring at approximately two hours. Effects of 2C-I can last up to 10 hours. Various users reported delayed desired effects compared to related drugs, which may result in some users taking additional doses or other drugs, which may increase the risk of toxicity or accidental overdose. 2C-I has been reported to cause a wide range of effects, including visual, auditory and thought process alterations, euphoria, relaxation, anxiety, paranoia, fear, dyspnea (breathing difficulty), nausea, vomiting, and mydriasis (dilation of pupils). Further, there have been some mentions of hospitalization from the abuse of 2C-I.

The radioimmunoassay-detection system that is commonly used for testing amphetamine and hallucinogens is not expected to detect 2C-I. In the Marquis Reagent Field Test, 2C-I produces a dark green to black color. 2C-I can be detected in blood or urine samples using Gas chromatography-mass spectrometric (GS-MS) techniques.

Illicit Uses of 4-Iodo-2,5-Dimethoxyphenethylamine

2C-I is abused for its hallucinogenic effects. 2C-I is taken orally in tablet or capsule forms or snorted in its powder form. It has also been found impregnated on small squares of blotter paper for oral administration, which is a technique often seen for the distribution and abuse of lysergic acid diethylamide (LSD). The drug has been misrepresented by distributors and sold as other hallucinogens such as 3,4-methylenedioxymethamphetamine (MDMA) and LSD.

4-Iodo-2,5-Dimethoxyphenethylamine: User Population

2C-I is used by the same population as those using "Ecstasy" and other club drugs, high school and college students, and other young adults in dance and nightlife settings.

Illicit Distribution of 4-Iodo-2,5-Dimethoxyphenethylamine

2C-I is distributed as capsules, tablets, in powder form, or in liquid form. U.S. Drug Enforcement Administration (DEA) identified occurrences of the drug being purchased through Internet retailers. In one instance, it was purchased in powder form through the Internet and encapsulated for retail, at a street value of $6 per capsule. In Europe, 2C-I has often been seized in tablet form with an 'i' logo which may be to signify that it is not ecstasy (MDMA).

The National Forensic Laboratory Information System (NFLIS) is a DEA database that collects scientifically verified data on drug items and cases submitted to and analyzed by federal, state, and local forensic laboratories. The System to Retrieve Information from Drug Evidence (STRIDE)/STARLiMS provides information on drug seizures reported to and analyzed by DEA laboratories. From 2007 to 2018, 529 exhibits have been identified as 2C-I by federal, state, and local forensic laboratories in 38 states. In 2010, there were 61 2C-I reports. There were 95 2C-I reports in 2011 and 73 in 2012. There have been 19 reports of 2C-I in 2016, 24 reports in 2017, and two reports in 2018.

Control Status of 4-Iodo-2,5-Dimethoxyphenethylamine

The Controlled Substances Act (CSA) lists 2C-I in Schedule I.

Section 24.3

Alpha-Methyltryptamine (Spirals)

This section includes text excerpted from "Alpha-Methyltryptamine,"
DEA Diversion Control Division, October 2018.

Alpha-methyltryptamine (AMT) is a tryptamine derivative and shares many pharmacological similarities with those of Schedule I hallucinogens such as alpha-ethyltryptamine, N, N-dimethyltryptamine, psilocybin, and lysergic acid diethylamide (LSD). Since 1999, AMT has become popular among drug abusers for its hallucinogenic-like effects. In the 1960s, following extensive clinical studies on AMT as a possible antidepressant drug, the Upjohn Company concluded that AMT was a toxic substance and produces psychosis.

AMT has no accepted medical uses in treatment in the United States.

Chemistry and Pharmacology of Alpha-Methyltryptamine

AMT has the molecular formula $C_{11}H_{14}N_2$ and a molecular weight of 174.74 g/mol. The hydrochloride salt of AMT is a white crystalline powder.

AMT, similar to several other Schedule I hallucinogens, binds with moderate affinities to serotonin (5-HT) receptors (5-HT1 and 5-HT2). AMT inhibits the uptake of monoamines especially 5-HT and is a potent inhibitor of monoamine oxidase (MAO) (especially MAOA), an enzyme critical for the metabolic degradation of monoamines, the brain chemicals important for sensory, emotional, and other behavioral functions. AMT has been shown to produce locomotor stimulant effects in animals. It has been hypothesized that both 5-HT and dopamine systems mediate the stimulant effects of AMT. In animals, AMT produces behavioral effects that are substantially similar to those of 1-(2,5-dimethoxy-4-methylphenyl)-2-aminopropane (DOM) and methylenedioxymethamphetamine (MDMA), both Schedule I hallucinogens, in animals.

In humans, AMT elicits subjective effects including hallucinations. It has an onset of action of about three to four hours and a duration of about 12 to 24 hours, but may produce an extended duration of two days in some subjects. Subjects report uncomfortable feelings, muscular tension, nervous tension, irritability, restlessness, an unsettled feeling in stomach, and the inability to relax and sleep. AMT can alter sensory perception and judgment and can pose serious health risks to the user and the general public. Abuse of AMT led to two emergency department admissions and one death. AMT increases blood pressure and heart rate, dilates pupils, and causes deep tendon reflexes and impairs coordination.

Illicit Uses of Alpha-Methyltryptamine

AMT is abused for its hallucinogenic effects and is used as a substitute for MDMA. It is often administered orally as either powder or capsules at doses ranging from 15–40 mg. Other routes of administration include smoking and snorting.

User Population: Alpha-Methyltryptamine

Youth and young adults are the main abusers of AMT. Internet websites are a source that high-school students and United States soldiers have used to obtain and abuse AMT.

Illicit Distribution of Alpha-Methyltryptamine

The National Forensic Laboratory Information System (NFLIS) is a U.S. Drug Enforcement Administration (DEA) database that collects scientifically verified data on drug items and cases submitted to and analyzed by federal, state, and local forensic laboratories. The System to Retrieve Information from Drug Evidence (STRIDE), integrated into STARLiMS, a web-based, commercial laboratory information-management system, since October 1, 2014 has replaced STRIDE as the DEA laboratory drug evidence data system of record. In which provides information on drug seizures reported to and analyzed by DEA laboratories. According to STRIDE/STARLiMS, the first recorded submission by law enforcement to DEA laboratories of a drug exhibit containing AMT occurred in 1999.

NFLIS and STRIDE/STARLiMS indicate that reports of AMT by federal, state, and local forensic laboratories increased from 35 in 2002 to 76 in 2003. In the years after temporary scheduling of AMT in 2003, the number of reports declined. In 2004, there were 57 reports and in 2005, there were 41 reports. From 2006 to 2011, NFLIS and STRIDE/STARLiMS indicated a total of five AMT reports in those databases. However, in 2012, the number of AMT reports in NFLIS and STRIDE/STARLiMS increased to 85. And, the number of drug reports has dramatically decreased to three in 2016 and one in 2017. AMT has been illicitly available from the United States and foreign chemical companies and from Internet websites. Additionally, there is evidence of attempted clandestine production of AMT.

Control Status of Alpha-Methyltryptamine

AMT is controlled in Schedule I substance under of the Controlled Substances Act (CSA).

Section 24.4

Blue Mystic (2C-T-7)

This section includes text excerpted from "2,5-Dimethoxy-4-(n)-Propylthiophenethylamine," DEA Diversion Control Division, October 2018.

Street names: 2C-T-7, Blue Mystic, T7, Beautiful, Tripstay, Tweety-Bird Mescaline

Licit Uses of Blue Mystic

2C-T-7 is not approved for marketing by the U.S. Food and Drug Administration (FDA) and is not sold legally in the United States.

Chemistry and Pharmacology of Blue Mystic

2,5-Dimethoxy-4-(n)-propylthiophenethylamine (2CT-7), is a phenethylamine hallucinogen that is structurally related to the Schedule I phenethylamine hallucinogens, 4-bromo-2, 5-dimethoxy-phenethylamine (2C-B, Nexus), and mescaline. Based on structural similarity to these compounds, the pharmacological profile of 2C-T-7 is expected to be qualitatively similar to these hallucinogens.

Drug discrimination studies in animals indicate that 2C-T-7 produces discriminative stimulus effects similar to those of several Schedule I hallucinogens. In rats trained to discriminate 2,5-dimethoxy-4-methylamphetamine (DOM), 2C-T-7 fully substituted for DOM and was slightly less potent than 2C-B in eliciting DOM like effects. 2C-T-7 was also shown to share some commonality with lysergic acid diethylamide (LSD); it partially substituted for LSD up to doses that severely disrupted performance in rats trained to discriminate LSD. 2C-T-7 can also function as a discriminative stimulus in rats. Rats readily learned to discriminate 2C-T-7 from saline. When either 2C-B or LSD was substituted for 2C-T-7, each elicited 2C-T-7- like discriminative stimulus effects.

The subjective effects of 2C-T-7, like those of 2C-B and DOM, appear to be mediated through central serotonin receptors. 2C-T-7 selectively binds to the 5- HT receptor system.

According to one published case report, 2C-T-7 abuse has been associated with convulsions in humans.

Illicit Uses Blue Mystic

2C-T-7 is abused orally and intranasally for its hallucinogenic effects. Information from a website about a variety of illicit drugs has suggested that 2C-T-7 produce effects similar to those of 2C-B. This information is based on individuals self-administering 2C-T-7 illicitly and self-reporting the effects. Its effects include visual hallucination, mood lifting, sense of well being, emotionality, volatility, increased appreciation of music, and psychedelic ideation. The oral and intranasal doses recommended on this website are 10 to 50 mg and 5 to 10 mg, respectively. 2C-T-7's onset and duration of actions are dependent upon the route of administration. Following oral administration, onset and duration of effects are 1 to 2.5 hours and 5 to 7 hours, respectively. After intranasal administration, the onset of action and duration of effects are 5 to 15 minutes and 2 to 4 hours, respectively.

User Population: Blue Mystic

Young adults are the main abusers of 2C-T-7.

Illicit Distribution of Blue Mystic

The National Forensic Laboratory Information System (NFLIS) is a DEA database that collects scientifically verified data on drug items and cases submitted to and analyzed by federal, state, and local forensic laboratories. The System to Retrieve Information from Drug Evidence (STRIDE) provides information on drug seizures reported to and analyzed by DEA laboratories. From January 2007 to December 2017, 61 reports, identified as 2C-T-7, were submitted to federal, state, and local forensic laboratories. During this time, law enforcement officials encountered 2C-T-7 in 16 states; 28 of the 61 reports were encountered in the state of Florida.

2C-T-7 was being purchased over the Internet from a company located in Indiana. This site was traced to an individual who had been selling large quantities of this substance since January 2000. Sales through this Internet site were thought to be the major sources of 2CT-7 in the United States. One clandestine laboratory was identified in Las Vegas, Nevada as the supplier of 2C-T-7 to the individual in Indiana. 2C-T-7 has been sold under the street names Blue Mystic, T7, Beautiful, Tweety-Bird Mescaline or Tripstay.

Control Status of Blue Mystic

2C-T-7 has been placed in Schedule I of the Controlled Substances Act (CSA).

Section 24.5

DMT

This section includes text excerpted from "N,N-Dimethyltryptamine," DEA Diversion Control Division, November 2016.

N,N-dimethyltryptamine (DMT) is the prototypical indolethylamine hallucinogen. The history of human experience with DMT probably goes back several hundred years since DMT usage is associated with a number of religious practices and rituals. As a naturally occurring substance in many species of plants, DMT is present in a number of South American snuffs and brewed concoctions, such as Ayahuasca. In addition, DMT can be produced synthetically. The original synthesis was conducted by a British chemist, Richard Manske, in 1931.

DMT gained popularity as a drug of abuse in the 1960s and was placed under federal control in Schedule I when the Controlled Substances Act (CSA) was passed in 1971. Today, it is still encountered on the illicit market along with a number of other tryptamine hallucinogens.

Licit Use of N,N-Dimethyltryptamine

DMT has no approved medical use in the United States but can be used by researchers under a Schedule I research registration that requires approval from both the U.S. Drug Enforcement Administration (DEA) and the U.S. Food and Drug Administration (FDA).

Chemical Structure and Pharmacology of N,N-Dimethyltryptamine

Like other indolethylamine hallucinogens, DMT consists of the tryptamine core structure. DMT is formed by substituting two The radioimmunoassay (CH_3) groups for the two hydrogen atoms (H) on the terminal nitrogen of the ethylamine side chain of tryptamine.

Administered alone, DMT is usually snorted, smoked or injected because the oral bioavailability of DMT is very poor unless it is combined with a substance that inhibits its metabolism. For example, in ayahuasca, the presence of harmala alkaloids (harmine, harmaline, tetrahydroharmaline (THH)) inhibits the enzyme, monoamine oxidase which normally metabolizes DMT. As a consequence, DMT remains intact long enough to be absorbed in sufficient amounts to affect brain function and produce psychoactive effects.

Administered alone, DMT is usually snorted, smoked or injected because the oral bioavailability of DMT is very poor unless it is combined with a substance that inhibits its metabolism. For example, in ayahuasca, the presence of harmala alkaloids (harmine, harmaline, THH) inhibits the enzyme, monoamine oxidase which normally metabolizes DMT. As a consequence, DMT remains intact long enough to be absorbed in sufficient amounts to affect brain function and produce psychoactive effects.

In clinical studies, DMT administered intravenously was fully hallucinogenic at doses between 0.2 and 0.4 mg/kg. The onset of DMT effects is very rapid but usually resolves within 30 to 45 minutes. Psychological effects include intense visual hallucinations, depersonalization, auditory distortions, and an altered sense of time and body image. Physiological effects include hypertension, increased heart rate, agitation, seizures, dilated pupils, nystagmus (involuntary rapid rhythmic movement of the eye), dizziness, and ataxia (muscular incoordination). According to the American Association of Poison Control Centers (AAPCC) data, coma and respiratory arrest have been associated with DMT exposures.

Illicit Use of N,N-Dimethyltryptamine

DMT is used for its psychoactive effects. The intense effects and short duration of action are attractive to individuals who want the psychedelic experience but do not choose to experience the mind-altering perceptions over an extended period of time as occurs with other hallucinogens, such as lysergic acid diethylamide (LSD).

DMT is generally smoked or consumed orally in brews like Ayahuasca.

Illicit Distribution of N,N-Dimethyltryptamine

DMT is found in a number of plant materials and can be extracted or synthetically produced in clandestine labs. Like other hallucinogens, Internet sales and distribution have served as the source of drug supply in this country. According to the National Forensic Laboratory Information System (NFLIS), there were 586 DMT reports from federal, state, and local forensic laboratories in 2015. From January to June 2016, there were 243 DMT reports. According to NFLIS, illicit use of DMT has been encountered in all states.

Control Status of N,N-Dimethyltryptamine

DMT is controlled in Schedule I of the Controlled Substances Act (CSA).

Section 24.6

Ecstasy (MDMA)

This section includes text excerpted from "MDMA (Ecstasy/Molly),"
National Institute on Drug Abuse (NIDA), June 2018.

What Is 3,4-Methylenedioxymethamphetamine?

3,4-methylenedioxymethamphetamine (MDMA) is a synthetic drug
that alters mood and perception (awareness of surrounding objects
and conditions). It is chemically similar to both stimulants and hallucinogens, producing feelings of increased energy, pleasure, emotional
warmth, and distorted sensory and time perception.

MDMA was initially popular in the nightclub scene and at all-night
dance parties ("raves"), but the drug now affects a broader range of
people who more commonly call the drug ecstasy or Molly.

How Do People Use
3,4-Methylenedioxymethamphetamine?

People who use MDMA usually take it as a capsule or tablet, though
some swallow it in liquid form or snort the powder. The popular nick-
name Molly (slang for "molecular") often refers to the supposedly "pure"
crystalline powder form of MDMA, usually sold in capsules. However,
people who purchase powder or capsules sold as Molly often actually
get other drugs such as synthetic cathinones ("bath salts") instead.

Some people take MDMA in combination with other drugs such as
alcohol or marijuana.

How Does 3,4-Methylenedioxymethamphetamine
Affect the Brain?

MDMA increases the activity of three brain chemicals:

- **Dopamine**—produces increased energy/activity and acts in the
  reward system to reinforce behaviors

- **Norepinephrine**—increases heart rate and blood pressure,
  which are particularly risky for people with heart and blood
  vessel problems

- **Serotonin**—affects mood, appetite, sleep, and other functions.
  It also triggers hormones that affect sexual arousal and
  trust. The release of large amounts of serotonin likely causes

emotional closeness, elevated mood, and empathy felt by those who use MDMA.

Other health effects include:

- Nausea
- Muscle cramping
- Involuntary teeth clenching
- Blurred vision
- Chills
- Sweating

MDMA's effects last about three to six hours, although many users take a second dose as the effects of the first dose begin to fade. Over the course of the week following moderate use of the drug, a person may experience:

- Irritability
- Impulsiveness and aggression
- Depression
- Sleep problems
- Anxiety
- Memory and attention problems
- Decreased appetite
- Decreased interest in and pleasure from sex

It's possible that some of these effects may be due to the combined use of MDMA with other drugs, especially marijuana.

What Are Other Health Effects of 3,4-Methylenedioxymethamphetamine?

High doses of MDMA can affect the body's ability to regulate temperature. This can lead to a spike in body temperature that can occasionally result in liver, kidney, or heart failure or even death.

In addition, because MDMA can promote trust and closeness, its use—especially combined with sildenafil (Viagra®)—may encourage unsafe sexual behavior. This increases people's risk of contracting or transmitting human immunodeficiency virus (HIV)/acquired immunodeficiency syndrome (AIDS) or hepatitis.

Added Risk of 3,4-Methylenedioxymethamphetamine

Adding to MDMA's risks is that pills, capsules, or powders sold as ecstasy and supposedly "pure" Molly may contain other drugs instead of or in addition to MDMA. Much of the Molly seized by the police contain additives such as cocaine, ketamine, methamphetamine, over-the-counter (OTC) cough medicine, or synthetic cathinones ("bath salts"). These substances may be extremely dangerous if the person does not know what he or she is taking. They may also be dangerous when combined with MDMA. People who purposely or unknowingly combine such a mixture with other substances, such as marijuana and alcohol, may be putting themselves at even higher risk for harmful health effects.

Is 3,4-Methylenedioxymethamphetamine Addictive?

Research results vary on whether MDMA is addictive. Experiments have shown that animals will self-administer MDMA—an important indicator of a drug's abuse potential—although to a lesser degree than some other drugs such as cocaine.

Some people report signs of addiction, including the following withdrawal symptoms:

- Fatigue
- Loss of appetite
- Depression
- Trouble concentrating

Does 3,4-Methylenedioxymethamphetamine Have Value in Therapy?

MDMA was first used in the 1970s as an aid in psychotherapy (mental-disorder treatment using "talk therapy"). The drug didn't have the support of clinical trials (studies using humans) or approval from the U.S. Food and Drug Administration (FDA). In 1985, The U.S. Drug Enforcement Administration (DEA) labeled MDMA as an illegal drug with no recognized medicinal use. Some researchers remain interested in its value in psychotherapy when given to patients under carefully controlled conditions. MDMA is in clinical trials as a possible treatment aid for posttraumatic stress disorder (PTSD) and anxiety in terminally ill patients, and for social anxiety in autistic adults.

How Can People Get Treatment for Addiction to MDMA?

There are no specific medical treatments for MDMA addiction. Some people seeking treatment for MDMA addiction have found behavioral therapy to be helpful.

Section 24.7

Foxy

This section includes text excerpted from "5-Methoxy-N,N-Diisopropyltryptamine," DEA Diversion Control Division, April 2013. Reviewed January 2019.

Street names: Foxy, or Foxy methoxy

5-methoxy-N, N-diisopropyltryptamine (5-MeO-DIPT) is a tryptamine derivative and shares many similarities with Schedule I tryptamine hallucinogens such as alpha-ethyltryptamine, N, N-dimethyltryptamine, N, N-diethyltryptamine, bufotenine, psilocybin, and psilocin. Since 1999, 5-MeO-DIPT has become popular among drug abusers. This substance is abused for its hallucinogenic effects.

5-MeO-DIPT has no accepted medical uses in treatment in the United States.

Chemistry and Pharmacology of 5-Methoxy-N,N-Diisopropyltryptamine

5-MeO-DIPT is a tryptamine derivative. The hydrochloride salt of 5-MeO-DIPT is a white crystalline powder. In animal behavioral studies, 5-MeO-DIPT has been shown to produce behavioral effects that are substantially similar to those of 1-(2,5-dimethoxy-4- methylphenyl)-2-aminopropane (DOM) and lysergic acid diethylamide (LSD), both Schedule I hallucinogens.

In humans, 5-MeO-DIPT elicits subjective effects including hallucinations similar to those produced by several Schedule I hallucinogens such as 2C-B and 4- ethyl-2,5-dimethoxyphenyl-isopropylamine (DOET). The threshold dose of 5-MeO-DIPT to produce psychoactive effects is 4 mg, while effective doses range from 6 to 20 mg. 5-MeO-DIPT produces effects with an onset of 20 to 30 minutes and with peak effects occurring between 1 to 1.5 hours after administration. Effects last about 3 to 6 hours. Initial effects include mild nausea, muscular hyperreflexia, and dilation of pupils. Other effects include relaxation associated with emotional enhancement, talkativeness, and behavioral disinhibition. High doses of 5-MeO-DIPT produce abstract eyes closed imagery. 5-MeO-DIPT alters sensory perception and judgment and can pose serious health risks to the user and the general public. Abuse of 5-MeO-DIPT led to at least one emergency department admission.

Illicit Uses of 5-Methoxy-N,N-Diisopropyltryptamine

5-MeO-DIPT is abused for its hallucinogenic-like effects and is used as a substitute for MDMA. It is often administered orally as either powder, tablets, or capsules at doses ranging from 6–20 mg. Other routes of administration include smoking and snorting. Tablets often bear imprints commonly seen on MDMA tablets (spider and alien head logos) and vary in color. Powder in capsules was found to vary in colors.

User Population: 5-Methoxy-N,N-Diisopropyltryptamine

Youth and young adults are the main abusers of 5- MeO-DIPT.

Illicit Distribution of 5-Methoxy-N,N-Diisopropyltryptamine

The National Forensic Laboratory Information System (NFLIS) is a U.S. Drug Enforcement Administration (DEA) database that collects scientifically verified data on drug items and cases submitted to and analyzed by state and local forensic laboratories. The System to Retrieve Information from Drug Evidence (STRIDE) provides information on drug seizures reported to and analyzed by DEA laboratories. According to NFLIS and STRIDE, 5-MeO-DIPT drug reports increased sharply from 72 in 2010 to 3,271 in 2011 and then decreased to 1,525 in 2012.

5-MeO-DIPT has been illicitly available from the United States and foreign chemical companies and from individuals through the Internet. There is some evidence of the attempted clandestine production of 5-MeO-DIPT.

Control Status of 5-Methoxy-N,N-Diisopropyltryptamine

The DEA temporarily placed 5-MeO-DIPT in Schedule I of the Controlled Substances Act (CSA) on April 4, 2003, pursuant to the temporary scheduling provisions of the CSA (68 FR 16427). On September 29, 2004, 5-MeO-DIPT was permanently controlled as a Schedule I substance under the CSA (69 FR 58050).

Section 24.8

LSD

This section includes text excerpted from "D-Lysergic Acid Diethylamide," DEA Diversion Control Division, August 2018.

Street names: LSD, Acid, Blotter Acid, Window Pane

Lysergic acid diethylamide (LSD), commonly referred to as "acid," is a synthetic hallucinogen. LSD is very potent, only microgram amounts are required to produce overt hallucinations. LSD has been abused since the 1960s. LSD's availability has declined significantly since 2001.

There is no legitimate medical use for LSD in the United States.

Chemistry and Pharmacology of Lysergic Acid Diethylamide

LSD's physiological effects are mediated primarily through the serotonergic neuronal system.

LSD induces a heightened awareness of sensory input that is accompanied by an enhanced sense of clarity but reduced ability to control what is experienced. The LSD trip is made up of perceptual and psychic effects. A user may experience the following perceptual effects: visual distortion in the size and shape of objects, movements, color, sound, touch and the user's own body image. The user may report "hearing colors" or "seeing sounds." The psychic effects experienced by the user may include a feeling of obtaining true insight, intensified emotions, sudden and dramatic mood swings, impairment of attention, concentration and motivation, distortion of time, and depersonalization.

The adverse effects experienced with LSD use are dependent on the dose taken by the users. Some of the adverse effects reported are dilated pupils, raised body temperature, increased heart rate and blood pressure, profuse sweating, loss of appetite, sleeplessness, dry mouth, and tremors.

High doses of LSD can induce a "bad trip" characterized by intense anxiety or panic, confusion, and combative behaviors. After an LSD trip, a user may also experience fatigue, acute anxiety, or depression for 12 to 24 hours.

Illicit Uses of Lysergic Acid Diethylamide

LSD is abused for its hallucinogenic effects. LSD is sold in a variety of forms, tablets, capsules, and liquid. The average effective oral dose is from 20 to 80 micrograms. Following ingestion, effects occur within 30 to 60 minutes and last 10 to 12 hours.

The 2017 Monitoring the Future (MTF) report indicated that the annual prevalence of LSD use among students in eighth, tenth, and twelfth grades was 0.9 percent, 2.1 percent, and 3.3 percent, respectively. According to the American Association of Poison Control Centers (AAPCC), 981 case mentions, 575 single exposures, and 21 major medical outcomes and no deaths related to LSD were reported to the National Poison Data System (NPDS) in 2016. The 2011 National Survey on Drug Use and Health (NSDUH) indicated that 23.0 million people in the United States population, age 12 and older, used LSD in their lifetime. The Drug Abuse Warning Network (DAWN ED) reports that an estimated 4,819 emergency department visits were associated with LSD in 2011.

User Population: Lysergic Acid Diethylamide

LSD is abused by teenagers and young adults in connection with raves, nightclubs, and concert settings.

Illicit Distribution of Lysergic Acid Diethylamide

According to the DEA, the number of LSD items seized decreased dramatically in 2002 due to the seizure of a large LSD lab in Kansas City in 2000. With the arrest of clandestine chemists and with the dismantling of their laboratory, the availability of LSD in the United States was reduced by 95 percent within two years. In subsequent years, seizures of LSD increased, and seizures have once again decreased.

According to the National Forensic Laboratory Information System (NFLIS) reporting from federal, state, and local forensic laboratories have increased since 2011 (1,177 LSD reports), after a brief low reporting period in 2013 and 2014 (861 vs. 788), to 3,561 LSD reports in 2016 and 3,795 reports in 2017. From January to May 2018, there were 373 reports from forensic laboratories identified as LSD.

LSD is odorless, colorless, and tasteless. It is sold in a variety of formulations. Some of the streets names include acid, battery acid, blotter, window pane, microdots, Loony toons, Sunshine, and Zen. Prices range from 2 to $5 per unit or "hit."

LSD is most commonly found in the form of small squares of paper called blotter; that paper is generally decorated with artwork or designs, perforated, soaked in a liquid LSD solution, and dried. Each square represents one dose of LSD. There have been some instances of blotter paper being found impregnated with hallucinogens other than LSD. The hallucinogens, 2,5-dimethoxyamphetamine (DMA), 4-bromo-2,5-dimethoxyamphetamine (DOB), 4-iodo-2,5- The radioimmunoassay (2C-I), and 4-iodo-2,5- dimethoxyamphetamine (DOI) have been found on blotter paper passed off as LSD.

Other forms of LSD include tablets (known as microdots), gelatin squares (known as window pane), and impregnated sugar cubes. LSD has also been available in gel wraps which look like "bubblewrap" packing material and are blue in color. LSD is also distributed in liquid form, which often is packaged in small bottles typically sold as breath drops. Additionally, LSD has been embedded in candy such as "Gummy Worms," "Sweet Tarts," "Smartie," and "Pez." The most common venues for retail LSD distribution are raves, dance clubs, and concerts.

Control Status of Lysergic Acid Diethylamide

Lysergic acid diethylamide acid is controlled in Schedule I of the Controlled Substances Act (CSA). Its two precursors lysergic acid and lysergic acid amide, are both Schedule III substances under the CSA. The LSD precursors ergotamine and ergonovine are List I chemicals.

Section 24.9

Mescaline (Peyote)

This section includes text excerpted from "Drugs of Abuse," U.S. Drug Enforcement Administration (DEA), September 5, 2018.

Peyote is a small, spineless cactus. The active ingredient in peyote is the hallucinogen mescaline. From the earliest recorded time, peyote has been used by indigenous people in northern Mexico and the southwestern United States as a part of their religious rites. Mescaline can be extracted from peyote or produced synthetically.

Other Questions on Mescaline
What Are Common Street Names?

Common street names include:

• Buttons, Cactus, Mesc, and Peyote

What Does It Look Like?

The top of the peyote cactus is referred to as the "crown" and consists of disc-shaped buttons that are cut off.

How Is It Abused?

The fresh or dried buttons are chewed or soaked in water to produce an intoxicating liquid. Peyote buttons may also be ground into a powder that can be placed inside gelatin capsules to be swallowed, or smoked with a leaf material such as *Cannabis* or tobacco.

What Is Its Effect on the Mind?

Abuse of peyote and mescaline will cause varying degrees of:

- Illusions, hallucinations, altered perception of space and time, and altered body image

Users may also experience euphoria, which is sometimes followed by feelings of anxiety.

What Is Its Effect on the Body?

Following the consumption of peyote and mescaline, users may experience:

- Intense nausea, vomiting, dilation of the pupils, increased heart rate, increased blood pressure, a rise in body temperature that causes heavy perspiration, headaches, muscle weakness, and impaired motor coordination

Which Drugs Cause Similar Effects

Other hallucinogens like lysergic acid diethylamide (LSD), psilocybin (mushrooms), and phencyclidine (PCP)

What Is Its Legal Status in the United States?

Peyote and mescaline are Schedule I substances under the Controlled Substances Act (CSA), meaning that they have a high potential for abuse, not accepted medical use in treatment in the United States, and a lack of accepted safety for use under medical supervision.

Section 24.10

Psilocybin

This section includes text excerpted from "Drugs of Abuse," U.S. Drug Enforcement Administration (DEA), September 5, 2018.

What Is Psilocybin?

Psilocybin is a chemical obtained from certain types of fresh or dried mushrooms. Psilocybin mushrooms are found in Mexico, Central America, and the United States.

Other Questions on Psilocybin
What Are Common Street Names?

Common street names include:

- Magic Mushrooms, Mushrooms, and Shrooms

What Does It Look Like?

Mushrooms containing psilocybin are available fresh or dried and have long, slender stems topped by caps with dark gills on the underside. Fresh mushrooms have white or whitish-gray stems; the caps are dark brown around the edges and light brown or white in the center. Dried mushrooms are usually rusty brown with isolated areas of off-white.

How Is It Abused?

Psilocybin mushrooms are ingested orally. They may also be brewed as a tea or added to other foods to mask their bitter flavor.

What Is Its Effect on the Mind?

The psychological consequences of psilocybin use include hallucinations and an inability to discern fantasy from reality. Panic reactions and psychosis also may occur, particularly if a user ingests a large dose.

What Is Its Effect on the Body?

The physical effects include:

- Nausea, vomiting, muscle weakness, and lack of coordination

What Are Its Overdose Effects?

Effects of overdose include:

- Longer, more intense "trip" episodes, psychosis, and possible death

Abuse of psilocybin mushrooms could also lead to poisoning if one of the many varieties of poisonous mushrooms is incorrectly identified as a psilocybin mushroom.

Which Drugs Cause Similar Effects

Psilocybin effects are similar to other hallucinogens, such as mescaline and peyote.

What Is Its Legal Status in the United States?

Psilocybin is a Schedule I substance under the Controlled Substances Act (CSA), meaning that it has a high potential for abuse, not accepted medical use in treatment in the United States, and a lack of accepted safety for use under medical supervision.

Section 24.11

Toonies (Nexus, 2C-B)

This section includes text excerpted from "4-Bromo-2,5-Dimethoxyphenethylamine," DEA Diversion Control Division, August 2018.

Street names: 2C-B, Nexus, 2's, Toonies, Bromo, Spectrum, Venus 4-Bromo-2,5-dimethoxyphenethylamine (2C-B, 4- bromo-2,5-DMPEA) is a synthetic Schedule I hallucinogen. It is abused for its hallucinogenic effects primarily as a club drug in the rave culture and circuit party scene.

2C-B has no approved medical uses in the United States.

Chemistry and Pharmacology of 4-Bromo-2,5-Dimethoxyphenethylamine

4-Bromo-2,5-dimethoxyphenethylamine is closely related to the phenylisopropylamine hallucinogen 1-(4-bromo 2, 5-dimethoxy-phenyl)-2-aminopropane (DOB) and is referred to as alpha-desmethyl DOB. 2C-B produces effects similar to 2,5-dimethoxy-4-methylamphet-amine (DOM) and DOB. 2C-B displays high affinity for central sero-tonin receptors. 2C-B produces dose-dependent psychoactive effects. Threshold effects are noted at approximately 4 mg of an oral dose; the user becomes passive and relaxed and is aware of integration of sensory perception with emotional states. There is euphoria with increased body awareness and enhanced receptiveness of visual, audi-tory, olfactory, and tactile sensation. Oral doses of 8 to 10 mg produce stimulant effects and cause a full intoxicated state. Doses in the range of 20 to 40 mg produce LSD-like hallucinations. Doses greater than 50 mg have produced extremely fearful hallucinations and morbid delu-sions. Onset of subjective effects following 2C-B ingestion is between 20 to 30 minutes with peak effects occurring at 1.5 to 2 hours. Effects of 2C-B can last up to eight hours.

The radioimmunoassay detection system that is commonly used for testing amphetamine and hallucinogens does not detect 2C-B. In the Marquis Reagent Field Test-902, 2C-B produces a bright green color. 2C-B is the only known drug to produce a bright green color when using this test.

Illicit Uses of 4-Bromo-2,5-Dimethoxyphenethylamine

2C-B is abused for its hallucinogenic effects. 2C-B is abused orally in tablet or capsule forms or snorted in its powder form. The drug has been misinterpreted by distributors and sold as other hallucinogens such as 3,4-methylenedioxymethamphetamine (MDMA) and lysergic acid diethylamide (LSD). Some user's abuse 2C-B in combination with LSD (referred to as a "banana split") or MDMA (called a "party pack").

User Population: 4-Bromo-2,5-Dimethoxyphenethylamine

2C-B is used by the same population as those using "ecstasy" and other club drugs, high-school and college students, and other young adults who frequent "rave" or "techno" parties.

Illicit Distribution of 4-Bromo-2,5-Dimethoxyphenethylamine

2C-B is distributed as tablets, capsules, or in powder form. Usually sold as MDMA, a single dosage unit of 2CB typically sells for $10 to $30 per tablet. The illicit source of 2C-B available on the street has not been identified by the U.S. Drug Enforcement Administration (DEA). Prior to its control, DEA seized both clandestine laboratories and illicit "repacking shops." As the name implies, these shops would repackage and reformulate the doses of the tablets prior to illicit sales.

According to the System to Retrieve Information from Drug Evidence (STRIDE) data, the first recorded submission by law enforcement to DEA forensic laboratories of a drug exhibit containing 2C-B occurred in 1986.

The National Forensic Laboratory Information System (NFLIS) is a DEA database that collects scientifically verified data on drug items and cases submitted to and analyzed by federal, state, and local forensic laboratories. The STRIDE database, integrated into STARLiMS, a web-based, commercial laboratory information-management system, since October 1, 2014 has replaced STRIDE as the DEA laboratory drug evidence data system of record which provides information on drug seizures reported to and analyzed by DEA laboratories. Since 2007, 2C-B has been encountered by law enforcement in 42 states. Law enforcement officials submitted 89 exhibits identified as 2C-B to federal, state, and local forensic laboratories in 2010, 64 exhibits in 2011, and 85 exhibits in 2012. There have been 52 2C-B exhibits in 2015, 83 in 2016, 54 in 2017, and preliminary 8 exhibits for 2018, so far.

Control Status of 4-Bromo-2,5-Dimethoxyphenethylamine

The U.S. Drug Enforcement Administration placed 2C-B in Schedule I of the Controlled Substances Act (CSA).

Chapter 25

Inhalants

What Are Inhalants?

Although other substances that are misused can be inhaled, the term "inhalants" refers to the various substances that people typically take only by inhaling. These substances include:

- Solvents (liquids that become gas at room temperature)

- Aerosol sprays

- Gases

- Nitrites (prescription medicines for chest pain)

Inhalants are various products easily bought and found in the home or workplace—such as spray paints, markers, glues, and cleaning fluids. They contain dangerous substances that have psychoactive (mind-altering) properties when inhaled. People don't typically think of these products as drugs because they're not intended for getting "high," but some people use them for that purpose. When these substances are used for getting high, they are called inhalants. Inhalants are mostly used by young kids and teens and are the only class of substance used more by younger than by older teens.

This chapter includes text excerpted from "Inhalants," National Institute on Drug Abuse (NIDA), February 2017.

How Do People Use Inhalants?

People who use inhalants breathe in the fumes through their noses or mouths, usually by "sniffing," "snorting," "bagging," or "huffing." It's called different names depending on the substance and equipment they use.

Although the high that inhalants produce usually lasts just a few minutes, people often try to make it last by continuing to inhale again and again over several hours.

Products Used as Inhalants
Solvents

- Industrial or household products, including:
- Paint thinners or removers
- Dry-cleaning fluids
- Gasoline
- Lighter fluid
- Art or office supply solvents, including:
- Correction fluids
- Felt-tip marker fluid
- Electronic contact cleaners
- Glue

Aerosols

- Household aerosol items, including:
- Spray paints
- Hair or deodorant sprays
- Aerosol computer cleaning products
- Vegetable oil sprays

Gases

- Found in household or commercial products, including:
- Butane lighters
- Propane tanks

- Whipped cream aerosols or dispensers (whippets)
- Used as anesthesia (to make patients lose sensation during surgery/procedures), including:
- Ether
- Chloroform
- Nitrous oxide

Nitrites

- Often sold in small brown bottles labeled as:
- Video head cleaner
- Room odorizer
- Leather cleaner
- Liquid aroma

How Do Inhalants Affect the Brain?

Most inhalants affect the central nervous system (CNS) and slow down brain activity. Short-term effects are similar to alcohol and include:

- Slurred or distorted speech
- Lack of coordination (control of body movement)
- Euphoria (feeling "high")
- Dizziness

People may also feel light-headed or have hallucinations (images/sensations that seem real but aren't) or delusions (false beliefs). With repeated inhalations, many people feel less self-conscious and less in control. Some may start vomiting, feel drowsy for several hours, or have a headache that lasts a while.

Unlike other types of inhalants, nitrites, which are often prescribed to treat chest pain, are misused in order to improve sexual pleasure by expanding and relaxing blood vessels.

What Are the Other Health Effects of Inhalants?

Long-term effects of inhalant use may include:

- Liver and kidney damage

- Hearing loss

- Bone marrow damage

- Loss of coordination and limb spasms (from nerve damage)

- Delayed behavioral development (from brain problems)

- Brain damage (from cut-off oxygen flow to the brain)

In addition, because nitrites are misused for sexual pleasure and performance, they can lead to unsafe sexual practices or other risky behavior. This increases the chance of getting or spreading infectious diseases such as human immunodeficiency virus (HIV)/acquired immunodeficiency syndrome (AIDS) or hepatitis.

Can a Person Overdose on Inhalants?

Yes, a person can overdose on inhalants. An overdose occurs when a person uses too much of a drug and has a toxic reaction that results in serious and harmful symptoms or death.

These symptoms can cause seizures and coma. They can even be deadly. Many solvents and aerosol sprays are highly concentrated, meaning they contain a large amount of chemicals with a lot of active ingredients. Sniffing these products can cause the heart to stop within minutes. This condition, known as sudden sniffing death, can happen to an otherwise healthy young person the first time he or she uses an inhalant. Using inhalants with a paper or plastic bag or in a closed area may cause death from suffocation (being unable to breathe).

How Can an Inhalant Overdose Be Treated?

Because inhalant overdose can lead to seizures or cause the heart to stop, first responders and emergency room doctors try to treat the overdose by treating these conditions. They will try to stop the seizure or restart the heart.

Can Inhalants Cause Addiction, a Form of Substance-Use Disorder?

Although it's not very common, repeated use of inhalants can lead to addiction, a form of substance-use disorder (SUD). An SUD develops when continued use of the drug causes issues, such as health problems and failure to meet responsibilities at work, school, or home. An SUD can range from mild to severe, the most severe form being addiction.

Those who try to quit inhalants may have withdrawal symptoms that include:

- Nausea

- Loss of appetite

- Sweating

- Problems sleeping

- Mood changes

How Can People Get Treatment for Addiction to Inhalants?

Some people seeking treatment for use of inhalants have found behavioral therapy to be helpful:

- **Cognitive-behavioral therapy (CBT)** helps patients recognize, avoid, and cope with the situations in which they are most likely to use drugs.

- **Motivational incentives use** vouchers or small cash rewards for positive behaviors such as staying drug-free.

Chapter 26

Narcotics (Opioids)

Chapter Contents

Section 26.1

Introduction to Narcotics

This section includes text excerpted from "Drugs of Abuse,"
U.S. Drug Enforcement Administration (DEA), August 26, 2018.

What Are Narcotics?

Also known as "opioids," the term "narcotic" comes from the Greek word for "stupor" and originally referred to a variety of substances that dulled the senses and relieved pain. Though some people still refer to all drugs as "narcotics," nowadays "narcotic" refers to opium, opium derivatives, and their semi-synthetic substitutes. A more current term for these drugs, with less uncertainty regarding its meaning, is "opioid." Examples include the illicit drug heroin and pharmaceutical drugs like OxyContin®, Vicodin, codeine, morphine, methadone, and fentanyl.

The poppy *Papaver somniferum* is the source for all natural opioids, whereas synthetic opioids are made entirely in a lab and include meperidine, fentanyl, and methadone. Semi-synthetic opioids are synthesized from naturally occurring opium products, such as morphine and codeine, and include heroin, oxycodone, hydrocodone, and hydromorphone. Teens can obtain narcotics from friends, family members, medicine cabinets, pharmacies, nursing homes, hospitals, hospices, doctors, and the Internet.

Other Questions on Narcotics
What Are Common Street Names?

Street names for various narcotics/opioids include Smack, Horse, Mud, Brown Sugar, Junk, Black Tat, Big H, Paregoric, Dover's Powder, MPTP (New Heroin), Hillbilly Heroin, Lean or Purple Drank, OC, Ox, Oxy, OxyContin®, and Sippin Syrup.

What Do They Look Like?

Narcotics/opioids come in various forms, including tablets, capsules, skin patches, powder, chunks in varying colors (from white to shades of brown and black), liquid form for oral use and injection, syrups, suppositories, and lollipops.

How Are They Abused?

Narcotics/opioids can be swallowed, smoked, sniffed, or injected.

What Is Their Effect on the Mind?

Besides their medical use, narcotics/opioids produce a general sense of well-being by reducing tension, anxiety, and aggression. These effects are helpful in a therapeutic setting but contribute to the drugs' abuse. Narcotic/opioid use comes with a variety of unwanted effects, including drowsiness, an inability to concentrate, and apathy.

Psychological Dependence

Use can create psychological dependence. Long after the physical need for the drug has passed, the addict may continue to think and talk about using drugs and feel overwhelmed coping with daily activities. Relapse is common if there are no changes to the physical environment or the behavioral motivators that prompted the abuse in the first place.

What Is Their Effect on the Body?

Narcotics/opioids are prescribed by doctors to treat pain, suppress cough, cure diarrhea, and put people to sleep. Effects depend heavily on the dose, how it's taken, and previous exposure to the drug. Negative effects include slowed physical activity, constriction of the pupils, flushing of the face and neck, constipation, nausea, vomiting, and slowed breathing.

As the dose is increased, both the pain relief and the harmful effects become more pronounced. Some of these preparations are so potent that a single dose can be lethal to an inexperienced user. However, except in cases of extreme intoxication, there is no loss of motor coordination or slurred speech.

Physical Dependence and Withdrawal

Physical dependence is a consequence of chronic opioid use, and withdrawal takes place when drug use is discontinued. The intensity and character of the physical symptoms experienced during withdrawal are directly related to the particular drug used, the total daily dose, the interval between doses, the duration of use, and the health and personality of the user. These symptoms usually appear shortly before the time of the next scheduled dose.

Early withdrawal symptoms often include watery eyes, runny nose, yawning, and sweating.

As the withdrawal worsens, symptoms can include restlessness, irritability, loss of appetite, nausea, tremors, drug craving, severe depression, vomiting, increased heart rate, and blood pressure, and chills alternating with flushing and excessive sweating.

However, without intervention, the withdrawal usually runs its course, and most physical symptoms disappear within days or weeks, depending on the particular drug.

What Are Their Overdose Effects?

Overdoses of narcotics are not uncommon and can be fatal. Physical signs of narcotics/opioid overdose include constricted (pinpoint) pupils, cold clammy skin, confusion, convulsions, extreme drowsiness, and slowed breathing.

Which Drugs Cause Similar Effects

With the exception of pain relief and cough suppression, most central nervous system depressants (such as barbiturates, benzodiazepines, and alcohol) have similar effects, including slowed breathing, tolerance, and dependence.

What Is Their Legal Status in the United States?

Narcotics/opioids are controlled substances that vary from Schedule I to Schedule V, depending on their medical usefulness, abuse potential, safety, and drug dependence profile. Schedule I narcotics, like heroin, have no medical use in the United States and are illegal to distribute, purchase, or use outside of medical research.

Section 26.2

Buprenorphine

This section includes text excerpted from "Buprenorphine,"
U.S. Drug Enforcement Administration (DEA),
July 2013, Reviewed January 2019.

Buprenorphine was first marketed in the United States in 1985 as a schedule V narcotic analgesic. Initially, the only available buprenorphine product in the United States had been a low-dose (0.3 mg/ml) injectable formulation under the brand name, Buprenex®. Diversion, trafficking and abuse of other buprenorphine products have occurred in Europe and other areas of the world.

In October 2002, the U.S. Food and Drug Administration (FDA) approved two buprenorphine products (Suboxone® and Subutex®) for the treatment of narcotic addiction. Both products are high dose (2 mg and 8 mg) sublingual (under the tongue) tablets: Subutex® is a single entity buprenorphine product and Suboxone® is a combination product with buprenorphine and naloxone in a 4:1 ratio, respectively. After reviewing the available data and receiving a Schedule III recommendation from the Department of Health and Human Services (DHHS), the U.S. Drug Enforcement Administration (DEA) placed buprenorphine and all products containing buprenorphine into Schedule III in 2002. Since 2003, diversion, trafficking and abuse of buprenorphine have become more common in the United States. In June 2010, FDA approved an extended-release transdermal film containing buprenorphine (Butrans®) for the management of moderate to severe chronic pain in patients requiring a continuous, extended period, around-the-clock opioid analgesic.

Licit Uses of Buprenorphine

Buprenorphine is intended for the treatment of pain (Buprenex®) and opioid addiction (Suboxone® and Subutex®). In 2001, 2005, and 2006, the Narcotic Addict Treatment Act (NATA) was amended to allow qualified physicians, under certification of the DHHS, to prescribe Schedule III-V narcotic drugs (FDA approved for the indication of narcotic treatment) for narcotic addiction, up to 30 patients per physician at any time, outside the context of clinic-based narcotic treatment programs. This limit was increased to 100 patients per physician, who meet the specified criteria, under the Office of National

Drug Control Policy Reauthorization Act (ONDCPRA), which became effective on December 29, 2006.

Suboxone® and Subutex® are the only treatment drugs that meet the requirement of this exemption. Currently, nearly 15,700 physicians have been approved by the Substance Abuse and Mental Health Services Administration (SAMHSA) and the DEA for office-based narcotic buprenorphine treatment. Of those physicians, approximately 13,150 were approved to treat up to 30 patients per provider and about 2,500 were approved to treat up to 100 patients. More than 3,000 physicians have submitted their intention to treat up to 100 patients per provider.

IMS Health National Prescription Audit (NPA) Plus indicates that 9.3 million buprenorphine prescriptions were dispensed in the U.S. in 2012. From January to March 2013, 2.5 million buprenorphine prescriptions were dispensed.

Chemistry and Pharmacology of Buprenorphine

Buprenorphine has a unique pharmacological profile. It produces the effects typical of both pure mu agonists (e.g., morphine) and partial agonists (e.g., pentazocine) depending on dose, pattern of use and population taking the drug. It is about 20 to 30 times more potent than morphine as an analgesic; and like morphine it produces dose-related euphoria, drug liking, papillary constriction, respiratory depression and sedation. However, acute, high doses of buprenorphine have been shown to have a blunting effect on both physiological and psychological effects due to its partial opioid activity.

Buprenorphine is a long-acting (24 to 72 hours) opioid that produces less respiratory depression at high doses than other narcotic treatment drugs. However, severe respiratory depression can occur when buprenorphine is combined with other central-nervous-system depressants, especially benzodiazepines. Deaths have resulted from this combination.

The addition of naloxone in the Suboxone® product is intended to block the euphoric high resulting from the injection of this drug by norbuprenorphine maintained narcotic abusers

User Population of Buprenorphine

In countries where buprenorphine has gained popularity as a drug of abuse, it is sought by a wide variety of narcotic abusers: young naive individuals, nonaddictive opioid abusers, heroin addicts, and buprenorphine-treatment clients.

Illicit Uses of Buprenorphine

Like other opioids commonly abused, buprenorphine is capable of producing significant euphoria. Data from other countries indicate that buprenorphine has been abused by various routes of administration (sublingual, intranasal, and injection) and has gained popularity as a heroin substitute and as a primary drug of abuse. Large percentages of the drug-abusing populations in some areas of France, Ireland, Scotland, India, Nepal, Bangladesh, Pakistan, and New Zealand have reported abusing buprenorphine by injection and in combination with a benzodiazepine.

The National Forensic Laboratory Information System (NFLIS) is a DEA database that collects scientifically verified data on drug items and cases submitted to and analyzed by state and local forensic laboratories. The System to Retrieve Information from Drug Evidence (STRIDE) provides information on drug seizures reported to and analyzed by DEA laboratories. In 2012, federal, state, and local forensic laboratories identified 10,804 known drug seizures. In the first quarter of 2013, 1,905 buprenorphine exhibits were identified.

According to the Drug Abuse Warning Network (DAWN ED), an estimated 21,483 emergency department (ED) visits were associated with nonmedical use of buprenorphine in 2011, nearly five times the 4,440 estimated number of buprenorphine ED visits in 2006. The American Association of Poison Control Centers (AAPCC) Annual Report indicates that U.S. poison centers recorded 3,625 case mentions and three deaths involving toxic exposure from buprenorphine in 2011.

Control Status of Buprenorphine

Buprenorphine and all products containing buprenorphine are controlled in Schedule III of the Controlled Substances Act (CSA).

Section 26.3

Fentanyl

This section includes text excerpted from "Fentanyl,"
DEA Diversion Control Division, October 2018.

Fentanyl is a potent synthetic opioid. It was introduced into medical practice as an intravenous anesthetic under the trade name of "Sublimaze" in the 1960s.

Licit Uses of Fentanyl

In 2015, there were 6.5 million fentanyl prescriptions dispensed in the United States. Similarly, during the height of the opioid epidemic, in 2016 and 2017, 5.96 million and 5.05 million fentanyl prescriptions were dispensed (IMS Health™). Fentanyl pharmaceutical products are currently available as oral transmucosal lozenges, commonly referred to as the fentanyl "lollipops" (Actiq®), effervescent buccal tablets (Fentora™), sublingual tablet (Abstral®), sublingual spray (Subsys™), nasal spray (Lazanda®), transdermal patches (Duragesic®), and injectable formulations. Oral transmucosal lozenges and effervescent buccal tablets are used for the management of breakthrough cancer pain in patients who are already receiving opioid medication for their underlying persistent pain. Transdermal patches are used in the management of chronic pain in patients who require continuous opioid analgesia. Fentanyl citrate injections are administered intravenously, intramuscularly, or as a spinal or epidural for potent analgesia and anesthesia. Because of a concern about deaths and overdoses resulting from fentanyl transdermal patches (Duragesic® and generic versions), on July 15, 2005, the U.S. Food and Drug Administration (FDA) issued safety warnings and reiterated the importance of strict adherence to the guidelines for the proper use of these products.

Chemistry and Pharmacology of Fentanyl

Fentanyl (N-(1-phenethylpiperidin-4-yl)-N-phenylpropionamide) is a water-soluble solid substance that exists in a crystal or crystalline powder form.

Fentanyl is about 100 times more potent than morphine as an analgesic. It is a μ-opioid receptor agonist with high lipid solubility

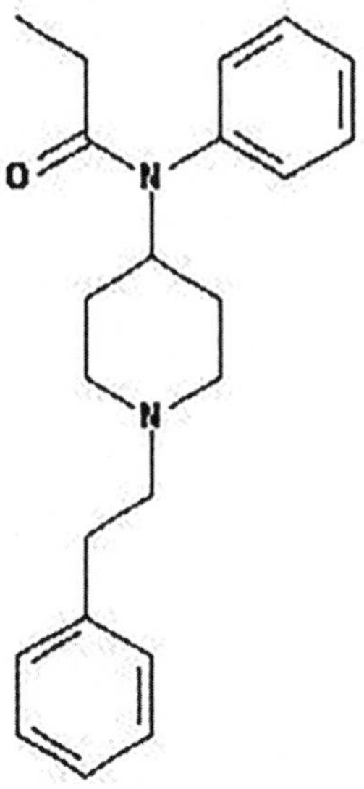

Figure 26.1. *Chemical Structure of Fentanyl*

and rapid onset and short duration of effects. Fentanyl rapidly crosses the blood-brain barrier (BBB). It is similar to other μ-opioid receptor agonists (like morphine or oxycodone) in its pharmacological effects and produces analgesia, sedation, nausea, vomiting, itching, and respiratory depression. Fentanyl appears to produce muscle rigidity with greater frequency than other opioids. Unlike some μ-opioid receptor agonists, fentanyl does not cause histamine release and has minimal depressant effects on the heart.

Illicit Uses of Fentanyl

Fentanyl is abused for its intense euphoric effects. Fentanyl can serve as a direct substitute for heroin in opioid-dependent individuals. However, fentanyl is a very dangerous substitute for heroin because it is much more potent than heroin and results in frequent overdoses that can lead to respiratory depression and death.

Fentanyl patches are abused by removing the gel contents from the patches and then injecting or ingesting these contents. Patches have also been frozen, cut into pieces, and placed under the tongue or in the cheek cavity for drug absorption through the oral mucosa. Used patches are attractive to abusers as a large percentage of fentanyl remains in these patches even after a three-day use. Fentanyl oral transmucosal lozenges and fentanyl injectables are also diverted and abused.

Abuse of fentanyl initially appeared in the mid-1970s and has increased in recent years. There have been reports of deaths associated with abuse of fentanyl products.

According to the Centers for Disease Control and Prevention (CDC), a 73 percent increase in synthetic opioid deaths occurred in the United States, from 5,544 in 2014 to 9,580 in 2015. In 2016, the nationwide synthetic opioid death toll rose to 103 percent, with 19,413 recorded fatalities. While the synthetic opioid category does include other substances such as Tramadol®, fentanyl largely dominates the category. Also, as annually reported by the U.S. Drug Enforcement Administration (DEA) National Drug Threat Assessment (NDTA), in October 2017, there is a strong relationship between the number of synthetic opioid deaths and the number of fentanyl exhibits encountered by forensic laboratories; demonstrating when the number of fentanyl exhibits in the National Forensic Laboratory Information System (NFLIS) increase, so too does the number of synthetic opioid deaths recorded by the CDC.

Illicit Distribution of Fentanyl

Licit fentanyl is diverted via theft, fraudulent prescriptions, and illicit distribution by patients, physicians, and pharmacists. Illicitly manufactured fentanyl is chiefly responsible for the current domestic crisis. According to the NFLIS, which does not distinguish between pharmaceutical and illicitly manufactured fentanyl, there were 5,533 reports/exhibits of fentanyl for 2014 and 15,427 in 2015 (a 179% increase) by federal, state and local forensic laboratories in the United States. In 2016, 37,158 fentanyl reports/exhibits were identified by forensic laboratories (a 141% increase from 2015). Preliminary findings indicate at least a 52 percent increase with 56,517 reports/exhibits of fentanyl identified in 2017.

Clandestine Manufacture of Fentanyl

From April 2005 to March 2007, an outbreak of fentanyl overdoses and deaths occurred. The CDC/DEA surveillance system reported 1,013 confirmed nonpharmaceutical fentanyl-related deaths. Most of these deaths occurred in Delaware, Illinois, Maryland, Michigan, Missouri, New Jersey, and Pennsylvania. Consequently, DEA immediately undertook the development of regulations to control the precursor chemicals used by the clandestine laboratories to illicitly manufacture fentanyl. In 2007, DEA published an Interim Final Rule to designate N-phenethyl-4-piperidone (NPP)—a precursor to fentanyl, as a List 1 chemical. DEA also completed a scheduling action of designating another chemical precursor, 4-anilino-N-phenethyl-4-piperidine (ANPP) as a Schedule II immediate precursor in 2010. After the control of ANPP, the number of fentanyl-related deaths declined until 2013.

Control Status of Fentanyl

Fentanyl is controlled in Schedule II of the Controlled Substances Act (CSA).

Section 26.4

Heroin

This section includes text excerpted from "Heroin,"
National Institute on Drug Abuse (NIDA), June 2018.

What Is Heroin?

Heroin is an opioid drug made from morphine, a natural substance taken from the seed pod of various opium poppy plants grown in Southeast and Southwest Asia, Mexico, and Colombia. Heroin can be a white or brown powder, or a black sticky substance known as black tar heroin. Other common names for heroin include Big H, Horse, Hell Dust, and Smack.

How Do People Use Heroin?

People inject, sniff, snort, or smoke heroin. Some people mix heroin with crack cocaine, a practice called "speedballing."

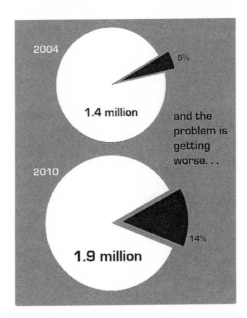

Figure 26.2. *Number of People Who Abused or Were Dependent on Pain Medications and Percentage of Them That Use Heroin.* (Source: "Abuse of Prescription Pain Medications Risks Heroin Use," National Institute on Drug Abuse (NIDA).)

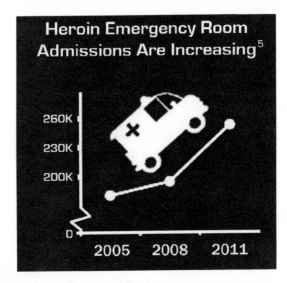

Figure 26.3. *Heroin Emergency Room Admissions Are Increasing.* (Source: "Abuse of Prescription Pain Medications Risks Heroin Use," National Institute on Drug Abuse (NIDA).)

What Are the Effects of Heroin?

Heroin enters the brain rapidly and binds to opioid receptors on cells located in many areas, especially those involved in feelings of pain and pleasure and in controlling heart rate, sleeping, and breathing.

Short-Term Effects

People who use heroin report feeling a "rush" (a surge of pleasure, or euphoria). However, there are other common effects, including:

- Dry mouth
- Warm flushing of the skin
- Heavy feeling in the arms and legs
- Nausea and vomiting
- Severe itching
- Clouded mental functioning
- Going "on the nod," a back-and-forth state of being conscious and semiconscious

Long-Term Effects

People who use heroin over the long term may develop:

- Insomnia
- Collapsed veins for people who inject the drug
- Damaged tissue inside the nose for people who sniff or snort it
- Infection of the heart lining and valves
- Abscesses (swollen tissue filled with pus)
- Constipation and stomach cramping
- Liver and kidney disease
- Lung complications, including pneumonia
- Mental disorders such as depression and antisocial personality disorder
- Sexual dysfunction for men
- Irregular menstrual cycles for women

Other Potential Effects

Heroin often contains additives, such as sugar, starch, or powdered milk, that can clog blood vessels leading to the lungs, liver, kidneys, or brain, causing permanent damage. Also, sharing drug injection equipment and having impaired judgment from drug use can increase the risk of contracting infectious diseases such as human immunodeficiency virus (HIV) and hepatitis.

Prescription Opioids and Heroin

Prescription opioid pain medicines such as OxyContin® and Vicodin® have effects similar to heroin. Research suggests that misuse of these drugs may open the door to heroin use. Nearly 80 percent of Americans using heroin (including those in treatment) reported misusing prescription opioids first.

While prescription opioid misuse is a risk factor for starting heroin use, only a small fraction of people who misuse pain relievers switch to heroin. According to a national survey, less than four percent of people who had misused prescription pain medicines started using heroin within five years. This suggests that prescription opioid misuse is just one factor leading to heroin use.

Injection Drug Use, Human Immunodeficiency Virus (HIV), and Hepatitis

People who inject drugs such as heroin are at high risk of contracting the HIV and hepatitis C (HCV) virus. These diseases are transmitted through contact with blood or other bodily fluids, which can occur when sharing needles or other injection drug use equipment. HCV is the most common bloodborne infection in the United States. HIV (and less often HCV) can also be contracted during unprotected sex, which drug use makes more likely.

Can a Person Overdose on Heroin?

Yes, a person can overdose on heroin. A heroin overdose occurs when a person uses enough of the drug to produce a life-threatening reaction or death. Heroin overdoses have increased in recent years.

When people overdose on heroin, their breathing often slows or stops. This can decrease the amount of oxygen that reaches the brain, a condition called hypoxia. Hypoxia can have short- and long-term mental effects and effects on the nervous system, including comma and permanent brain damage.

How Can a Heroin Overdose Be Treated?

Naloxone is a medicine that can treat an opioid overdose when given right away. It works by rapidly binding to opioid receptors and blocking the effects of heroin and other opioid drugs. Sometimes more than one dose may be needed to help a person start breathing again, which is why it's important to get the person to an emergency department or a doctor to receive additional support if needed.

Naloxone is available as an injectable (needle) solution, a hand-held auto-injector (EVZIO®), and a nasal spray (NARCAN® Nasal Spray). Friends, family, and others in the community can use the auto-injector and nasal spray versions of naloxone to save someone who is overdosing.

The rising number of opioid overdose deaths has led to an increase in public health efforts to make naloxone available to at-risk persons and their families, as well as first responders and others in the community. Some states have passed laws that allow pharmacists to dispense naloxone without a prescription from a person's personal doctor.

Is Heroin Addictive?

Heroin is highly addictive. People who regularly use heroin often develop a tolerance, which means that they need higher and/or more frequent doses of the drug to get the desired effects. A substance-use disorder (SUD) is when continued use of the drug causes issues, such as health problems and failure to meet responsibilities at work, school, or home. An SUD can range from mild to severe, the most severe form being addiction.

Those who are addicted to heroin and stop using the drug abruptly may have severe withdrawal. Withdrawal symptoms—which can begin as early as a few hours after the drug was last taken—include:

- Restlessness
- Severe muscle and bone pain
- Sleep problems
- Diarrhea and vomiting
- Cold flashes with goosebumps ("cold turkey")

- Uncontrollable leg movements ("kicking the habit")

- Severe heroin cravings

Researchers are studying the long-term effects of opioid addiction on the brain. Studies have shown some loss of the brain's white matter associated with heroin use, which may affect decision-making, behavior control, and responses to stressful situations.

How Is Heroin Addiction Treated?

A range of treatments including medicines and behavioral therapies are effective in helping people stop heroin use. It's important to match the best treatment approach to meet the particular needs of each individual patient.

There are medicines being developed to help with the withdrawal process. The U.S. Food and Drug Administration (FDA) approved lofexidine, a nonopioid medicine designed to reduce opioid withdrawal symptoms.

Medicines to help people stop using heroin include buprenorphine and methadone. They work by binding to the same opioid receptors in the brain as heroin, but more weakly, reducing cravings and withdrawal symptoms. Another treatment is naltrexone, which blocks opioid receptors and prevents opioid drugs from having an effect. A National Institute on Drug Abuse (NIDA) study found that, once treatment is initiated, both a buprenorphine/naloxone combination and an extended-release naltrexone formulation are similarly effective in addiction. Because full detoxification is necessary for treatment with naloxone, initiating treatment among active users was difficult, but once detoxification was complete, both medications had similar effectiveness.

Behavioral therapies for heroin addiction include methods called cognitive-behavioral therapy (CBT) and contingency management. CBT helps modify the patient's drug-use expectations and behaviors, and helps effectively manage triggers and stress. Contingency management provides motivational incentives, such as vouchers or small cash rewards for positive behaviors such as staying drug-free. These behavioral treatment approaches are especially effective when used along with medicines.

Section 26.5

Hydrocodone

This section includes text excerpted from "Hydrocodone,"
DEA Diversion Control Division, October 2018.

Since 2009, hydrocodone has been the second most frequently
encountered opioid pharmaceutical in drug evidence submitted to
federal, state, and local forensic laboratories as reported by U.S. Drug
Enforcement Administration's (FDA) National Forensic Laboratory
Information System (NFLIS) and System to Retrieve Information from
Drug Evidence (STRIDE)/STARLiMS databases.

Licit Uses of Hydrocodone

Hydrocodone is an antitussive (cough suppressant) and narcotic
analgesic agent for the treatment of moderate to moderately severe
pain. Studies indicate that hydrocodone is as effective, or more effective, than codeine for cough suppression and nearly equipotent to
morphine for pain relief.

Hydrocodone is the most frequently prescribed opiate in the United
States with more than 136.7 million prescriptions for hydrocodone-con-
taining products dispensed in 2013 and with 93.7 million and 83.6 million dispensed recently in 2016 and 2017, respectively (IMS Health™).
There are several hundred brand name and generic hydrocodone products marketed, most of which are combination products. The most
frequently prescribed combination is hydrocodone and acetaminophen
(Vicodin®, Lortab®).

Chemistry and Pharmacology of Hydrocodone

Hydrocodone (4,5α-epoxy-3-methoxy-17-methylmorphinan-6-one
tartrate (1:1) hydrate (2:5), dihydrocodeinone) Hydrocodone (4,5α-ep-
oxy-3-methoxy-17- methylmorphinan-6-one tartrate (1:1) hydrate (2:5),
dihydrocodeinone) is a semi-synthetic opioid most closely related to
codeine in structure and morphine in producing opiate-like effects.
The first report, that hydrocodone produces euphoria and habituation
symptoms, was published in 1923. The first report of hydrocodone
dependence and addiction was published in 1961.

Hydrocodone exerts its principle pharmacological effects through
agonistic binding to opioid receptors. Hydrocodone primarily binds and

activates the mu-opioid receptor in the central nervous system (CNS) and possesses analgesic and antitussive effects. Binding of hydrocodone to this receptor also results in analgesia, euphoria, respiratory depression, decreased gastrointestinal motility and physical dependence. Additionally, hydrocodone is converted to hydromorphone by the cytochrome P 450 enzyme *CYP2D6*.

Illicit Uses of Hydrocodone

Hydrocodone is abused for its opioid effects. Widespread diversion via bogus call-in prescriptions, altered prescriptions, theft, and illicit purchases from Internet sources are made easier by the present controls placed on hydrocodone products. Hydrocodone pills are the most frequently encountered dosage form in illicit traffic. Hydrocodone is generally abused orally, often in combination with alcohol.

Of particular concern is the prevalence of illicit use of hydrocodone among school-aged children. The 2016 Monitoring the Future Survey reports that 0.8 percent, 1.7 percent and 2.9 percent of eighth, tenth, and twelfth graders, respectively, used Vicodin® for nonmedical purposes in the past year.

The American Association of Poison Control Centers (AAPCC) reports that in 2016, there were 1,826 total exposures, 832 single exposures, and 2 deaths associated with hydrocodone in the United States. The 2016 National Survey on Drug Use and Health (NSDUH) reports that 11.5 million people in the United States population, age 12 and older, misused hydrocodone in the past year compared to 12.5 million in 2015, a significant difference decrease.

As with most opiates, abuse of hydrocodone is associated with tolerance, dependence, and addiction. The co-formulation with acetaminophen carries an additional risk of liver toxicity when high, acute doses are consumed. Some individuals who abuse very high doses of acetaminophen-containing hydrocodone products may be spared this liver toxicity if they have been chronically taking these products and have escalated their dose slowly over a long period of time.

User Population: Hydrocodone

Every age group has been affected by the relative ease of hydrocodone availability and the perceived safety of these products by medical prescribers. Sometimes viewed as a "white collar" addiction, hydrocodone abuse has increased among all ethnic and economic groups.

Illicit Distribution of Hydrocodone

Hydrocodone has been encountered in tablets, capsules, and liquid form in the illicit market. However, hydrocodone tablets with the co-ingredient, acetaminophen, is the most frequently encountered form. Hydrocodone is not typically found to be clandestinely produced; diverted pharmaceuticals are the primary source of the drug for abuse purposes. Doctor shopping, altered or fraudulent prescriptions, bogus call-in prescriptions, diversion by some physicians and pharmacists, and drug theft are also major sources of the diverted drug.

The National Forensic Laboratory Information System (NFLIS) is a DEA database that collects scientifically verified data on drug items and cases submitted to and analyzed by federal, state, and local forensic laboratories. The System to Retrieve Information from Drug Evidence (STRIDE)/STARLiMS provides information on drug seizures reported to and analyzed by DEA laboratories. In 2017, there were 19,718 4 hydrocodone reports identified in the NFLIS, a decrease from 24,934 reports in 2016.

Control Status of Hydrocodone

Hydrocodone is controlled in Schedule II of the Controlled Substances Act (CSA).

Section 26.6

Hydromorphone

This section includes text excerpted from "Drugs of Abuse," U.S.
Drug Enforcement Administration (DEA), 2017.

What Is Hydromorphone?

Hydromorphone belongs to a class of drugs called "opioids," which includes morphine. It has an analgesic potency of two to eight times greater than that of morphine and has a rapid onset of action.

Hydromorphone is legally manufactured and distributed in the United States. However, users can obtain hydromorphone from forged prescriptions, "doctor shopping," theft from pharmacies, and from friends and acquaintances.

Other Questions on Hydromorphone
What Are the Street Names?

Common street names include D, Dillies, Dust, Footballs, Juice, and Smack.

What Does It Look Like?

Hydromorphone comes in tablets, capsules, oral solutions, and injectable formulations.

How Is It Abused?

Users may abuse hydromorphone tablets by ingesting them. Injectable solutions, as well as tablets that have been crushed and dissolved in a solution, may be injected as a substitute for heroin.

What Is Its Effect on the Mind?

When used as a drug of abuse, and not under a doctor's supervision, hydromorphone is taken to produce feelings of euphoria, relaxation, sedation, and reduced anxiety. It may also cause mental clouding, changes in mood, nervousness, and restlessness. It works centrally (in the brain) to reduce pain and suppress cough. Hydromorphone use is associated with both physiological and psychological dependence.

What Is Its Effect on the Body?

Hydromorphone may cause constipation, pupillary constriction, urinary retention, nausea, vomiting, respiratory depression, dizziness, impaired coordination, loss of appetite, rash, slow or rapid heartbeat, and changes in blood pressure.

What Are Its Overdose Effects?

Acute overdose of hydromorphone can produce severe respiratory depression, drowsiness progressing to stupor or coma, lack of skeletal muscle tone, cold and clammy skin, constricted pupils, and reduction in blood pressure and heart rate.

Severe overdose may result in death due to respiratory depression.

Which Drugs Cause Similar Effects

Drugs that have similar effects include heroin, morphine, hydrocodone, fentanyl, and oxycodone.

What Is Its Legal Status in the United States?

Hydromorphone is a Schedule II drug under the Controlled Substances Act (CSA) with an accepted medical use as a pain reliever. Hydromorphone has a high potential for abuse and use may lead to severe psychological or physical dependence.

Section 26.7

Methadone

This section includes text excerpted from "Methadone,"
U.S. Drug Enforcement Administration (DEA), 2017.

What Is Methadone?

Methadone is a synthetic (manufactured) narcotic.

German scientists synthesized methadone during World War II because of a shortage of morphine. Methadone was introduced into the United States in 1947 as an analgesic (Dolophine).

Other Questions on Methadone
What Are Common Street Names?

Common street names include Amidone, Chocolate Chip Cookies, Fizzies, Maria, Pastora, Salvia, Street Methadone, and Wafer.

What Does It Look Like?

Methadone is available as a tablet, oral solution, or injectable liquid. Tablets are available in 5 mg and 10 mg formulations. As of January 1, 2008, manufacturers of methadone hydrochloride tablets 40 mg (dispersible) have voluntarily agreed to restrict distribution of this formulation to only those facilities authorized for detoxification and maintenance treatment of opioid addiction, and hospitals. Manufacturers will instruct their wholesale distributors to discontinue supplying this formulation to any facility not meeting the above criteria.

How Is It Abused?

Methadone can be swallowed or injected.

What Is Its Effect on the Mind?

Abuse of methadone can lead to psychological dependence.

What Is Its Effect on the Body?

When an individual uses methadone, he/she may experience physical symptoms such as sweating, itchy skin, or sleepiness. Individuals who abuse methadone risk becoming tolerant of and physically dependent on the drug.

When use is stopped, individuals may experience withdrawal symptoms including anxiety, muscle tremors, nausea, diarrhea, vomiting, and abdominal cramps.

What Are Its Overdose Effects?

The effects of a methadone overdose are slow and shallow breathing, blue fingernails and lips, stomach spasms, clammy skin, convulsions, weak pulse, coma, and possible death.

Which Drugs Cause Similar Effects

Although chemically unlike morphine or heroin, methadone produces many of the same effects.

What Is Its Legal Status in the United States?

Methadone is a Schedule II drug under the Controlled Substances Act (CSA). While it may legally be used under a doctor's supervision, its nonmedical use is illegal.

Section 26.8

Oxycodone

This section includes text excerpted from "Drugs of Abuse," U.S. Drug Enforcement Administration (DEA), 2017.

What Is Oxycodone?

Oxycodone is a semi-synthetic narcotic analgesic and historically has been a popular drug of abuse among the narcotic abusing population.

Oxycodone is synthesized from thebaine, a constituent of the poppy plants.

Other Questions on Oxycodone
What Are Common Street Names?

Common street names include Hillbilly Heroin, Kicker, OC, Ox, Roxy, Perc, and Oxy.

What Does It Look Like?

Oxycodone is marketed alone as OxyContin® in 10, 20, 40, and 80 mg extended-release tablets and other immediate-release capsules like 5 mg OxyIR. It is also marketed in combination products with aspirin such as Percodan or acetaminophen such as Roxicet.

How Is It Abused?

Oxycodone is abused orally or intravenously. The tablets are crushed and sniffed or dissolved in water and injected. Others heat a tablet that has been placed on a piece of foil then inhale the vapors.

What Is Its Effect on the Mind?

Euphoria and feelings of relaxation are the most common effects of oxycodone on the brain, which explains its high potential for abuse.

What Is Its Effect on the Body?

Physiological effects of oxycodone include pain relief, sedation, respiratory depression, constipation, papillary constriction, and cough suppression. Extended or chronic use of oxycodone containing acetaminophen may cause severe liver damage.

What Are Its Overdose Effects?

Overdose effects include extreme drowsiness, muscle weakness, confusion, cold and clammy skin, pinpoint pupils, shallow breathing, slow heart rate, fainting, coma, and possible death.

Which Drugs Cause Similar Effects

Drugs that cause similar effects to Oxycodone include opium, codeine, heroin, methadone, hydrocodone, fentanyl, and morphine.

What Is Its Legal Status in the United States?

Oxycodone products are in Schedule II of the Controlled Substances Act (CSA).

Chapter 27

Sedatives (Depressants)

Chapter Contents

Section 27.1

Introduction to Depressants

This section includes text excerpted from "Drugs of Abuse," U.S. Drug Enforcement Administration (DEA), August 26, 2018.

What Are Depressants?

Depressants will put you to sleep, relieve anxiety and muscle spasms, and prevent seizures. Barbiturates are older drugs and include butalbital (Fiorina), phenobarbital, Pentothal, Seconal, and Nembutal. A person can rapidly develop a dependence on and tolerance to barbiturates, meaning a person needs more and more of them to feel and function normally. This makes them unsafe, increasing the likelihood of coma or death. Benzodiazepines were developed to replace barbiturates, though they still share many of the undesirable side effects, including tolerance and dependence. Some examples are Valium, Xanax, Halcion, Ativan, Klonopin, and Restoril. Rohypnol is a benzodiazepine that is not manufactured or legally marketed in the United States, but it is used illegally. Lunesta, Ambien, and Sonata are sedative-hypnotic medications approved for the short-term treatment of insomnia that shares many of the properties of benzo-diazepines. Other central nervous system (CNS) depressants include meprobamate, methaqualone (Quaalude), and the illicit drug gamma-hydroxybutyrate (GHB).

Origin of Depressants

Generally, legitimate pharmaceutical products are diverted to the illicit market. Teens can obtain depressants from the family medicine cabinet, friends, family members, the Internet, doctors, and hospitals.

Other Questions on Depressants
What Are Common Street Names?

Common street names for depressants include Barbs, Benzos, Downers, Georgia Home Boy, GHB, Grievous Bodily Harm (GBH), Liquid X, Nerve Pills, Phennies, R2, Reds, Roofies, Rophies, Tranks, and Yellows.

What Do They Look Like?

Depressants come in the form of pills, syrups, and injectable liquids.

How Are They Abused?

Individuals abuse depressants to experience euphoria. Depressants are also used with other drugs to add to the other drugs' high or to deal with their side effects. Users take higher doses than people taking the drugs under a doctor's supervision for therapeutic purposes. Depressants like GHB and Rohypnol are also misused to facilitate sexual assault.

What Is Their Effect on the Mind?

Depressants used therapeutically do what they are prescribed for inducing sleep, relieving anxiety and muscle spasms, and preventing seizures.

They also cause amnesia, leaving no memory of events that occur while under the influence, reduce reaction time, impair mental functioning and judgment, and cause confusion.

Long-term use of depressants produces psychological dependence and tolerance.

What Is Their Effect on the Body?

Some depressants can relax the muscles. Unwanted physical effects include slurred speech, loss of motor coordination, weakness, headache, lightheadedness, blurred vision, dizziness, nausea, vomiting, low blood pressure, and slowed breathing.

Prolonged use of depressants can lead to physical dependence even at doses recommended for medical treatment. Unlike barbiturates, large doses of benzodiazepines are rarely fatal unless combined with other drugs or alcohol. But unlike the withdrawal syndrome seen with most other drugs of abuse, withdrawal from depressants can be life-threatening.

What Is Their Legal Status in the United States?

Most depressants are controlled substances that range from Schedule I to Schedule IV under the Controlled Substances Act (CSA), depending on their risk for abuse and whether they currently have an accepted medical use. Many of the depressants have U.S. Food and Drug Administration (FDA)-approved medical uses. Rohypnol and Quaaludes are not manufactured or legally marketed in the United States.

Section 27.2

Barbiturates

This section includes text excerpted from "Drugs of Abuse,"
U.S. Drug Enforcement Administration (DEA), August 26, 2018.

What Are Barbiturates?

Barbiturates are depressants that produce a wide spectrum of central nervous system depression from mild sedation to coma. They also have been used as sedatives, hypnotics, anesthetics, and anticonvulsants. Barbiturates are classified as Ultrashort, Short, Intermediate, and Long-acting.

Barbiturates were first introduced for medical use in the 1900s, and nowadays about 12 substances are in medical use.

Other Questions on Barbiturates
What Are Common Street Names?

Common street names include Barbs, Block Busters, Christmas Trees, Goof Balls, Pinks, Red Devils, Reds and Blues, and Yellow Jackets.

What Do They Look Like?

Barbiturates come in a variety of multicolored pills and tablets. Users prefer the short-acting and intermediate barbiturates such as Amytal and Seconal.

How Are They Abused?

Barbiturates are abused by swallowing a pill or injecting a liquid form. Barbiturates are generally abused to reduce anxiety, decrease inhibitions, and treat unwanted effects of illicit drugs. Barbiturates can be extremely dangerous because overdoses can occur easily and lead to death.

What Is Their Effect on the Mind?

Barbiturates cause mild euphoria, lack of inhibition, relief of anxiety, and sleepiness.

Higher doses cause impairment of memory, judgment, and coordination; irritability; and paranoid and suicidal ideation.

Tolerance develops quickly and larger doses are then needed to produce the same effect, increasing the danger of an overdose.

What Is Their Effect on the Body?

Barbiturates slow down the central nervous system (CNS) and cause sleepiness.

What Are Their Overdose Effects?

Effects of overdose include shallow respiration, clammy skin, dilated pupils, weak and rapid pulse, coma, and possible death.

Which Drugs Cause Similar Effects

Drugs with similar effects include alcohol, benzodiazepines like Valium and Xanax, tranquilizers, sleeping pills, Rohypnol, and gamma-hydroxybutyrate (GHB).

What Is Their Legal Status in the United States?

Barbiturates are Schedule II, III, and IV depressants under the Controlled Substances Act (CSA).

Section 27.3

Benzodiazepines

This section includes text excerpted from "Drugs of Abuse," U.S. Drug Enforcement Administration (DEA), August 26, 2018.

What Are Benzodiazepines?

Benzodiazepines are depressants that produce sedation and hypnosis, relieve anxiety and muscle spasms, and reduce seizures.

Benzodiazepines are only legally available through prescription. Many users maintain their drug supply by getting prescriptions from several doctors, forging prescriptions, or buying them illicitly. Alprazolam and diazepam are the two most frequently encountered benzodiazepines on the illicit market.

Other Questions on Benzodiazepines
What Are Common Street Names?

Common street names include Benzos and Downers.

What Do They Look Like?

The most common benzodiazepines are the prescription drugs Valium, Xanax, Halcion, Ativan, and Klonopin. Tolerance can develop, although at variable rates and to different degrees. Shorter-acting benzodiazepines used to manage insomnia include estazolam (ProSom), flurazepam (Dalmane), temazepam (Restoril), and triazolam (Halcion). Midazolam (Versed), a short-acting benzodiazepine, is utilized for sedation, anxiety, and amnesia in critical care settings and prior to anesthesia. It is available in the United States as an injectable preparation and as a syrup (primarily for pediatric patients). Benzodiazepines with a longer duration of action are utilized to treat insomnia in patients with daytime anxiety. These benzodiazepines include alprazolam (Xanax), chlordiazepoxide (Librium), clorazepate (Tranxene), diazepam (Valium), halazepam (Paxipam), Lorazepam (Ativan), oxazepam (Serax), prazepam (Centrax), and quazepam (Doral). Clonazepam (Klonopin), diazepam, and clorazepate are also used as anticonvulsants.

How Are They Abused?

Abuse is frequently associated with adolescents and young adults who take the drug orally or crush it up and snort it to get high. Abuse is particularly high among heroin and cocaine users.

What Is Their Effect on the Mind?

Benzodiazepines are associated with amnesia, hostility, irritability, and vivid or disturbing dreams.

What Is Their Effect on the Body?

Benzodiazepines slow down the central nervous system and may cause sleepiness.

286

What Are Their Overdose Effects?

Effects of overdose include shallow respiration, clammy skin, dilated pupils, weak and rapid pulse, coma, and possible death.

Which Drugs Cause Similar Effects

Drugs that cause similar effects include alcohol, barbiturates, sleeping pills, and gamma-hydroxybutyrate (GHB).

What Is Their Legal Status in the United States?

Benzodiazepines are controlled in Schedule IV of the Controlled Substances Act (CSA).

Section 27.4

Kava

This section includes text excerpted from "Kava," DEA Diversion Control Division, January 2013, Reviewed January 2019.

Kava, also known as *Piper methysticum* (intoxicating pepper), is a perennial shrub native to the South Pacific Islands, including Hawaii. It is harvested for its rootstock, which contains the pharmacologically active compounds kavalactones.

The term "kava" also refers to the nonfermented, psychoactive beverage prepared from the rootstock. For many centuries, Pacific Island societies have consumed kava beverages for social, ceremonial, and medical purposes. Traditionally, kava beverages are prepared by chewing or pounding the rootstock to produce a cloudy, milky pulp that is then soaked in water before the liquid is filtered to drink.

There is an increasing use of kava for recreational purposes. The reinforcing effects of kava include mild euphoria, muscle relaxation, sedation, and analgesia.

Licit Uses of Kava

In the United States, kava is sold as dietary supplements promoted as natural alternatives to antianxiety drugs and sleeping pills. An analysis of six kava clinical trials found that kava (60 to 200 mg of kavalactones/day) produced a significant reduction in anxiety compared to placebo. However, the U.S. Food and Drug Administration (FDA) has not made a determination about the ability of dietary supplements containing kava to provide such benefits.

Kava dietary supplements are commonly formulated as tablets and capsules (30 to 90% kavalactones; 50 to 250 mg per capsule). Kava is also available as whole root, powdered root, extracts (powder, paste, and liquid), tea bags, and instant powdered drink mix. Kava is frequently found in products containing a variety of herbs or vitamins, or both.

A number of cases of liver damage (hepatitis and cirrhosis), and liver failure have been associated with commercial extract preparations of kava. In 2002, the FDA issued an advisory alerting consumers and healthcare providers to the potential risk of liver-related injuries associated with the use of kava dietary supplements.

Chemistry and Pharmacology of Kava

The pharmacologically active kavalactones are found in the lipid-soluble resin of the kava rootstock. Of the 18 isolated and identified, yangonin, methysticin, dihydromethysticin, dihydrokavain, kavain, and desmethoxyyangonin are the six major kavalactones. Different varieties of kava plants possess varying concentrations of kavalactones.

The pharmacokinetics of the kavalactones has not been extensively studied. Kavalactones are thought to be relatively quickly absorbed in the gut. There may be differences in the bioavailability between each kavalactone.

The limbic structures, amygdala complex, and reticular formation of the brain appear to be the preferential sites of action of kavalactones. However, the exact molecular mechanisms of action are not clear.

Kava has the potential for causing drug interactions through the inhibition of CYP450 enzymes that are responsible for the metabolism of many pharmaceutical agents and other herbal remedies. Chronic use of kava in large quantities may cause a dry scaly skin or yellow skin discoloration known as kava dermopathy. It may also cause liver toxicity, and extrapyramidal effects (e.g., tremor and abnormal body movement).

Individuals may experience a numbing or tingling of the mouth upon drinking kava due to its local anesthetic action. High doses of kavalactones can also produce central nervous system (CNS) depressant effects (e.g., sedation and muscle weakness) that appear to be transient.

Illicit Uses of Kava

Information on the illicit use of kava in the United States is anecdotal. Based on information on the Internet, kava is being used recreationally to relax the body and achieve a mild euphoria. It is typically consumed as a beverage made from dried kava root powder, flavored and unflavored powdered extracts, and liquid extract dissolved in pure grain alcohol and vegetable glycerin. Individuals may consume 25 grams of kavalactones, which is about 125 times the daily dose in kava dietary supplements.

Intoxicated individuals typically have sensible thought processes and comprehensive conversations, but have difficulty coordinating movement and often fall asleep. Kava users do not exhibit the generalized confusion and delirium that occurs with high levels of alcohol intoxication. While kava alone does not produce the motor and cognitive impairments caused by alcohol, kava does potentiate both the perceived and measured impairment produced by alcohol.

The American Association of Poison Control Centers (AAPCC) reported 42 case mentions and 21 single exposures associated with kava in 2010.

User Population: Kava

Information on user population in the United States (U.S.) is very limited. In the 1980s, kava was introduced to Australian Aboriginal communities where it quickly became a drug of abuse. It has become a serious social problem in regions of Northern Australia.

Distribution of Kava

Kava is widely available on the Internet. Some websites promoting and selling kava products also sell other uncontrolled psychoactive products such as *Salvia divinorum* and kratom. Several kava bars and lounges in the United States sell kava drinks. The National Forensic Laboratory Information System (NFLIS) and the System to Retrieve Information from Drug Evidence (STRIDE) do not indicate any kava reports.

Control Status of Kava

Kava is not a controlled substance in the United States. Due to concerns of liver toxicity, many countries including Australia, Canada, France, Germany, Malaysia, Singapore, Switzerland, and the United Kingdom have placed regulatory controls on kava. These controls range from warning consumers of the dangers of taking kava to removing kava products from the marketplace.

Chapter 28

Stimulants

Chapter Contents

Section 28.1

Introduction to Stimulants

This section includes text excerpted from "Drugs of Abuse,"
U.S. Drug Enforcement Administration (DEA), August 26, 2018.

What Are Stimulants?

Stimulants speed up the body's systems. This class of drugs includes prescription drugs such as amphetamines (Adderall and dexedrine), methylphenidate (Concerta and Ritalin), diet aids (such as Didrex, Bontril, Preludin, Fastin, Adipex P, Ionamin, and Meridia), and illicitly produced drugs such as methamphetamine, cocaine, and methcathinone.

Origin of Stimulants

Stimulants are diverted from legitimate channels and clandestinely manufactured exclusively for the illicit market.

Other Questions on Stimulants

What Are Common Street Names?

Common street names for stimulants include Bennies, Black Beauties, Cat, Coke, Crank, Crystal, Flake, Ice, Pellets, R-Ball, Skippy, Snow, Speed, Uppers, and Vitamin R.

What Do They Look Like?

Stimulants come in the form of pills, powder, rocks, and injectable liquids.

How Are They Abused?

Stimulants can be pills or capsules that are swallowed. Smoking, snorting, or injecting stimulants produces a sudden sensation known as a "rush" or a "flash."

Abuse is often associated with a pattern of binge use—sporadically consuming large doses of stimulants over a short period of time. Heavy users may inject themselves every few hours, continuing until they have depleted their drug supply or reached a point of delirium, psychosis, and physical exhaustion. During heavy use, all other interests become secondary to recreating the initial euphoric rush.

What Is Their Effect on the Mind?

When used as drugs of abuse and not under a doctor's supervision, stimulants are frequently taken to produce a sense of exhilaration, enhance self-esteem, improve mental and physical performance, increase activity, reduce appetite, extend wakefulness for a prolonged period, and "getting high"

Chronic, high-dose use is frequently associated with agitation, hostility, panic, aggression, and suicidal or homicidal tendencies.

Paranoia, sometimes accompanied by both auditory and visual hallucinations, may also occur.

Tolerance, in which more and more drug is needed to produce the usual effects, can develop rapidly, and psychological dependence occurs. In fact, the strongest psychological dependence observed occurs with the more potent stimulants, such as amphetamine, methylphenidate, methamphetamine, cocaine, and methcathinone.

Abrupt cessation is commonly followed by depression, anxiety, drug craving, and extreme fatigue, known as a "crash."

What Is Their Effect on the Body?

Stimulants are sometimes referred to as uppers and reverse the effects of fatigue on both mental and physical tasks. Therapeutic levels of stimulants can produce exhilaration, extended wakefulness, and loss of appetite. These effects are greatly intensified when large doses of stimulants are taken. Taking too large a dose at one time or taking large doses over an extended period of time may cause such physical side effects as dizziness, tremors, headache, flushed skin, chest pain with palpitations, excessive sweating, vomiting, and abdominal cramps.

What Are Their Overdose Effects?

In overdose, unless there is medical intervention, high fever, convulsions, and cardiovascular collapse may precede death. Because accidental death is partially due to the effects of stimulants on the body's cardiovascular and temperature-regulating systems, physical exertion increases the hazards of stimulant use.

Which Drugs Cause Similar Effects

Some hallucinogenic substances, such as ecstasy, have a stimulant component to their activity.

What Is Their Legal Status in the United States?

A number of stimulants have no medical use in the United States but have a high potential for abuse. These stimulants are controlled in Schedule I. Some prescription stimulants are not controlled, and some stimulants like tobacco and caffeine don't require a prescription—though society's recognition of their adverse effects has resulted in a proliferation of caffeine-free products and efforts to discourage cigarette smoking.

Stimulant chemicals in over-the-counter (OTC) products, such as ephedrine and pseudoephedrine, can be found in allergy and cold medicine. As required by the Combat Methamphetamine Epidemic Act (CMEA) of 2005, a retail outlet must store these products out of reach of customers, either behind the counter or in a locked cabinet. Regulated sellers are required to maintain a written or electronic form of a logbook to record sales of these products. In order to purchase these products, customers must now show a photo identification issued by a state or federal government. They are also required to write or enter into the logbook: their name, signature, address, date, and time of sale. In addition to the above, there are daily and monthly sales limits set for customers.

Section 28.2

Amphetamine

This section includes text excerpted from "Drugs of Abuse,"
U.S. Drug Enforcement Administration (DEA), August 26, 2018.

What Are Amphetamines?

Amphetamines are stimulants that speed up the body's system. Many are legally prescribed and used to treat attention deficit hyperactivity disorder (ADHD).

Origin of Amphetamines

Amphetamine was first marketed in the 1930s as Benzedrine in an over-the-counter (OTC) inhaler to treat nasal congestion. By 1937 amphetamine was available by prescription in tablet form and was used in the treatment of the sleeping disorder narcolepsy and ADHD.

Over the years, the use and abuse of clandestinely produced amphetamines have spread. Nowadays, clandestine laboratory production of amphetamines has mushroomed, and the abuse of the drug has increased dramatically.

Other Questions on Amphetamines
What Are Common Street Names?

Common street names include Bennies, Black Beauties, Crank, Ice, Speed, and Uppers.

What Do They Look Like?

Amphetamines can look like pills or powder. Common prescription amphetamines include methylphenidate (Ritalin or Ritalin SR), amphetamine and dextroamphetamine (Adderall), and dextroamphetamine (Dexedrine).

How Are They Abused?

Amphetamines are generally taken orally or injected. However, the addition of "Ice," the slang name of crystallized methamphetamine hydrochloride, has promoted smoking as another mode of administration. Just as "Crack" is smokable cocaine, "Ice" is smokable methamphetamine.

What Is Their Effect on the Mind?

The effects of amphetamines and methamphetamine are similar to cocaine, but their onset is slower and their duration is longer. In contrast to cocaine, which is quickly removed from the brain and is almost completely metabolized, methamphetamine remains in the central nervous system longer, and a larger percentage of the drug remains unchanged in the body, producing prolonged stimulant effects.

Chronic abuse produces a psychosis that resembles schizophrenia and is characterized by paranoia, picking at the skin, preoccupation with one's own thoughts, and auditory and visual hallucinations. Violent and erratic behavior is frequently seen among chronic users of amphetamines and methamphetamine.

What Is Their Effect on the Body?

Physical effects of amphetamine use include increased blood pressure and pulse rates, insomnia, loss of appetite, and physical exhaustion.

What Are Their Overdose Effects?

Overdose effects include agitation, increased body temperature, hallucinations, convulsions, and possible death.

Which Drugs Cause Similar Effects

Drugs that cause similar effects include dexmethylphenidate, phentermine, benzphetamine, phendimetrazine, cocaine, crack, methamphetamine, and khat.

What Is Their Legal Status in the United States?

Amphetamines are Schedule II stimulants, which means that they have a high potential for abuse and a currently acceptable medical use (in U.S. Food and Drug Administration (FDA)-approved products). Pharmaceutical products are available only through a prescription that cannot be refilled.

Section 28.3

BZP

This section includes text excerpted from "N-Benzylpiperazine," DEA Diversion Control Division, March 2014. Reviewed January 2019.

N-Benzylpiperazine (BZP) was first synthesized in 1944 as a potential antiparasitic agent. It was subsequently shown to possess antidepressant activity and amphetamine-like effects, but was not developed for marketing. The amphetamine-like effects of BZP attracted the attention of drug abusers. Since 1996, BZP has been abused by drug abusers; as evidenced by the encounters of this substance by law enforcement officials in various states and the District of Columbia (DC) The U.S. Drug Enforcement Administration (DEA) placed BZP in Schedule I of the Controlled Substances Act (CSA) because of its high abuse potential and lack of accepted medical use or safety.

Licit Uses of N-Benzylpiperazine

BZP is used as an intermediate in chemical synthesis. It has no known medical use in the United States.

Chemistry and Pharmacology of N-Benzylpiperazine

BZP is an N-monosubstituted piperazine derivative available as either base or the hydrochloride salt. The base form is a slightly yellowish-green liquid. The hydrochloride salt is a white solid. BZP base is corrosive and causes burns. The salt form of BZP is an irritant to eyes, respiratory system, and skin.

Both animal studies and human clinical studies have demonstrated that the pharmacological effects of BZP are qualitatively similar to those of amphetamine. BZP has been reported to be similar to amphetamine in its effects on chemical transmission in the brain. BZP fully mimics discriminative stimulus effects of amphetamine in animals. BZP is self-administered by monkeys indicating reinforcing effects. Subjective effects of BZP were amphetamine-like in drug-naive volunteers and in volunteers with a history of stimulant dependence. BZP acts as a stimulant in humans and produces euphoria and cardiovascular effects, namely increases in heart rate and systolic blood pressure. BZP is about 10 to 20 times less potent than amphetamine in producing these effects. Experimental studies demonstrate that the abuse, dependence potential, pharmacology, and toxicology of BZP are similar to those of amphetamine. Public-health risks of BZP are similar to those of amphetamine.

Illicit Uses of N-Benzylpiperazine

BZP is often abused in combination with 1-(3 (trifluoro-methyl) phenyl) piperazine (TFMPP), a noncontrolled substance. This combination has been promoted to the youth population as a substitute for 3,4-methylenedioxymethamphetamine (MDMA) at raves (all-night dance parties). However, there are no clinical studies that directly compared the behavioral effects of BZP to those of MDMA. BZP may also be abused alone for its stimulant effects. BZP is generally administered orally as either powder or tablets and capsules. Other routes of administration included smoking and snorting. There have also been several life-threatening incidents that resulted in emergency department admissions following the ingestion of BZP.

User Population: N-Benzylpiperazine

Youth and young adults are the main abusers of BZP.

Illicit Distribution of N-Benzylpiperazine

According to DEA's System to Retrieve Information from Drug Evidence (STRIDE) and National Forensic Laboratory Information System (NFLIS), the number of reports submitted to federal, state, and local forensic laboratories and identified as BZP peaked in 2009 at 15,174 and decreased each year thereafter. In 2013, there were 2,548 BZP reports identified.

Illicit distributions occur through smuggling of bulk powder through drug trafficking organizations with connections to overseas sources of supply. The bulk powder is then processed into capsules and tablets. BZP is encountered as pink, white, off-white, purple, orange, tan, and mottle orange-brown tablets. These tablets bear imprints commonly seen on MDMA tablets such as housefly, crown, heart, butterfly, smiley face or bull's head logos and are often sold as "ecstasy." BZP has been found in powder or liquid form which is packaged in small convenience sizes and sold on the Internet.

Control Status of N-Benzylpiperazine

BZP was temporarily placed into Schedule I of the CSA on September 20, 2002 (67 FR 59161). On March 18, 2004, the DEA published a Final Rule in the Federal Register permanently placing BZP in Schedule I.

Section 28.4

Cocaine

This section includes text excerpted from "Cocaine," National Institute on Drug Abuse (NIDA), July 2018.

What Is Cocaine?

Cocaine is a powerfully addictive stimulant drug made from the leaves of the coca plant native to South America. Although, healthcare providers can use it for valid medical purposes, such as local anesthesia for some surgeries, recreational cocaine use is illegal. As a street drug, cocaine looks like a fine and white crystal powder. Street dealers often mix it with things like cornstarch, talcum powder, or flour to increase profits. They may also mix it with other drugs such as the stimulant amphetamine, or synthetic opioids, including fentanyl. Adding synthetic opioids to cocaine is especially risky when people using cocaine don't realize it contains this dangerous additive. Increasing numbers of overdose deaths among cocaine users might be related to this tampered cocaine.

Popular nicknames for cocaine include:

- Blow

- Coke

- Crack

- Rock

- Snow

How Do People Use Cocaine?

People snort cocaine powder through the nose, or they rub it into their gums. Others dissolve the powder and inject it into the bloodstream. Some people inject a combination of cocaine and heroin, called a Speedball.

Another popular method of use is to smoke cocaine that has been processed to make a rock crystal (also called "freebase cocaine"). The crystal is heated to produce vapors that are inhaled into the lungs. This form of cocaine is called Crack, which refers to the crackling sound of the rock as it's heated. Some people also smoke Crack by sprinkling it on marijuana or tobacco and smoke it like a cigarette.

People who use cocaine often take it in binges—taking the drug repeatedly within a short time, at increasingly higher doses—to maintain their high.

How Does Cocaine Affect the Brain?

Cocaine increases levels of the natural chemical messenger dopamine in brain circuits related to the control of movement and reward.

Normally, dopamine recycles back into the cell that released it, shutting off the signal between nerve cells. However, cocaine prevents dopamine from being recycled, causing large amounts to build up in the space between two nerve cells, stopping their normal communication. This flood of dopamine in the brain's reward circuit strongly reinforces drug-taking behaviors, because the reward circuit eventually adapts to the excess of dopamine caused by cocaine, and becomes less sensitive to it. As a result, people take stronger and more frequent doses in an attempt to feel the same high and to obtain relief from withdrawal.

Short-Term Effects

Short-term health effects of cocaine include:

- Extreme happiness and energy
- Mental alertness
- Hypersensitivity to sight, sound, and touch
- Irritability
- Paranoia—extreme and unreasonable distrust of others

Some people find that cocaine helps them perform simple physical and mental tasks more quickly, although others experience the opposite effect. Large amounts of cocaine can lead to bizarre, unpredictable, and violent behavior.

Cocaine's effects appear almost immediately and disappear within a few minutes to an hour. How long the effects last and how intense they are depend on the method of use. Injecting or smoking cocaine produces a quicker and stronger but shorter-lasting high than snorting. The high from snorting cocaine may last 15 to 30 minutes. The high from smoking may last 5 to 10 minutes.

What Are the Other Health Effects of Cocaine Use?

Other health effects of cocaine use include:

- Constricted blood vessels

- Dilated pupils

- Nausea

- Raised body temperature and blood pressure

- Fast or irregular heartbeat

- Tremors and muscle twitches

- Restlessness

Long-Term Effects

Some long-term health effects of cocaine depend on the method of use and include the following:

- **Snorting.** loss of smell, nosebleeds, frequent runny nose, and problems with swallowing

- **Smoking.** cough, asthma, respiratory distress, and higher risk of infections such as pneumonia

- **Consuming by mouth.** severe bowel decay from reduced blood flow

- **Needle injection.** higher risk for contracting human immunodeficiency virus (HIV), hepatitis C, and other bloodborne diseases, skin or soft tissue infections, as well as scarring or collapsed veins

However, even people involved with nonneedle cocaine use place themselves at a risk for HIV because cocaine impairs judgment, which can lead to risky sexual behavior with infected partners.

Other long-term effects of cocaine use include being malnourished, because cocaine decreases appetite, and movement disorders, including Parkinson disease (PD), which may occur after many years of use. In addition, people report irritability and restlessness from cocaine binges, and some also experience severe paranoia, in which they lose touch with reality and have auditory hallucinations—hearing noises that aren't real.

Cocaine, Human Immunodeficiency Virus, and Hepatitis

Studies have shown that cocaine use speeds up HIV infection. According to research, cocaine impairs immune cell function and promotes the reproduction of the HIV virus. Research also suggests that people who use cocaine and are infected with HIV may be more susceptible to contracting other viruses, such as hepatitis C, a virus that affects the liver.

Can a Person Overdose on Cocaine?

Yes, a person can overdose on cocaine. An overdose occurs when a person uses enough of a drug to produce serious adverse effects, life-threatening symptoms, or death. An overdose can be intentional or unintentional.

Death from overdose can occur on the first use of cocaine or unexpectedly thereafter. Many people who use cocaine also drink alcohol at the same time, which is particularly risky and can lead to overdose. Others mix cocaine with heroin, another dangerous—and deadly—combination.

Some of the most frequent and severe health consequences of overdose are irregular heart rhythm, heart attacks, seizures, and strokes. Other symptoms of cocaine overdose include difficulty breathing, high blood pressure, high body temperature, hallucinations, and extreme agitation or anxiety.

How Can a Cocaine Overdose Be Treated?

There is no specific medication that can reverse a cocaine overdose. Management involves supportive care and depends on the symptoms present. For instance, because cocaine overdose often leads to a heart attack, stroke, or seizure, first responders and emergency room doctors try to treat the overdose by treating these conditions, with the intent of:

- Restoring blood flow to the heart (heart attack)
- Restoring oxygen-rich blood supply to the affected part of the brain (stroke)
- Stopping the seizure

How Does Cocaine Use Lead to Addiction?

As with other drugs, repeated use of cocaine can cause long-term changes in the brain's reward circuit and other brain systems, which may lead to addiction. The reward circuit eventually adapts to the extra dopamine caused by the drug, becoming steadily less sensitive to it. As a result, people take stronger and more frequent doses to feel the same high they did initially and to obtain relief from withdrawal.

Withdrawal symptoms include:

- Depression
- Fatigue
- Increased appetite
- Unpleasant dreams and insomnia
- Slowed thinking

How Can People Get Treatment for Cocaine Addiction?

Behavioral therapy may be used to treat cocaine addiction. Examples include:

- Cognitive-behavioral therapy (CBT)
- Contingency management or motivational incentives—providing rewards to patients who remain substance free
- Therapeutic communities—drug-free residences in which people in recovery from substance-use disorders help each other to understand and change their behaviors
- Community-based recovery groups, such as 12-step programs

While no government-approved medicines are available as of now to treat cocaine addiction, researchers are testing some treatments that have been used to treat other disorders, including:

- Disulfiram (used to treat alcoholism)

- Modafinil (used to treat narcolepsy—a disorder characterized by uncontrollable episodes of deep sleep)

- Lorcaserin (used to treat obesity)

- Buprenorphine (used to treat opioid addiction)

Section 28.5

Khat

This section includes text excerpted from "Drugs of Abuse," U.S. Drug Enforcement Administration (DEA), August 26, 2018.

What Is Khat?

Khat is a flowering evergreen shrub that is abused for its stimulant-like effect. Khat has two active ingredients, cathine and cathinone.

Origin of Khat

Khat is native to East Africa and the Arabian Peninsula, where the use of it is an established cultural tradition for many social situations.

Other Questions on Khat
What Are Common Street Names?

Common street names for khat include Abyssinian Tea, African Salad, Catha, Chat, Kat, and Oat.

What Does It Look Like?

Khat is a flowering evergreen shrub. Khat that is sold and abused is usually just the leaves, twigs, and shoots of the khat shrub.

How Is It Abused?

Khat is typically chewed like tobacco, then retained in the cheek and chewed intermittently to release the active drug, which produces a stimulant-like effect. Dried khat leaves can be made into tea or a chewable paste, and khat can also be smoked and even sprinkled on food.

What Is Its Effect on the Mind?

Khat can induce manic behavior with grandiose delusions, paranoia, nightmares, hallucinations, and hyperactivity chronic khat abuse can result in violence and suicidal depression.

What Is Its Effect on the Body?

Khat causes an immediate increase in blood pressure and heart rate. Khat can also cause brown staining of the teeth, insomnia, and gastric disorders. Chronic abuse of khat can cause physical exhaustion.

What Are Its Overdose Effects?

The dose needed to constitute an overdose is not known, however, it has been historically associated with those who are long-term chewers of the leaves. Symptoms of toxicity include delusions, loss of appetite, difficulty breathing, and increases in both blood pressure and heart rate.

Additionally, there are reports of liver damage (chemical hepatitis) and of cardiac complications, specifically myocardial infarctions. This mostly occurs among long-term chewers of khat or those who have chewed too large a dose.

Which Drugs Cause Similar Effects

Khat's effects are similar to other stimulants, such as cocaine, amphetamine, and methamphetamine

What Is Its Legal Status in the United States?

The chemicals found in khat are controlled under the Controlled Substances Act (CSA). Cathine is a Schedule IV stimulant, and cathinone is a Schedule I stimulant under the CSA, meaning that it has a high potential for abuse, as of now there is no accepted medical use of khat in treatment in the United States, and a lack of accepted safety for use under medical supervision.

Section 28.6

Kratom

This section includes text excerpted from "Kratom," National Institute on Drug Abuse (NIDA), September 2018.

What Is Kratom?

Kratom is a tropical tree *(Mitragyna speciosa)* native to Southeast Asia, with leaves that contain compounds that can have psychotropic (mind-altering) effects.

Kratom, as of now, is not an illegal substance and has been easy to order on the Internet. It is sometimes sold as a green powder in packets labeled "not for human consumption." It is also sometimes sold as an extract or gum.

Kratom sometimes goes by the following names:

- Biak
- Ketum
- Kakuam
- Ithang
- Thom

How Do People Use Kratom?

Most people take kratom as a pill, capsule, or extract. Some people chew kratom leaves or brew the dried or powdered leaves as a tea. Sometimes the leaves are smoked or eaten in food.

How Does Kratom Affect the Brain?

Kratom can cause effects similar to both opioids and stimulants. Two compounds in kratom leaves, *mitragynine* and

7-α-hydroxymitragynine, interact with opioid receptors in the brain, producing sedation, pleasure, and decreased pain, especially when users consume large amounts of the plant. Mitragynine also interacts with other receptor systems in the brain to produce stimulant effects. When kratom is taken in small amounts, users report increased energy, sociability, and alertness instead of sedation. However, kratom can also cause uncomfortable and sometimes dangerous side effects.

What Are the Health Effects of Kratom?

Reported health effects of kratom use include:

- Nausea

- Itching

- Sweating

- Dry mouth

- Constipation

- Increased urination

- Loss of appetite

- Seizures

- Hallucinations

Symptoms of psychosis have been reported in some users.

Can a Person Overdose on Kratom?

In 2017, the U.S. Food and Drug Administration (FDA) began issuing a series of warnings about kratom and now identifies at least 44 deaths related to its use, with at least one case being investigated as possible use of pure kratom. Most kratom associated deaths appear to have resulted from adulterated products (other drugs mixed in with the kratom) or taking kratom along with other potent substances, including illicit drugs, opioids, benzodiazepines, alcohol, gabapentin, and over-the-counter (OTC) medications, such as cough syrup. Also, there have been some reports of kratom packaged as dietary supplements or dietary ingredients that were laced with other compounds that caused deaths.

Is Kratom Addictive?

Like other drugs with opioid-like effects, kratom might cause dependence, which means users will feel physical withdrawal symptoms when they stop taking the drug. Some users have reported becoming addicted to kratom. Withdrawal symptoms include:

- Muscle aches
- Insomnia
- Irritability
- Hostility
- Aggression
- Emotional changes
- Runny nose
- Jerky movements

How Is Kratom Addiction Treated?

There are no specific medical treatments for kratom addiction. Some people seeking treatment have found behavioral therapy to be helpful. Scientists need more research to determine how effective this treatment option is.

Does Kratom Have Value as a Medicine?

In recent years, some people have used kratom as an herbal alternative to medical treatment in attempts to control withdrawal symptoms and cravings caused by addiction to opioids or to other addictive substances such as alcohol. There is no scientific evidence that kratom is effective or safe for this purpose; further research is needed.

Section 28.7

Methamphetamine

This section includes text excerpted from "Methamphetamine,"
National Institute on Drug Abuse (NIDA), June 2018.

What Is Methamphetamine?

Methamphetamine is a stimulant drug usually used as a white, bitter-tasting powder or a pill. Crystal methamphetamine is a form of the drug that looks like glass fragments or shiny, bluish-white rocks. It is chemically similar to amphetamine (a drug used to treat attention deficit hyperactivity disorder (ADHD) and narcolepsy, a sleep disorder).

Other common names for methamphetamine include Chalk, Crank, Crystal, Ice, Meth, and Speed.

How Do People Use Methamphetamine?

People can take methamphetamine by:

- Inhaling/smoking

- Swallowing (pill)

- Snorting

- Injecting the powder that has been dissolved in water/alcohol

Because the "high" from the drug both starts and fades quickly, people often take repeated doses in a "binge and crash" pattern. In some cases, people take methamphetamine in a form of binging known as a "run," giving up food and sleep while continuing to take the drug every few hours for up to several days.

How Does Methamphetamine Affect the Brain?

Methamphetamine increases the amount of natural chemical dopamine in the brain. Dopamine is involved in body movement, motivation, and reinforcement of rewarding behaviors. The drug's ability to rapidly release high levels of dopamine in reward areas of the brain strongly reinforces drug-taking behavior, making the user want to repeat the experience.

Short-Term Effects

Taking even small amounts of methamphetamine can result in many of the same health effects as those of other stimulants, such as cocaine or amphetamines. These include:

- Increased wakefulness and physical activity
- Decreased appetite
- Faster breathing
- Rapid and/or irregular heartbeat
- Increased blood pressure and body temperature

How Do Manufacturers Make Methamphetamine?

Manufacturers make most of the methamphetamine found in the United States in "superlabs" here or, more often, in Mexico. But some also make the drug in small, secret labs with inexpensive over-the-counter (OTC) ingredients such as pseudoephedrine, a common ingredient in cold medicines. To curb production, the law requires pharmacies and other retail stores to keep a purchase record of products containing pseudoephedrine. A person may only buy a limited amount of those products on a single day.

What Are Other Health Effects of Methamphetamine?
Long-Term Effects

People who inject methamphetamine are at increased risk of contracting infectious diseases such as human immunodeficiency virus (HIV) and hepatitis B and C. These diseases are transmitted through contact with blood or other bodily fluids. Methamphetamine use can also alter judgment and decision-making leading to risky behaviors, such as unprotected sex, which also increases the risk of infection.

Methamphetamine use may worsen the progression of HIV, acquired immunodeficiency syndrome (AIDS), and its consequences. Studies indicate that HIV causes more injury to nerve cells and more cognitive problems in people who have HIV and use methamphetamine than it does in people who have HIV and don't use the drug. Cognitive problems are those involved with thinking, understanding, learning, and remembering.

Long-term methamphetamine use has many other negative consequences, including:

- Extreme weight loss
- Severe dental problems ("meth mouth")
- Intense itching, leading to skin sores from scratching
- Anxiety
- Confusion
- Sleeping problems
- Violent behavior
- Paranoia—extreme and unreasonable distrust of others
- Hallucinations—sensations and images that seem real though they aren't

In addition, continued methamphetamine use causes changes in the brain's dopamine system that are associated with reduced coordination and impaired verbal learning. In studies of people who used methamphetamine over the long term, severe changes also affected areas of the brain involved with emotion and memory. This may explain many of the emotional and cognitive problems observed in those who use methamphetamine.

Although some of these brain changes may reverse after being off the drug for a year or more, other changes may not recover even after a long period of abstinence. A study suggests that people who used methamphetamine have an increased risk of developing Parkinson disease (PD), a disorder of the nerves that affect movement.

Are There Health Effects from Exposure to Secondhand Methamphetamine Smoke?

Researchers don't yet know whether people breathing in secondhand methamphetamine smoke can get high or have other health effects. What they do know is that people can test positive for methamphetamine after exposure to secondhand smoke.

Can a Person Overdose on Methamphetamine?

Yes, a person can overdose on methamphetamine. An overdose occurs when the person uses too much of a drug and has a toxic reaction that results in serious, harmful symptoms or death.

Methamphetamine overdose can lead to stroke, heart attack, or organ problems—such as kidney failure—caused by overheating. These conditions can result in death.

How Can a Methamphetamine Overdose Be Treated?

Because methamphetamine overdose often leads to a stroke, heart attack, or organ problems, first responders and emergency room doctors try to treat the overdose by treating these conditions, with the intent of:

- Restoring blood flow to the affected part of the brain (stroke)

- Restoring blood flow to the heart (heart attack)

- Treating organ problems

Is Methamphetamine Addictive?

Yes, methamphetamine is highly addictive. When people stop taking it, withdrawal symptoms can include:

- Anxiety

- Fatigue

- Severe depression

- Psychosis

- Intense drug cravings

How Can People Get Treatment for Methamphetamine Addiction?

The most effective treatments for methamphetamine addiction so far are behavioral therapies, such as:

- **Cognitive-behavioral therapy (CBT)**, which helps patients recognize, avoid, and cope with the situations in which they are most likely to use drugs

- **Motivational incentives**, which uses vouchers or small cash rewards to encourage patients to remain drug-free

While research is underway, there are no government-approved medications to treat methamphetamine addiction as of now.

Section 28.8

Methylphenidate

This section includes text excerpted from "Methylphenidate," DEA
Diversion Control Division, May 2013. Reviewed January 2019.

Methylphenidate (methyl-alpha-phenyl-2-piperidine-acetate hydrochloride) is a central nervous system (CNS) stimulant that has been
marketed in the United States since the 1950s. For many years, Rit-
alin® (immediate release (IR) product), was the only brand-name
product available. In recent years, other IR, extended release (ER),
and long-acting methylphenidate products have entered the market.
These products are primarily prescribed to children for the treatment
of attention deficit hyperactivity disorder (ADHD).

Domestic and worldwide use of methylphenidate has increased
dramatically since 1990. According to the United Nations' (UN) International Narcotic Control Board (INCB) report, the United States is
the main consumer of methylphenidate accounting for about 69 percent
of the global medical use of methylphenidate in 2011.

Licit Use of Methylphenidate

Methylphenidate is used almost exclusively for the treatment of
ADHD. There is a considerable body of literature on the short-term
efficacy of methylphenidate pharmacotherapy for the treatment of
ADHD. However, attentional improvement is not diagnostic of ADHD.
There is no diagnostic test that can confirm an ADHD diagnosis.

Data suggests that some children may continue to have significant
ADHD-symptoms into adulthood. As a consequence, the prescription
of methylphenidate for individuals 18 and older is the most rapidly
growing market. Longer-acting products, primarily Concerta®, have
gained a significant share of the total methylphenidate market. The
IMS Health National Prescription Audit (NPA) Plus™ reported 15.7
million methylphenidate prescriptions dispensed in 2011 and 16.3
million dispensed in 2012.

Chemistry and Pharmacology of Methylphenidate

Methylphenidate is a CNS stimulant and produces a number of effects including appetite suppression, increased alertness,
and increases in blood pressure, heart rate, respiration, and body

temperature. Almost complete absorption of immediate release (IR) methylphenidate occurs after oral administration with peak plasma levels in about two hours. It is extensively metabolized and about 80 percent of the dose is excreted in the urine as ritalinic acid. Only 20 percent of the administered oral dose is bioavailable due to extensive first-pass metabolism.

Biochemically, methylphenidate enhances the release and blocks the reuptake of dopamine (DA) and norepinephrine (NE) in the mammalian brain. Pharmacologically methylphenidate is most closely related to cocaine. In human subjects, methylphenidate binds to the same receptor sites as cocaine in the brain and produces effects that are indistinguishable from cocaine.

Illicit Use of Methylphenidate

Like other potent stimulants, methylphenidate is abused for its "feel good" stimulant effects. The occasional abuser may use methylphenidate as a study aid to increase attention and stay awake. Others may use methylphenidate recreationally and combine it with alcohol or some other depressant to feel more alert or less drunk. Serious methylphenidate abusers often snort or inject methylphenidate for its intense euphoric effects or to alleviate the severe depression and craving associated with a stimulant withdrawal syndrome.

Monitoring the Future (MTF) is a National Institute on Drug Abuse (NIDA) funded study conducted by the University of Michigan (UM). In 2012, the Monitoring the Future (MTF) survey indicated that 0.7 percent of eighth-grade students, 1.9 percent of tenth-grade students and 2.6 percent of twelfth-grade students reported nonmedical use of Ritalin®.

The National Survey on Drug Use and Health (NSDUH) is a database that measures drug use by noninstitutionalized people age 12 or older living in the United States. In 2011, 4.9 percent of 18- to 25-year olds reported nonmedical use of methylphenidate or Ritalin® in their lifetime. An estimated 4.9 million people (1.9% of the population) age 12 years or older used methylphenidate or Ritalin® for nonmedical purposes in their lifetime, according to the 2011 NSDUH report.

The American Association of Poison Control Centers (AAPCC) report indicates that in 2011, there were a total of 9,798 methylphenidate exposures. Of this total, 5,341 were unintentional exposures and 1,189 were intentional. According to the Drug Abuse Warning Network (DAWN ED), nonmedical use of methylphenidate accounted for an estimated 4,778 visits to the emergency department (ED) in

2010. The number of ED visits associated with nonmedical use of methylphenidate increased to 6,395 in 2011.

The National Forensic Laboratory Information System (NFLIS) is a DEA database that collects scientifically verified data on drug items and cases submitted to and analyzed by state and local forensic laboratories. The System to Retrieve Information from Drug Evidence (STRIDE) provides information on drug seizures reported to and analyzed by DEA laboratories. Of the substance exhibits submitted to federal, state and local forensic laboratories in 2010, there were 2,224 identified as methylphenidate. There were 2,300 exhibits in 2011 and 2,164 exhibits in 2012 which were identified as methylphenidate.

User Population: Methylphenidate

While a wide spectrum of the population has abused methylphenidate products, the primary abusers are individuals younger than 25 years of age; who often obtain methylphenidate from a friend or classmate and use this drug as a study aid or to party.

Illicit Distribution of Methylphenidate

Unlike other potent stimulants, there is no clandestine production of methylphenidate and diverted pharmaceutical products are the only source for abuse purposes. Methylphenidate is obtained from fraudulent prescriptions, doctor shopping, pharmacy theft and from friends or associates who have obtained the drug through.

Control Status of Methylphenidate

Methylphenidate is a Schedule II substance under the Controlled Substances Act (CSA).

Chapter 29

Synthetic Drugs

Chapter Contents

Section 29.1

What Are Synthetic Drugs?

This section includes text excerpted from "About
Synthetic Drugs," DEA Diversion Control Division,
October 20, 2015. Reviewed January 2019.

Drug Enforcement Administration Warning

The U.S. Drug Enforcement Administration (DEA) is warning the
public about the dangers of designer synthetic drugs, also referred
to as "New Psychoactive Substances (NPS)." These substances have
no legitimate industrial or medical use and the misuse and abuse of
these substances represent an emerging and ongoing public-health
and safety threat in the United States. Law enforcement has encountered over 300 NPS, the most prevalent being synthetic cannabinoids
and synthetic cathinones. The manufacture and distribution of these
dangerous substances may result in a prosecutable offense.

Synthetic Cannabinoids

Synthetic cannabinoids are substances that have been encountered
laced on plant material and in liquid form and misused and abused
for their psychoactive effects. They are often sold under names such
as Joker, Green Giant, Scooby Snax, and many others. The misuse
and abuse of these substances may result in serious adverse health
effects including severe agitation and anxiety, racing heartbeat and
high blood pressure, intense hallucinations, and psychotic episodes.
Synthetic cannabinoids have also been connected to overdose deaths.
These products are generally sold over the Internet, in head shops,
tobacco/smoke shops, convenience stores, and gas stations and are
often packaged in shiny plastic bags with bright logos.

Synthetic Cathinones

Synthetic cathinones have stimulant properties related to cathinone, the psychoactive substance found in the khat shrub, and produce
pharmacological effects similar to methamphetamine, cocaine, and
3,4-methylenedioxymethamphetamine (MDMA), to name a few. They
have been sold as "bath salts," and sold over the Internet, at convenience stores, tobacco/smoke shops, and gas stations and packaged
in shiny plastic bags and bright logos. Of late, the cathinone market

has been pushed underground, and is being sold in "traditional drug packaging" such as little baggies, and can be found in tablet, capsule, or powder form. Users can experience symptoms such as nausea, vomiting, paranoia, hallucinations, delusions, suicidal thoughts, seizures, chest pains, increased blood pressure and heart rate, and violent outbursts. These drugs have also resulted in overdose deaths.

One of the synthetic cathinone product encountered is Flakka; sometimes called "Gravel." Flakka is sold as a street deal, like other illegal drugs, not in stores, and can be sold in capsule form or in small baggies. Laboratory analysis has identified the Schedule I controlled substance alpha-pyrrolidinopentiophenone (alpha-PVP) in some of these encounters.

Synthetic Phenethylamines

Synthetic phenethylamines, which mimic hallucinogens, have been encountered as powders, liquid solutions, laced on edible items, and soaked onto blotter papers. Two of the known street names are N-bomb and Smiles. Like Flakka, phenethylamines are not sold over-the-counter (OTC) and are sold like other illegal drugs. The ingestion of extremely small amounts of these substances may result in seizures, cardiac and respiratory arrest, and death.

The DEA continues to monitor and respond to the emergence of new synthetic drugs to protect the public.

Section 29.2

Bath Salts

This section includes text excerpted from "Bath Salts," National Institute on Drug Abuse (NIDA) for Teens, March 2017.

What Are Synthetic Cathinones (Bath Salts)?

Also known as:

- Bloom
- Cloud nine
- Flakka
- Scarface
- Vanilla sky
- White lightning

"Bath salts" is the name given to synthetic cathinones, a class of drugs that have one or more human-made chemicals related to cathinone. Cathinone is a stimulant found naturally in the khat plant, grown in East Africa and southern Arabia. Chemically, cathinones are similar to amphetamines such as methamphetamine and to 3,4-methylenedioxymethamphetamine (MDMA) (Ecstasy or Molly). Common man-made cathinones found in bath salts include 3,4-methylenedioxypyrovalerone (MDPV), mephedrone (Drone, Meph, or Meow Meow), and methylone, but there are many others. These man-made cathinones can be much stronger than the natural product and can be very dangerous.

Bath salts are usually white or brown crystal-like powder and are sold in small plastic or foil packages labeled "Not for Human Consumption." Sometimes labeled as "plant food"—or "jewelry cleaner" or "phone screen cleaner"—they are sold online and in drug product stores. These names or descriptions have nothing to do with the product. It's a way for the drug makers to avoid detection by the U.S. Drug Enforcement Administration (DEA) or local police.

The human-made cathinone products sold as "bath salts" should not be confused with products such as Epsom salts (the original bath salts) that people add to bathwater to help ease stress and relax muscles. Epsom salts are made of a mineral mixture of magnesium and sulfate.

How Bath Salts Are Used

Use of "bath salts" (the drugs) sometimes causes severe intoxication (a person seems very drunk or "out of it") and dangerous health effects. There are also reports of people becoming psychotic (losing touch with reality) and violent. Although it is rare, there have been several cases in which bath salts have been the direct cause of death.

In addition, people who believe they are taking drugs such as MDMA (Molly or ecstasy) may be getting "bath salts" instead. Methylone, a common chemical in bath salts, has been substituted for MDMA in capsules sold as Molly in some areas.

Bath salts can be swallowed, snorted through the nose, inhaled, or injected with a needle. Snorting or injecting is the most harmful.

Banning Bath Salts

At the end of the last decade, bath salts began to be gain in popularity in the United States and Europe as "legal highs." In October 2011, the DEA put an emergency ban on three common human-made cathinones until officials knew more about them. In July 2012, former U.S. President Barack Obama signed legislation permanently banning two of them—mephedrone and MDPV, along with several other human-made drugs often sold as marijuana substitutes (like Spice).

Although the law also bans chemically similar versions of the named drugs, manufacturers have responded by making new drugs different enough from the banned substances to get around the law.

What Happens to Your Brain When You Use Synthetic Cathinones (Bath Salts)?

The human-made cathinones in bath salts can produce:

- Feelings of joy

- Increased social interaction

- Increased sex drive

- Paranoia

- Nervousness

- Hallucinations (see or hear things that are not real)

It is still not known how the different chemicals in bath salts affect the brain. Researchers do know that bath salts are chemically similar to amphetamines, cocaine, and MDMA. Therefore, some of the effects of bath salts—feeling energetic and agitated—are similar. These drugs raise the level of dopamine in brain circuits that control reward and movement. Dopamine is the main neurotransmitter (a substance that passes messages between nerve cells) that makes people feel good when they do something they enjoy. A rush of dopamine causes feelings of joy and increased activity and can also raise heart rate and blood pressure.

A study in animals found that MDPV raises brain dopamine in the same way as cocaine but is at least ten times stronger. If this is also true in people, it may account for the reason that MDPV is the most common man-made cathinone found in the blood and urine of patients admitted to emergency rooms after taking bath salts.

Additionally, the hallucinations often reported by users of bath salts are similar to the effects caused by other drugs such as MDMA or lysergic acid diethylamide (LSD). These drugs raise levels of the neurotransmitter serotonin.

What Happens to Your Body When You Use Synthetic Cathinones (Bath Salts)?

People who take bath salts can experience nosebleeds, sweating, and nausea. But, some of the effects of bath salts are much more serious.

In 2011, bath salts were reported in close to 23,000 emergency room visits. Reports show bath salts users have needed help for heart problems (such as racing heart, high blood pressure, and chest pains) and symptoms like paranoia, hallucinations, and panic attacks.

Some people experience a syndrome known as "excited delirium" after taking bath salts. They may also have dehydration, breakdown of muscle tissue attached to bones, and kidney failure. Intoxication from several man-made cathinones including MDPV, mephedrone, methedrone, and butylone has caused death among some users. Snorting or needle injection of bath salts seems to cause the most harm.

Can You Overdose or Die If You Use Synthetic Cathinones (Bath Salts)?

Yes. Intoxication from several man-made cathinones, including MDPV, mephedrone, methedrone, and butylone, has caused death among some users.

Are Synthetic Cathinones (Bath Salts) Addictive?

Yes. Research shows bath salts are highly addictive. Users have reported that the drugs cause an intense urge to use the drug again. Frequent use may cause tolerance (a person needs to take more to feel the same effects), dependence, and strong withdrawal symptoms when not taking the drug. Withdrawal symptoms may include:

- Depression

- Anxiety

- Tremors

- Problems sleeping

- Paranoia

How Many Teens Use Synthetic Cathinones (Bath Salts)?

Bath salts have been involved in thousands of visits to the emergency room. In 2011 alone, there were 22,904 reports of bath salts use during emergency room visits. About two-thirds of those visits involved bath salts in combination with other drugs.

In addition, poison centers took more than 6,000 calls about exposures to bath salts in 2011. In contrast, there were 266 reported exposures to bath salts in the first half of 2016.

Below is a chart showing the percentage of teens who use bath salts.

Table 29.1. Monitoring the Future Study: Trends in Prevalence of Bath Salts for Eighth Graders, Tenth Graders, and Twelfth Graders; 2018 (In Percent)

Drug	Time Period	Eighth Graders	Tenth Graders	Twelfth Graders
Bath Salts	2014	0.9	0.5	0.6

What Should You Do If Someone You Know Needs Help?

If you, or a friend, are in crisis and need to speak with someone now:

- Call National Suicide Prevention Lifeline (NSPL) at 800-273-8255 (they don't just talk about suicide—they cover a lot of issues and will help put you in touch with someone close by)

If you need information on drug treatment and where you can find it, the Substance Abuse and Mental Health Services Administration (SAMHSA) can help.

- Call Substance Abuse Treatment Facility Locator at 800-662-4357

- Visit the locator online at www.findtreatment.samhsa.gov

Chapter 30

Tobacco, Nicotine, and E-Cigarettes

What Are Tobacco, Nicotine, and E-Cigarette Products?

Also known as:

- **Cigarettes:** Butts, Cigs, and Smokes
- **Smokeless tobacco:** Chew, Dip, Snuff, Snus, and Spit Tobacco
- **Hookah:** Goza, Hubble-bubble, Narghile, Shisha, and Waterpipe

Tobacco is a leafy plant grown around the world, including in parts of the United States. There are many chemicals found in tobacco leaves or created by burning them (as in cigarettes), but nicotine is the ingredient that can lead to addiction. Other chemicals produced by smoking, such as tar, carbon monoxide, acetaldehyde, and nitrosamines, also can cause serious harm to the body. For example, tar causes lung cancer and other serious diseases that affect breathing, and carbon monoxide can cause heart problems.

Teens who are considering smoking for social reasons should keep this in mind:

This chapter includes text excerpted from "Tobacco, Nicotine, and E-Cigarettes," National Institute on Drug Abuse (NIDA) for Teens, December 2018.

- Tobacco use is the leading preventable cause of disease, disability, and death in the United States.

- According to the Centers for Disease Control and Prevention (CDC), cigarettes cause more than 480,000 premature deaths in the United States each year—from smoking or exposure to secondhand smoke—about 1 in every 5 U.S. deaths, or 1,300 deaths every day.

- An additional 16 million people suffer from a serious illness caused by smoking. So, for every 1 person who dies from smoking, 30 more suffer from at least 1 serious tobacco-related illness.

How Tobacco and Nicotine Products Are Used

Tobacco and nicotine products come in many forms. People can smoke, chew, sniff them, or inhale their vapors.

- **Smoked tobacco products.**

- **Cigarettes (regular, light, and menthol).** No evidence exists that "lite" or menthol cigarettes are safer than regular cigarettes.

- **Cigars and pipes.** Some small cigars are hollowed out to make room for marijuana, known as "blunts." Some young people do this to attempt to hid the fact that they are smoking marijuana. Either way, they are inhaling toxic chemicals.

- **Bidis and kreteks (clove cigarettes).** Bidis are small, thin, hand-rolled cigarettes primarily imported to the United States from India and other Southeast Asian countries. Kreteks— sometimes referred to as clove cigarettes—contain about 60 to 80 percent tobacco and 20 to 40 percent ground cloves. Flavored bidis and kreteks are banned in the United States because of the ban on flavored cigarettes.

- **Hookahs or water pipes.** Hookah tobacco comes in many flavors, and the pipe is typically passed around in groups. A study found that a typical hookah session delivers approximately 125 times the smoke, 25 times the tar, 2.5 times the nicotine, and 10 times the carbon monoxide as smoking a cigarette.

- **Smokeless tobacco products.** The tobacco is not burned with these products:

- **Chewing tobacco.** It is typically placed between the cheek and gums.

- **Snuff.** Ground tobacco that can be sniffed if dried or placed between the cheek and gums.

- **Dip.** Moist snuff that is used like chewing tobacco.

- **Snus.** A small pouch of moist snuff.

- **Dissolvable products** (including lozenges, orbs, sticks, and strips).

- **Electronic cigarettes** (also called e-cigarettes, electronic nicotine delivery systems, or e-cigs). Electronic cigarettes are battery-operated devices that deliver nicotine and flavorings without burning tobacco. In most e-cigarettes, puffing activates the battery-powered heating device, which vaporizes the liquid in the cartridge. The resulting vapor is then inhaled (called "vaping").

What Happens in the Brain When You Use Tobacco and Nicotine?

Like other drugs, nicotine increases levels of a neurotransmitter called dopamine. Dopamine is released normally when you experience something pleasurable like good food, your favorite activity, or spending time with people you care about. When a person uses tobacco products, the release of dopamine causes similar effects. This effect wears off quickly, causing people who smoke to get the urge to light up again for more of that good feeling, which can lead to addiction.

A typical smoker will take 10 puffs on a cigarette over the period of about 5 minutes that the cigarette is lit. So, a person who smokes about 1 pack (25 cigarettes) daily gets 250 "hits" of nicotine each day.

Studies suggest that other chemicals in tobacco smoke, such as acetaldehyde, may increase the effects of nicotine on the brain.

When smokeless tobacco is used, nicotine is absorbed through the mouth tissues directly into the blood, where it goes to the brain. Even after the tobacco is removed from the mouth, nicotine continues to be absorbed into the bloodstream. Also, the nicotine stays in the blood longer for users of smokeless tobacco than for smokers.

What Happens to Your Body When You Use Tobacco and Nicotine?

When nicotine enters the body, it initially causes the adrenal glands to release a hormone called adrenaline. The rush of adrenaline stimulates the body and causes an increase in blood pressure, heart rate, and breathing.

Most of the harm to the body is not from the nicotine, but from other chemicals in tobacco or those produced when burning it—including carbon monoxide, tar, formaldehyde, cyanide, and ammonia. Tobacco use harms every organ in the body and can cause many problems. The health effects of smokeless tobacco are somewhat different from those of smoked tobacco, but both can cause cancer.

Secondhand Smoke

People who do not smoke but live or hang out with smokers are exposed to secondhand smoke—exhaled smoke as well as smoke given off by the burning end of tobacco products. Just like smoking, this also increases the risk for many diseases. Each year, an estimated 58 million Americans are regularly exposed to secondhand smoke and more than 42,000 nonsmokers die from diseases caused by secondhand smoke exposure. 1 in 4 U.S. middle and high school students say they've been exposed to unhealthy secondhand aerosol from e-cigarettes.

The chart below lists the health problems people are at risk for when smoking or chewing tobacco or as a result of exposure to secondhand smoke.

Can You Die If You Use Tobacco and Nicotine Products?

Yes. Tobacco use (both smoked and smokeless) is the leading preventable cause of death in the United States. It is a known cause of cancer. Smoking tobacco also can lead to early death from heart disease, health problems in children, and accidental home and building fires caused by dropped cigarettes. In addition, the nicotine in smokeless tobacco may increase the risk for sudden death from a condition where the heart does not beat properly (ventricular arrhythmias); as a result, the heart pumps little or no blood to the body's organs.

According to the CDC, cigarette smoking results in more than 480,000 premature deaths in the United States each year—about 1 in every 5 deaths, or 1,300 deaths every day. On average, smokers die 10 years earlier than nonsmokers. People who smoke are at increased

Table 30.1. Increased Risk of Health Problems

Increased Risk of Health Problems			
Health Effect	**Smoking Tobacco**	**Secondhand Smoke**	**Smokeless Tobacco**
Cancer	Cancers: Cigarette smoking can be blamed for about one-third of all cancer deaths, including 90 percent of lung cancer cases. Tobacco use is also linked with cancers of the mouth, pharynx, larynx, esophagus, stomach, pancreas, cervix, kidney, ureter, bladder, and bone marrow (leukemia).	Lung cancer: People exposed to secondhand smoke increase their risk for lung cancer by 20 percent to 30 percent. About 7,300 lung cancer deaths occur per year among people who do not smoke.	Cancers: Close to 30 chemicals in smokeless tobacco have been found to cause cancer. People who use smokeless tobacco are at increased risk for oral cancer (cancers of the mouth, lip, tongue, and pharynx) as well as esophageal and pancreatic cancers.
Lung Problems	Breathing problems: Bronchitis (swelling of the air passages to the lungs), emphysema (damage to the lungs), and pneumonia have been linked with smoking. Lowered lung capacity: People who smoke can't exercise or play sports for as long as they once did.	Breathing problems: Secondhand smoke causes breathing problems in people who do not smoke, like coughing, phlegm, and lungs not working as well as they should.	
Heart Disease/ Stroke	Heart disease and stroke: Smoking increases the risk for stroke, heart attack, vascular disease (diseases that affect the circulation of blood through the body), and aneurysm (a balloon-like bulge in an artery that can rupture and cause death).	Heart disease: Secondhand smoke increases the risk for heart disease by 25 percent to 30 percent. It is estimated to contribute to as many as 34,000 deaths related to heart disease.	Heart disease and stroke: Research shows smokeless tobacco may play a role in causing heart disease and stroke.

Table 30.1. Continued

Increased Risk of Health Problems			
Health Effect	**Smoking Tobacco**	**Secondhand Smoke**	**Smokeless Tobacco**
Other Health Problems	Cataracts: People who smoke can get cataracts, which is clouding of the eye that causes blurred vision.		Mouth problems: Smokeless tobacco increases the chance of getting cavities, gum disease, and sores in the mouth that can make eating and drinking painful.
	Loss of sense of smell and taste		
	Aging skin and teeth: After smoking for a long time, people find their skin ages faster and their teeth discolor.		
Pregnant Women and Children	Pregnant women: Pregnant women who smoke are at increased risk for delivering their baby early or suffering a miscarriage, stillbirth, or experiencing other problems with their pregnancy. Smoking by pregnant women also may be associated with learning and behavior problems in children.	Health problems for children: Children exposed to secondhand smoke are at an increased risk for sudden infant death syndrome, lung infections, ear problems, and more severe asthma.	
Accidental Death	Fire-related deaths: Smoking is the leading cause of fire-related deaths—more than 600 deaths each year.		

risk of death from cancer, particularly lung cancer, heart disease, lung diseases, and accidental injury from fires started by dropped cigarettes.

The good news is that people who quit may live longer. A 24-year-old man who quits smoking will, on average, increase his life expectancy (how long he is likely to live) by 5 years.

Are Tobacco or Nicotine Products Addictive?

Yes. It is the nicotine in tobacco that is addictive. Each cigarette contains about 10 milligrams of nicotine. A person inhales only some of the smoke from a cigarette, and not all of each puff is absorbed in the lungs. The average person gets about 1 to 2 milligrams of the drug from each cigarette.

Studies of widely used brands of smokeless tobacco showed that the amount of nicotine per gram of tobacco ranges from 4.4 milligrams to 25.0 milligrams. Holding an average-size dip in your mouth for 30 minutes gives you as much nicotine as smoking 3 cigarettes. A 2-can-a-week snuff dipper gets as much nicotine as a person who smokes 1½ packs a day.

Whether a person smokes tobacco products or uses smokeless tobacco, the amount of nicotine absorbed in the body is enough to make someone addicted. When this happens, the person continues to seek out the tobacco even though he or she understands the harm it causes. Nicotine addiction can cause:

- **Tolerance.** Over the course of a day, someone who uses tobacco products develops tolerance—more nicotine is required to produce the same initial effects. In fact, people who smoke often report that the first cigarette of the day is the strongest or the "best."

- **Withdrawal.** When people quit using tobacco products, they usually experience uncomfortable withdrawal symptoms, which often drive them back to tobacco use. Nicotine withdrawal symptoms include:

  - Irritability

  - Problems with thinking and paying attention

  - Sleep problems

  - Increased appetite

  - Craving, which may last six months or longer, and can be a major stumbling block to quitting

What about E-Cigarettes?

E-cigarettes are fairly new products. They've only been around for about ten years, so researchers are in the early stage of studying how they affect your health.

How E-Cigarettes Work

E-cigarettes are designed to deliver nicotine without the other chemicals produced by burning tobacco leaves. Puffing on the mouthpiece of the cartridge activates a battery-powered inhalation device (called a vaporizer). The vaporizer heats the liquid inside the cartridge which contains nicotine, flavors, and other chemicals. The heated liquid turns into an aerosol (vapor) which the user inhales—referred to as "vaping."

How E-Cigarettes Affect the Brain

E-cigarettes may be less harmful than regular tobacco cigarettes because users do not inhale burning smoke, which has cancer-causing and other harmful ingredients. But we don't yet have enough research to show potential harmful effects of the vaping mist. Also, research shows that many teens start smoking regular cigarettes soon after being introduced to nicotine through electronic vaporizers. It is important to remember that nicotine in any form is a highly addictive drug. Health experts have raised many questions about the safety of these products, particularly for teens:

- Testing of some e-cigarette products found the aerosol (vapor) to contain known cancer-causing and toxic chemicals, and particles from the vaporizing mechanism that may be harmful. The health effects of repeated exposure to these chemicals are not yet clear.

- There is animal research which shows that nicotine exposure may cause changes in the brain that make other drugs more rewarding. If this is true in humans, as some experts believe, it would mean that using nicotine in any form would increase the risk of other drug use and for addiction.

- Some research suggests that e-cigarette use may serve as a "gateway" or introductory product for youth to try other tobacco products, including regular cigarettes, which are known to cause disease and lead to early death. A study showed that students who have used e-cigarettes by the time they start ninth grade are more likely than others to start smoking traditional cigarettes and other smoked tobacco products within the next year.

- The liquid in e-cigarettes can cause nicotine poisoning if someone drinks, sniffs, or touches it. Recently there has been a surge of poisoning cases in children under age 5. There is also a concern for users changing cartridges and for pets.

- Some research shows that secondhand e-cig vapor pollutes the air quality with particles that could harm the lungs and heart.

- Some research suggests that certain brands of e-cigs contain metals such as nickel and chromium, possibly coming from the heating of coils.

Regulation of E-Cigarettes

Yes. The U.S. Food and Drug Administration (FDA) announced in 2016 that the FDA will now regulate the sales of e-cigarettes, hookah tobacco, and cigars. Therefore:

- It is now illegal to sell e-cigarettes, hookah tobacco, or cigars in person or online to anyone under age 18

- Buyers have to show their photo identification (ID) to purchase e-cigarettes, hookah tobacco, or cigars, verifying that they are 18 years or older

- These products cannot be sold in vending machines (unless in an adult-only facility)

- It is illegal to hand out free samples

The FDA regulation also means that the federal government will now have a lot more information about what is in e-cigarettes, the safety or harms of the ingredients, how they are made, and what risks need to be communicated to the public (for example, on health warnings on the product and in advertisements). They will also be able to stop manufacturers from making statements about their products that are not scientifically proven.

Regulation does not mean that e-cigarettes are necessarily safe for all adults to use, or that all of the health claims currently being made in advertisements by manufactures are true. But it does mean that e-cigarettes, hookah tobacco, and cigars now have to follow the same type of rules as cigarette manufacturers.

How Many Teens Use Tobacco and Nicotine Products?

Smoking and smokeless tobacco use generally start during the teen years. Among people who use tobacco:

- Each day, nearly 3,200 people younger than 18 years of age smoke their first cigarette.

- Every day, an estimated 2,100 youth and young adults who have been occasional smokers become daily cigarette smokers.

- If smoking continues at the current rate among youth in this country, 5.6 million of Americans under the age of 18—or about 1 in every 13 young people—could die prematurely (too early) from a smoking-related illness.

- E-cigarettes are the most commonly used form of tobacco among youth in the United States.

- Young people who use e-cigs or smokeless tobacco may be more likely to also become smokers.

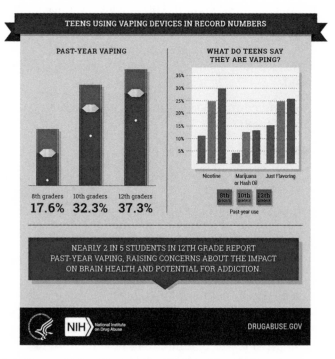

Figure 30.1. *Teens Using Vaping Devices in Record Numbers*

- Using smokeless tobacco remains a mostly male behavior. About 490,000 teens ages 12 to 17 are current smokeless tobacco users. For every 100 teens who use smokeless tobacco, 85 of them are boys.

A survey of teens in the United States shows nicotine vaping is on the rise, raising concerns about the impact of nicotine on brain health and the potential for addiction.

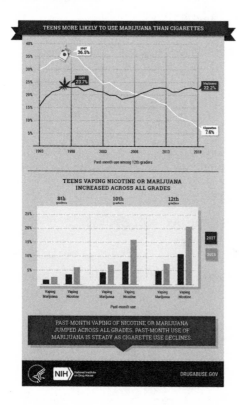

Figure 30.2. *Teens More Likely to Use Marijuana Than Cigarettes*

What Do I Do If I Want to Quit Using Tobacco and Nicotine Products?

Treatments can help people who use tobacco products manage these symptoms and improve the likelihood of successfully quitting. For now, teen and young adult smokers who want to quit have good options for help.

Nearly 70 percent of people who smoke want to quit. Most who try to quit on their own relapse (go back to smoking)—often within a week. Most former smokers have had several failed quit attempts before they finally succeed.

Some people believe e-cigarette products may help smokers lower nicotine cravings while they are trying to quit smoking cigarettes. However, several research studies show that using electronic devices to help quit cigarette smoking does not usually work in the long term, and might actually discourage people from quitting. One study showed that only nine percent of people using e-vaporizers to quit smoking cigarettes had actually stopped smoking a year later.

If you or someone you know needs more information or is ready to quit, check out these resources:

Teens

• Visit SmokeFree.gov.

Adults

• Call 800-QUIT-NOW (800-784-8669), a national toll-free number that can help people get the information they need to quit smoking.

• Visit SmokeFree.gov.

Table 30.2 shows the percentage of teens who use tobacco and nicotine products.

Table 30.2. Monitoring the Future Study: Trends in Prevalence of Various Drugs for Eighth Graders, Tenth Graders, and Twelfth Graders; 2018 (In Percent)*

Drug	Time Period	Eighth Graders	Tenth Graders	Twelfth Graders
Cigarettes (any use)	Lifetime	9.1	16	[23.8]
	Past month	2.2	4.2	[7.60]
	Daily	0.8	1.8	3.6
	1/2-pack+/day	0.3	0.7	1.5
Smokeless Tobacco	Lifetime	6.4	10	10.1
	Past month	2.1	3.9	4.2
	Daily	0.3	1	1.6
Any Vaping	Lifetime	[21.50]	[36.90]	[42.50]
	Past year	[17.60]	[32.30]	[37.30]
	Past month	[10.40]	[21.70]	[26.70]

* Data in brackets indicate statistically significant change from the previous year

Part Four

The Causes and Consequences of Drug Abuse and Addiction

Chapter 31

Drug Addiction Is a Chronic Disease

Sometimes it's hard for friends and family members to understand why their loved one can't just quit using the substance that is hurting them. The reason it's so difficult for people struggling with drug or alcohol addiction is that it isn't just a habit—it's a disease.

When a person takes drugs or drinks alcohol over a period of time, it can change their brain circuits. In fact, addiction changes the way that crucial parts of the brain function so much that the person has a very hard time stopping their use of drugs or alcohol—even when they want to do so.

Addiction Beats up Your Brain

Brain-science research has shown that addiction harms the brain in at least three ways:

- **It makes the brain's reward circuits less sensitive.**
  Addictive drugs cause the brain to release dopamine, a chemical that makes a person feel pleasure. If the person continues to take the drug over time, however, the circuit can become imbalanced. To get the same reward they got when they first used the drug, they need to take larger amounts of it. And

---

This chapter includes text excerpted from "Addiction Is a Disease," National Institute on Drug Abuse (NIDA) for Teens, March 29, 2016.

natural rewards no longer give the person pleasure, but instead cause them to lose interest in things they used to enjoy, such as spending time with friends.

- **It increases the brain's reaction to stress.** Some brain circuits control our responses to stressful situations. In the brain of a person with addiction, that system of circuits becomes overactive, making people feel very stressed when they aren't using drugs.

- **It weakens regions of the brain that help a person make good decisions.** Drug addiction also affects the prefrontal cortex (PFC), the part of the brain that helps a person make decisions and control their impulses. It's as if their car has worn-out brake pads: even if they try to stop using the drug, they may not be able to control their impulses and may take the drug anyway.

While many factors influence whether or not a person will become addicted to drugs or alcohol, teens are especially at risk. A person's brain doesn't stop developing until they're in their early twenties; until then, their brain's circuits are especially sensitive to the effects of drugs.

Treating the Disease

Understanding addiction as a disease that changes the brain is helping researchers develop better treatments for it. Many people need help to overcome addiction. This doesn't mean they're weak; it means they're fighting an illness that is tough (but not impossible!) to overcome.

Chapter 32

Common Risk and Protective Factors for Drug Use

Assessing the risk and protective factors that contribute to substance-use disorders (SUDs) helps practitioners select appropriate interventions.

Many factors influence a person's chance of developing a mental- or substance-use disorder. Effective prevention focuses on reducing those risk factors and strengthening protective factors that are most closely related to the problem being addressed. Applying the Strategic Prevention Framework (SPF) helps prevention professionals identify factors having the greatest impact on their target population.

- **Risk factors** are characteristics at the biological, psychological, family, community, or cultural level that precede and are associated with a higher likelihood of negative outcomes.

- **Protective factors** are characteristics associated with a lower likelihood of negative outcomes or that reduce a risk factor impact. Protective factors may be seen as positive countering events.

Some risk and protective factors are fixed; they don't change over time. Other risk and protective factors are considered variable and can change over time.

This chapter includes text excerpted from "Risk and Protective Factors," Substance Abuse and Mental Health Services Administration (SAMHSA), August 13, 2018.

- **Variable risk factors** include income level, peer group, adverse childhood experiences (ACEs), and employment status.

- **Individual-level risk factors** may include a person's genetic predisposition to addiction or exposure to alcohol prenatally.

- **Individual-level protective factors** might include positive self-image, self-control, or social competence.

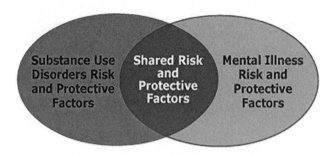

Figure 32.1. *Shared Risk and Protective Factors*

Key Features of Risk and Protective Factors

Prevention professionals should consider these key features of risk and protective factors when designing and evaluating prevention interventions. Then, prioritize the risk and protective factors that most impact your community.

Risk and Protective Factors Exist in Multiple Contexts

All people have biological and psychological characteristics that make them vulnerable to, or resilient in the face of, potential behavioral-health issues. Because people have relationships within their communities and larger society, each person's biological and psychological characteristics exist in multiple contexts. A variety of risk and protective factors operate within each of these contexts. These factors also influence one another.

Targeting only one context when addressing a person's risk or protective factors is unlikely to be successful because people don't exist in isolation. For example:

- **In relationships,** risk factors include parents who use drugs and alcohol or who suffer from mental illness, child abuse and maltreatment, and inadequate supervision. In this context, parental involvement is an example of a protective factor.

- **In communities,** risk factors include neighborhood poverty and violence. Here, protective factors could include the availability of faith-based resources and after-school activities.

- **In society,** risk factors can include norms and laws favorable to substance use, as well as racism and a lack of economic opportunity. Protective factors in this context would include hate-crime laws or policies limiting the availability of alcohol.

Risk and Protective Factors Are Correlated and Cumulative

Risk factors tend to be positively correlated with one another and negatively correlated to protective factors. In other words, people with some risk factors have a greater chance of experiencing even more risk factors, and they are less likely to have protective factors.

Risk and protective factors also tend to have a cumulative effect on the development—or reduced development—of behavioral-health issues. Young people with multiple risk factors have a greater likelihood of developing a condition that impacts their physical or mental health; young people with multiple protective factors are at a reduced risk.

These correlations underscore the importance of:

- Early intervention
- Interventions that target multiple, not single, factors

Individual Factors Can Be Associated with Multiple Outcomes

Though preventive interventions are often designed to produce a single outcome, both risk and protective factors can be associated with multiple outcomes. For example, negative life events are associated with substance use as well as anxiety, depression, and other behavioral-health issues. Prevention efforts targeting a set of risk or protective factors have the potential to produce positive effects in multiple areas.

Risk and Protective Factors Are Influential Over Time

Risk and protective factors can have influence throughout a person's entire lifespan. For example, risk factors such as poverty and family dysfunction can contribute to the development of mental and/or SUDs later in life. Risk and protective factors within one particular context—such as the family—may also influence or be influenced by factors in another context. Effective parenting has been shown to mediate the effects of multiple risk factors, including poverty, divorce, parental bereavement, and parental mental illness.

Universal, Selective, and Indicated Prevention Interventions

Not all people or populations are at the same risk of developing behavioral-health problems. Prevention interventions are most effective when they are matched to their target population's level of risk. Prevention interventions fall into three broad categories:

- **Universal preventive interventions** take the broadest approach and are designed to reach entire groups or populations. Universal prevention interventions might target schools, whole communities, or workplaces.

- **Selective interventions** target biological, psychological, or social risk factors that are more prominent among high-risk groups than among the wider population. Examples include prevention education for immigrant families with young children or peer support groups for adults with a family history of SUDs.

- **Indicated preventive interventions** target individuals who show signs of being at risk for a SUD. These types of interventions include referral to support services for young adults who violate drug policies or screening and consultation for families of older adults admitted to hospitals with potential alcohol-related injuries.

Chapter 33

Prescription and Over-the-Counter Drug Abuse

Chapter Contents

Section 33.1

Causes and Prevalence of Prescription-Drug Misuse

This Section includes text excerpted from "Misuse of Prescription Drugs," National Institute on Drug Abuse (NIDA), January 2018.

Misuse of prescription drugs means taking medication in a manner or dose other than prescribed; taking someone else's prescription, even if for a legitimate medical complaint such as pain; or taking a medication to feel euphoria (i.e., to get high). The phrase "nonmedical use of prescription drugs" also refers to these categories of misuse. The three classes of medication most commonly misused are:

- **Opioids**—usually prescribed to treat pain

- **Central nervous system (CNS) depressants** (this category includes tranquilizers, sedatives, and hypnotics)—used to treat anxiety and sleep disorders

- **Stimulants**—most often prescribed to treat attention deficit hyperactivity disorder (ADHD)

Prescription-drug misuse can have serious medical consequences. Increases in prescription-drug misuse over the last 15 years are reflected in increased emergency room visits, overdose deaths associated with prescription drugs, and treatment admissions for prescription-drug-use disorders, the most severe form of which is an addiction. Overdose deaths involving prescription opioids were 5 times higher in 2016 than in 1999.

What Is the Scope of Prescription-Drug Misuse?

Misuse of prescription opioids, CNS depressants, and stimulants is a serious public-health problem in the United States. Although most people take prescription medications responsibly, in 2017, an estimated 18 million people (more than 6% of those age 12 and older) misused such medications at least once in the past year. According to results from the 2017 National Survey on Drug Use and Health (NSDUH), an estimated 2 million Americans misused prescription pain relievers for the first time within the past year, which averages to approximately 5,480 initiates per day. Additionally, more than one million misused prescription stimulants, 1.5 million misused tranquilizers, and 271,000 misused sedatives for the first time.

The reasons for the high prevalence of prescription-drug misuse vary by age, gender, and other factors, but likely include ease of access. The number of prescriptions for some of these medications has increased dramatically since the early 1990s. Moreover, misinformation about the addictive properties of prescription opioids and the perception that prescription drugs are less harmful than illicit drugs are other possible contributors to the problem. Although misuse of prescription drugs affects many Americans, certain populations such as youth and older adults may be at particular risk.

Adolescents and Young Adults

Misuse of prescription drugs is highest among young adults age 18 to 25, with 14.4 percent reporting nonmedical use in the past year. Among youth age 12 to 17, 4.9 percent reported past-year nonmedical use of prescription medications.

After alcohol, marijuana, and tobacco, prescription drugs (taken nonmedically) are among the most commonly used drugs by twelfth graders. The National Institute on Drug Abuse (NIDA) Monitoring the Future survey of substance use and attitudes in teens found that about 6 percent of high-school seniors reported past-year nonmedical use of the prescription stimulant Adderall® in 2017, and 2 percent reported misusing the opioid pain reliever Vicodin®.

Although past-year nonmedical use of CNS depressants has remained fairly stable among twelfth graders since 2012, use of prescription opioids has declined sharply. For example, past-year nonmedical use of Vicodin among twelfth graders was reported by 9.6 percent in 2002 and declined to 2.0 percent in 2017. Nonmedical use of Adderall® increased between 2009 and 2013 but has decreased through 2017. When asked how they obtained prescription stimulants for nonmedical use, around 60 percent of the adolescents and young adults surveyed said they either bought or received the drugs from a friend or relative.

Youth who misuse prescription medications are also more likely to report the use of other drugs. Multiple studies have revealed associations between prescription-drug misuse and higher rates of cigarette smoking; heavy episodic drinking; and marijuana, cocaine, and other illicit-drug use among U.S. adolescents, young adults, and college students. In the case of prescription opioids,

347

receiving a legitimate prescription for these drugs during adolescence is also associated with a greater risk of future opioid misuse, particularly in young adults who have little to no history of drug use.

Older Adults

More than 80 percent of older patients (ages 57 to 85 years) use at least one prescription medication on a daily basis, with more than 50 percent taking more than five medications or supplements daily. This can potentially lead to health issues resulting from unintentionally using the prescription medication in a manner other than how it was prescribed, or from intentional nonmedical use. The high rates of multiple (comorbid) chronic illnesses in older populations, age-related changes in drug metabolism, and the potential for drug interactions make medication (and other substance) misuse more dangerous in older people than in younger populations. Further, a large percentage of older adults also use over-the-counter (OTC) medicines and dietary and herbal supplements, which could compound any adverse health consequences resulting from nonmedical use of prescription drugs.

Is It Safe to Use Prescription Drugs in Combination with Other Medications?

The safety of using prescription drugs in combination with other substances depends on a number of factors, including the types of medications, dosages, other substance use (e.g., alcohol), and individual patient-health factors. Patients should talk with their healthcare provider about whether they can safely use their prescription drugs with other substances, including prescription and OTC medications, as well as alcohol, tobacco, and illicit drugs. Specifically, drugs that slow down the breathing rate, such as opioids, alcohol, antihistamines, CNS depressants, or general anesthetics, should not be taken together because these combinations increase the risk of life-threatening respiratory depression. Stimulants should also not be used with other medications unless recommended by a physician. Patients should be aware of the dangers associated with mixing stimulants and OTC cold medicines that contain decongestants, as combining these substances may cause blood pressure to become dangerously high or lead to irregular heart rhythms.

What Classes of Prescription Drugs Are Commonly Misused?
What Are Opioids?

Opioids are medications that act on opioid receptors in both the spinal cord and brain to reduce the intensity of pain-signal perception. They also affect brain areas that control emotion, which can further diminish the effects of painful stimuli. They have been used for centuries to treat pain, cough, and diarrhea. The most common modern use of opioids is to treat acute pain. However, since the 1990s, they have been increasingly used to treat chronic pain, despite sparse evidence for their effectiveness when used long term. Indeed, some patients experience a worsening of their pain or increased sensitivity to pain as a result of treatment with opioids, a phenomenon known as "hyperalgesia."

Importantly, in addition to relieving pain, opioids also activate reward regions in the brain causing the euphoria—or high—that underlies the potential for misuse and substance-use disorder (SUD). Chemically, these medications are very similar to heroin, which was originally synthesized from morphine as a pharmaceutical in the late nineteenth century. These properties confer an increased risk of SUD even in patients who take their medication as prescribed.

Overdose is another significant danger with opioids, because these compounds also interact with parts of the brainstem that control breathing. Taking too much of an opioid can suppress breathing enough that the user suffocates. An overdose can be reversed (and fatality prevented) if the compound naloxone is administered quickly.

Prescription opioid medications include hydrocodone (e.g., Vicodin®), oxycodone (e.g., OxyContin®, Percocet®), oxymorphone (e.g., Opana®), morphine (e.g., Kadian®, Avinza®), codeine, fentanyl, and others. Hydrocodone products are the most commonly prescribed in the United States for a variety of indications, including dental- and injury-related pain. Oxycodone and oxymorphone are also prescribed for moderate to severe pain relief. Morphine is often used before and after surgical procedures to alleviate severe pain, and codeine is typically prescribed for milder pain. In addition to their pain-relieving properties, some of these drugs—codeine and diphenoxylate (Lomotil®), for example—are used to relieve coughs and severe diarrhea.

How Do Opioids Affect the Brain and Body?

Opioids act by attaching to and activating opioid-receptor proteins, which are found on nerve cells in the brain, spinal cord, gastrointestinal (GI) tract, and other organs in the body. When these drugs attach to their receptors, they inhibit the transmission of pain signals. Opioids can also produce drowsiness, mental confusion, nausea, constipation, and respiratory depression, and since these drugs also act on brain regions involved in reward, they can induce euphoria, particularly when they are taken at a higher-than-prescribed dose or administered in other ways than intended. For example, OxyContin® is an oral medication used to treat moderate to severe pain through a slow, steady release of the opioid. Some people who misuse OxyContin® intensify their experience by snorting or injecting it. This is a very dangerous practice, greatly increasing the person's risk for serious medical complications, including overdose.

What Are the Possible Consequences of Prescription Opioid Misuse?

When taken as prescribed, patients can often use opioids to manage pain safely and effectively. However, it is possible to develop a SUD when taking opioid medications as prescribed. This risk and the risk for overdose increase when these medications are misused. Even a single large dose of an opioid can cause severe respiratory depression (slowing or stopping of breathing), which can be fatal; taking opioids with alcohol or sedatives increases this risk.

When properly managed, short-term medical use of opioid pain relievers—taken for a few days following oral surgery, for instance—rarely leads to an opioid-use disorder or addiction. But regular (e.g., several times a day, for several weeks or more) or longer-term use of opioids can lead to dependence (physical discomfort when not taking the drug), tolerance (diminished effect from the original dose, leading to increasing the amount taken), and, in some cases, addiction (compulsive drug-seeking and use). With both dependence and addiction, withdrawal symptoms may occur if drug use is suddenly reduced or stopped. These symptoms may include restlessness, muscle and bone pain, insomnia, diarrhea, vomiting, cold flashes with goosebumps, and involuntary leg movements.

Misuse of prescription opioids is also a risk factor for transitioning to heroin use.

Understanding Dependence, Addiction, and Tolerance

Dependence occurs as a result of physiological adaptations to chronic exposure to a drug. It is often a part of addiction, but they are not equivalent. Addiction involves other changes to brain circuitry and is distinguished by compulsive drug-seeking and use despite negative consequences.

Those who are dependent on a medication will experience unpleasant physical withdrawal symptoms when they abruptly reduce or stop use of the drug. These symptoms can be mild to severe (depending on the drug) and can usually be managed medically or avoided by slowly tapering down the drug dosage.

Tolerance, or the need to take higher doses of a medication to get the same effect, often accompanies dependence. When tolerance occurs, it can be difficult for a physician to evaluate whether a patient is developing a drug problem or has a medical need for higher doses to control his or her symptoms. For this reason, physicians should be vigilant and attentive to their patients' symptoms and level of functioning and should screen for substance misuse when tolerance or dependence is present.

How Is Prescription Opioid Misuse Related to Chronic Pain?

Healthcare providers have long wrestled with how best to treat the more than 100 million Americans who suffer from chronic pain. Opioids have been the most common treatment for chronic pain since the late 1990s, but research has cast doubt both on their safety and their efficacy in the treatment of chronic pain when it is not related to cancer or palliative care. The potential risks involved with long-term opioid treatment, such as the development of drug tolerance, hyperalgesia, and addiction, present doctors with a dilemma, as there is limited research on alternative treatments for chronic pain. Patients themselves may even be reluctant to take an opioid medication prescribed to them for fear of becoming addicted.

Estimates of the rate of opioid misuse among chronic-pain patients vary widely as a result of differences in treatment duration, insufficient research on long-term outcomes, disparate study populations, and different outcome measures (e.g., dependence versus OUD or addiction). One study assessing current criteria for opioid-use disorder (OUD) in a large number of chronic pain patients receiving opioids found that 28.1 percent had mild OUD, 9.7 percent had moderate OUD, and 3.5 percent had severe OUD (addiction).

To mitigate addiction risk, physicians should adhere to the Centers for Disease Control and Prevention (CDC) Guideline for Prescribing Opioids for Chronic Pain. Before prescribing, physicians should assess pain and functioning, consider if nonopioid treatment options are appropriate, discuss a treatment plan with the patient, evaluate the patient's risk of harm or misuse, and co-prescribe naloxone to mitigate the risk for overdose. When first prescribing opioids, physicians should give the lowest effective dose for the shortest therapeutic duration. As treatment continues, the patient should be monitored at regular intervals, and opioid treatment should be continued only if meaningful clinical improvements in pain and functioning are seen without harm.

What Are Central Nervous System Depressants?

Central nervous system (CNS) depressants, a category that includes tranquilizers, sedatives, and hypnotics, are substances that can slow brain activity. This property makes them useful for treating anxiety and sleep disorders. The following are among the medications commonly prescribed for these purposes:

- **Benzodiazepines,** such as diazepam (Valium®), clonazepam (Klonopin®), and alprazolam (Xanax®), are sometimes prescribed to treat anxiety, acute stress reactions, and panic attacks. Clonazepam may also be prescribed to treat seizure disorders and insomnia. The more sedating benzodiazepines, such as triazolam (Halcion®) and estazolam (Prosom®) are prescribed for short-term treatment of sleep disorders. Usually, benzodiazepines are not prescribed for long-term use because of the high risk for developing tolerance, dependence, or addiction.

- **Nonbenzodiazepine sleep medications,** such as zolpidem (Ambien®), eszopiclone (Lunesta®), and zaleplon (Sonata®), known as z-drugs, have a different chemical structure but act on the same gamma-aminobutyric acid (GABA) type A receptors in the brain as benzodiazepines. They are thought to have fewer side effects and less risk of dependence than benzodiazepines.

- **Barbiturates,** such as mephobarbital (Mebaral®), phenobarbital (Luminal®), and pentobarbital sodium (Nembutal®), are used less frequently to reduce anxiety or to help with sleep problems because of their higher risk of overdose compared to benzodiazepines. However, they are still used in surgical procedures and to treat seizure disorders.

352

How Do Central Nervous System Depressants Affect the Brain and Body?

Most CNS depressants act on the brain by increasing activity at receptors for the inhibitory neurotransmitter GABA. Although the different classes of CNS depressants work in unique ways, it is through their ability to increase GABA signaling—thereby increasing inhibition of brain activity—that they produce a drowsy or calming effect that is medically beneficial to those suffering from anxiety or sleep disorders.

What Are the Possible Consequences of CNS Depressant Misuse?

Despite their beneficial therapeutic effects, benzodiazepines and barbiturates have the potential for misuse and should be used only as prescribed. The use of nonbenzodiazepine sleep aids, or Z-drugs, is less well-studied, but certain indicators have raised concern about their misuse potential as well.

During the first few days of taking a depressant, a person usually feels sleepy and uncoordinated, but as the body becomes accustomed to the effects of the drug and tolerance develops, these side effects begin to disappear. If one uses these drugs long term, he or she may need larger doses to achieve the therapeutic effects. Continued use can also lead to dependence and withdrawal when use is abruptly reduced or stopped. Because CNS depressants work by slowing the brain's activity, when an individual stops taking them, there can be a rebound effect, resulting in seizures or other harmful consequences.

Although withdrawal from benzodiazepines can be problematic, it is rarely life threatening, whereas withdrawal from prolonged use of barbiturates can have life-threatening complications. Therefore, someone who is thinking about discontinuing a CNS depressant or who is suffering withdrawal after discontinuing use should speak with a physician or seek immediate medical treatment.

What Are Stimulants?

Stimulants increase alertness, attention, and energy, as well as elevate blood pressure, heart rate, and respiration. Historically, stimulants were used to treat asthma and other respiratory problems, obesity, neurological disorders, and a variety of other ailments. But as their potential for misuse and addiction became apparent, the number of conditions treated with stimulants has decreased. Now, stimulants are prescribed for the treatment of only a few health conditions, including attention deficit hyperactivity disorder (ADHD), narcolepsy, and occasionally treatment-resistant depression.

How Do Stimulants Affect the Brain and Body?

Stimulants, such as dextroamphetamine (Dexedrine®, Adderall®) and methylphenidate (Ritalin®, Concerta®), act in the brain on the family of monoamine neurotransmitter systems, which include norepinephrine and dopamine. Stimulants enhance the effects of these chemicals. An increase in dopamine signaling from nonmedical use of stimulants can induce a feeling of euphoria, and these medications' effects on norepinephrine increase blood pressure and heart rate, constrict blood vessels, increase blood glucose, and open up breathing passages.

What Are the Possible Consequences of Stimulant Misuse?

As with other drugs in the stimulant category, such as cocaine, it is possible for people to become dependent on or addicted to prescription stimulants. Withdrawal symptoms associated with discontinuing stimulant use include fatigue, depression, and disturbed sleep patterns. Repeated misuse of some stimulants (sometimes within a short period) can lead to feelings of hostility or paranoia or even psychosis. Further, taking high doses of a stimulant may result in dangerously high body temperature and an irregular heartbeat. There is also the potential for cardiovascular failure or seizures.

Cognitive Enhancers

The dramatic increases in stimulant prescriptions over the last two decades have led to their greater availability and to increased risk for diversion and nonmedical use. When taken to improve properly diagnosed conditions, these medications can greatly enhance a patient's quality of life (QOL). However, because many perceive them to be generally safe and effective, prescription stimulants such as Adderall® and Modafinil® are being misused more frequently.

Stimulants increase wakefulness, motivation, and aspects of cognition, learning, and memory. Some people take these drugs in the absence of medical need in an effort to enhance mental performance. Militaries have long used stimulants to increase performance in the

354

face of fatigue, and the U.S. Armed Forces allow for their use in limited operational settings. The practice is now reported by some professionals to increase their productivity, by older people to offset declining cognition, and by both high-school and college students to improve their academic performance.

Nonmedical use of stimulants for cognitive enhancement poses potential health risks, including addiction, cardiovascular events, and psychosis. The use of pharmaceuticals for cognitive enhancement has also sparked debate over the ethical implications of the practice. Issues of fairness arise if those with access and willingness to take these drugs have a performance edge over others, and implicit coercion takes place if a culture of cognitive enhancement gives the impression that a person must take drugs in order to be competitive.

Section 33.2

Over-the-Counter Medicines and Their Misuse

This Section includes text excerpted from
"Over-the-Counter Medicines," National Institute on
Drug Abuse (NIDA), December 2017.

What Are Over-the-Counter Medicines?

Over-the-counter (OTC) medicines are those that can be sold directly to people without a prescription. OTC medicines treat a variety of illnesses and their symptoms including pain, coughs and colds, diarrhea, constipation, acne, and others. Some OTC medicines have active ingredients with the potential for misuse at higher-than-recommended dosages.

How Do People Use and Misuse Over-the-Counter Medicines?

Misuse of an OTC medicine means:

- Taking medicine in a way or dose other than directed on the package

- Taking medicine for the effect it causes- for example, to get high

- Mixing OTC medicines together to create new products

What Are Some of the Commonly Misused Over-the-Counter Medicines?

There are two OTC medicines that are most commonly misused.

Dextromethorphan (DXM) is a cough suppressant found in many OTC cold medicines. The most common sources of abused DXM are "extra-strength" cough syrup, tablets, and gel capsules. OTC medications that contain DXM often also contain antihistamines and decongestants. DXM may be swallowed in its original form or may be mixed with soda for flavor, called "robotripping" or "skittling." Users sometimes inject it. These medicines are often misused in combination with other drugs, such as alcohol and marijuana.

Loperamide is an antidiarrheal that is available in tablet, capsule, or liquid form. When misusing loperamide, people swallow large quantities of the medicine. It is unclear how often this drug is misused.

"Behind-the-Counter"

Pseudoephedrine, a nasal decongestant found in many OTC cold medicines, can be used to make methamphetamine. For this reason, products containing pseudoephedrine are sold "behind the counter" nationwide. A prescription is not needed in most states, but in states that do require a prescription, there are limits on how much a person can buy each month. In some states, only people 18 years of age or older can buy pseudoephedrine.

How Do These Over-the-Counter Medicines Affect the Brain?

DXM is an opioid without effects on pain reduction and does not act on the opioid receptors. When taken in large doses, DXM causes a depressant effect and sometimes a hallucinogenic effect, similar to Phencyclidine (PCP) and ketamine. Repeatedly seeking to experience that feeling can lead to addiction-a chronic relapsing brain condition characterized by inability to stop using a drug despite damaging consequences to a person's life and health.

Loperamide is an opioid designed not to enter the brain. However, when taken in large amounts and combined with other substances, it may cause the drug to act in a similar way to other opioids. Other opioids, such as certain prescription pain relievers and heroin, bind to and activate opioid receptors in many areas of the brain, especially those involved in feelings of pain and pleasure. Opioid receptors are also located in the brain stem, which controls important processes, such as blood pressure, arousal, and breathing.

What Are the Health Effects of These Over-the-Counter Medicines?

DXM—Short-term effects of DXM misuse can range from mild stimulation to alcohol- or marijuana-like intoxication. At high doses, a person may have hallucinations or feelings of physical distortion, extreme panic, paranoia, anxiety, and aggression.

Other health effects from DXM misuse can include the following:

- Hyperexcitability
- Poor motor control
- Lack of energy
- Stomach pain

- Vision changes
- Slurred speech
- Increased blood pressure
- Sweating

Misuse of DXM products containing acetaminophen can cause liver damage.

Loperamide—In the short-term, loperamide is sometimes misused to lessen cravings and withdrawal symptoms; however, it can cause euphoria, similar to other opioids.

Loperamide misuse can also lead to fainting, stomach pain, constipation, eye changes, and loss of consciousness. It can cause the heart to beat erratically or rapidly, or cause kidney problems. These effects may increase if taken with other medicines that interact with loperamide. Other effects have not been well studied and reports are mixed, but the physical consequences of loperamide misuse can be severe.

Opioid Withdrawal Symptoms

These symptoms include:

- Muscle and bone pain
- Sleep problems
- Diarrhea and vomiting

- Cold flashes with goosebumps
- Uncontrollable leg movements
- Severe cravings

Can a Person Overdose on These OTC Medicines?

Yes, a person can overdose on cold medicines containing DXM or loperamide. An overdose occurs when a person uses enough of the drug to produce a life-threatening reaction or death.

As with other opioids, when people overdose on DXM or loperamide, their breathing often slows or stops. This can decrease the amount of oxygen that reaches the brain, a condition called hypoxia. Hypoxia can have short- and long-term mental effects and effects on the nervous system, including coma and permanent brain damage and death.

How Can These Over-the-Counter Medicine Overdoses Be Treated?

A person who has overdosed needs immediate medical attention. Call 911. If the person has stopped breathing or if breathing is weak, begin cardiopulmonary resuscitation (CPR). DXM overdoses can also be treated with naloxone.

Certain medications can be used to treat heart rhythm problems caused by loperamide overdose. If the heart stops, healthcare providers will perform CPR and other cardiac support therapies.

Can Misuse of These Over-the-Counter Medicines Lead to Addiction?

Yes, misuse of DXM or loperamide can lead to addiction. An addiction develops when continued use of the drug causes issues, such as health problems and failure to meet responsibilities at work, school, or home.

The symptoms of withdrawal from DXM and loperamide have not been well studied.

How Can People Get Treatment for Addiction to These Over-the-Counter Medicines?

There are no medications approved specifically to treat DXM or loperamide addiction. Behavioral therapies, such as cognitive-behavioral therapy (CBT) and contingency management, may be helpful. CBT helps to modify the patient's drug-use expectations and behaviors, and effectively manage triggers and stress. Contingency management provides vouchers or small cash rewards for positive behaviors such as staying drug-free.

Section 33.3

Misuse of Over-the-Counter Cough and Cold Medicines

This Section includes text excerpted from "Cough and Cold Medicine (DXM and Codeine Syrup)," National Institute on Drug Abuse (NIDA) for Teens, May 2017.

What Are Cough and Cold Medicines?

Millions of Americans take cough and cold medicines each year to help with symptoms of colds, and when taken as instructed, these medicines can be safe and effective. However, several cough and cold medicines contain ingredients that are psychoactive (mind-altering) when taken in higher-than-recommended dosages, and some people misuse them. These products also contain other ingredients that can add to the risks. Many of these medicines are bought "over-the-counter" (OTC), meaning you do not need a prescription to have them.

Two commonly misused cough and cold medicines are:

- **Cough syrups and capsules containing dextromethorphan (DXM).** These OTC cough medicines are safe for stopping coughs during a cold if you take them as directed. Taking more than the recommended amount can produce euphoria (a relaxed pleasurable feeling) but also dissociative effects (like you are detached from your body).

- **Promethazine-codeine cough syrup.** These prescription medications contain an opioid drug called "codeine," which stops coughs, but when taken in higher doses produces a "buzz" or "high."

Also known as:

- Candy

- Dex

- Drank

- Lean

- Robo

- Robotripping

- Skittles

- Triple C

- Tussin

- Velvet

How Cough and Cold Medicines Are Misused

Cough and cold medicines are usually sold in liquid syrup, capsule, or pill form. They may also come in a powder. Drinking promethazine-codeine cough syrup mixed with soda (a combination called syrup, sizzurp, purple drank, barre, or lean) was referenced frequently in some popular music beginning in the late 1990s and has become increasingly popular among youth in several areas of the country.

Young people are often more likely to misuse cough and cold medicines containing DXM than some other drugs because these medicines can be purchased without a prescription.

What Happens to Your Brain When You Misuse Cough or Cold Medicines

When cough and cold medicines are taken as directed, they safely treat symptoms caused by colds and flu. But when taken in higher quantities or when such symptoms aren't present, they may affect the brain in ways very similar to illegal drugs, and can even lead to addiction.

DXM acts on the same brain cell receptors as drugs such as ketamine or PCP. A single high dose of DXM can cause hallucinations (imagined experiences that seem real). Ketamine and PCP are called "dissociative" drugs, which means they make you feel separated from your body or your environment, and they twist the way you think or feel about something or someone.

Codeine attaches to the same cell receptors as opioids such as heroin. High doses of promethazine-codeine cough syrup can produce euphoria similar to that produced by other opioid drugs. Also, both codeine and promethazine depress activities in the central nervous system (CNS) (brain and spinal cord), which produces calming effects.

Both codeine and DXM cause an increase in the amount of dopamine in the brain's reward pathway. Extra amounts of dopamine increase the feeling of pleasure and at the same time cause important messages to get lost, causing a range of effects from lack of motivation to serious health problems. Repeatedly seeking to experience that feeling can lead to addiction.

What Happens to Your Body When You Misuse Cough or Cold Medicines

DXM misuse can cause:

- Loss of coordination

- Numbness

- Feeling sick to the stomach

- Increased blood pressure

- Faster heartbeat

- In rare instances, lack of oxygen to the brain, creating lasting brain damage, when DXM is taken with decongestants

Promethazine-codeine cough syrup misuse can cause:

- Slowed heart rate

- Slowed breathing (high doses can lead to overdose and death)

Cough and cold medicines are even more dangerous when taken with alcohol or other drugs.

Are Cough and Cold Medicines Addictive?

Yes, high doses and repeated misuse of cough and cold medicines can lead to addiction. That's when a person seeks out and takes the drug over and over again, even though it is causing health or other problems.

Can You Overdose or Die If You Use Cough and Cold Medicines?

Yes. Misuse of promethazine-codeine cough syrup slows down the central nervous system (CNS), which can slow or stop the heart and lungs. Mixing it with alcohol greatly increases this risk. Promethazine-codeine cough syrup has been linked to the overdose deaths of a few prominent musicians.

How Many Teens Misuse Cough and Cold Medicines?

Table 33.1. Monitoring the Future Study: Trends in Prevalence of Cough Medicine (Nonprescription) for Eighth Graders, Tenth Graders, and Twelfth Graders; 2018 (In Percent)

Drug	Time Period	Eighth Graders	Tenth Graders	Twelfth Graders
Cough medicine (nonprescription)	Past Year	2.8	3.3	3.4

What Should You Do If Someone You Know Needs Help?

If you, or a friend, are in crisis and need to speak with someone now call National Suicide Prevention Lifeline (NSPL) at 800-273-8255. (They don't just talk about suicide—they cover a lot of issues and will help put you in touch with someone close by.)

If you need information on drug treatment and where you can find it, the Substance Abuse and Mental Health Services Administration (SAMHSA) can help.

- Call Substance Abuse Treatment Facility Locator at 800-662-4357

- Visit the locator online at www.findtreatment.samhsa.gov

Chapter 34

Legal, Financial, and Social Consequences of Drug Abuse

Chapter Contents

Section 34.1

Legal Consequences of Drug Abuse

This section includes text excerpted from "You Are Caught
with Drugs," Just Think Twice, U.S. Drug Enforcement
Administration (DEA), October 14, 2014. Reviewed January 2019.

When You Test Positive for Drugs

Testing positive for drugs can have many bad consequences. You
can be suspended from your sports team, lose the chance to participate
in other extracurricular activities, be fired from a job, or not be hired
for a job you really want. Drug testing has become a fact of life in many
high schools, sports settings, and in the workplace.

Why Do Schools Really Test for Drugs?

Yes, if your school chooses to and follows the directions set forth by
the Supreme Court. In 2002 the U.S. Supreme Court ruled to allow
random drug tests for all middle- and high-school students participating in competitive extracurricular activities.

Can Your School Really Test You for Drugs?

School drug testing is not done for disciplinary reasons. It is not
meant to punish, but to prevent students from using drugs in the first
place. For those using drugs, testing is meant to get them the help
they need to stop using.

What Is the Benefit to Students?

Schools with random drug tests are hoping that these tests will
keep students from using drugs and provide a reason to resist peer
pressure to take drugs. Schools also want to identify teens that have
started using drugs in hopes that early intervention or treatment will
help them. Using drugs interferes with the ability to learn and may
also disrupt others trying to learn. Schools recognize that drug testing alone won't necessarily change students' drug use—it takes many
different actions to reduce substance use.

Can You Beat a Drug Test?

Many students are aware of methods that supposedly detoxify the
system or mask drug use. Popular magazines and Internet sites give

advice on how to dilute urine samples, and some even sell products to dilute or alter your test results. Many of these products are costly, do not work, and can be identified in the testing process. Even if they mask a certain drug, the product itself will be detected, and another test will be given. Even in states where recreational marijuana is "legal," things are no different. School and workplace drug testing is still in place and you can still be fired from your job or suspended from school.

When You Are Caught with Drugs

If you're using drugs, selling drugs, or spending a lot of time around people who do, you may have to face legal consequences. A drug-related conviction can have a major impact on your future. With a drug-related offense on your record:

- You may not be able to get the job you want
- You may not be able to join the military
- You may not be able to keep your college loans
- You may get a criminal record
- You may spend time in jail—or worse, a state or federal prison

U.S. has clear, explicit drug laws at the federal, state, and local levels. Sometimes just being around drugs can justify an arrest and conviction, even if you're not using drugs and the drugs aren't yours. Depending on the laws in your area, even having drug paraphernalia may be cause for an arrest.

It's up to you to learn the legal consequences and consider all the facts before you make any decisions about drugs.

What Are the Federal Drug Laws?

The Controlled Substances Act (CSA) prohibits illegal manufacturing, distributing, or dispensing of controlled substances. It also prohibits their possession for the purpose of distributing and dispensing.

Controlled substances are drugs and other substances that are placed under government control based upon their accepted medical use, abuse potential, and likelihood of causing dependence when abused. They are controlled to protect the public from harm.

Federal law generally focuses on larger quantities of controlled substances than state and local laws. Federal law also focuses on interstate or international drug trafficking.

Federal penalties are usually much higher than those at the state and local level. For example, a crime that might bring one year in prison at the state level may bring ten years at the federal level because it involves much larger amounts of a controlled substance and impacts a larger area and more people.

What Are State and Local Drug Laws?

Although there are differences among the states, every state has specific drug laws and penalties regarding drugs. These laws deal with the manufacture, possession, distribution, use, and advertising and labeling drugs, as well as related behavior (like driving under the influence).

Drugs, Vehicles, and the Police

You and your friends are driving around and hanging out, just having fun. What would happen if you and your friends get stopped by the police, and the police have reason to search your car and they find drugs or drug paraphernalia?

Could you be arrested if drugs are found in the car? Could you be arrested if your friend has drugs? The answer is YES, you can be arrested along with your friend for the possession of a controlled substance. While every situation is different, the risk is the same. Even if the drugs aren't yours, you may still be charged with a crime, required to attend court, pay a fine, or even go to prison. Is it really worth taking the chance?

Section 34.2

Financial Consequences of Drug Abuse

This section includes text excerpted from "You Lose Your
Money to Drugs," Just Think Twice, U.S. Drug Enforcement
Administration (DEA), October 14, 2014. Reviewed January 2019.

At first, you might not have to spend any money on drugs. You may
get them for free from a friend or relative, or at a party. And that's
great if you do—but that may not always happen. What if you want
to use drugs more often? What if you get hooked?

For most of the people, friends and relatives don't have the money
to keep providing them with free drugs. And people in the drug business are in it to make money, so someone has to pay. Sooner or later
that will be you.

Using drugs costs money. It takes money to buy drugs. The more
you use drugs, the more you keep spending on them.

How much money depends on what drug you use and how often you
use it. You can spend as little as $100 a month to over $1,000 a month.

Depending on your income and how much is left after expenses can
help you determine how much it will hurt you.

If you start using more often, the costs can add up quickly. The
more often you use, the greater the chances that you will keep spending more and more.

What if the money you spent on rent, food, and gas is spent on the
drugs instead? How will you pay for these things?

You Lose Your Job Because of Drugs

Do you know how drug use can affect job performance and cause
you problems at work?

- Poor performance

- Inconsistent work quality

- Lack of concentration and focus

- Decreased productivity or erratic work patterns

- Increased absenteeism or when on the job or you're not mentally
  there while at work

- Unexplained disappearances while at work

- Poor judgment

- No regard for your safety or the safety of others

- Erratic behavior

- Borrowing money

- Customers and coworkers start complaining about you

- Inappropriate personal appearance

All these factors suggest that there is something negative going on in your life. All are factors that can lead to being fired.

Don't risk getting fired.

Section 34.3

Drugged Driving

This section contains text excerpted from the following sources: Text in this section begins with excerpts from "Impaired Driving: Get the Facts," Centers for Disease Control and Prevention (CDC), June 16, 2017; Text beginning with the heading "Why Is Drugged Driving Dangerous?" is excerpted from "Drugged Driving," National Institute on Drug Abuse (NIDA), June 2016.

Every day, 29 people in the United States die in motor-vehicle crashes that involve an alcohol-impaired driver. This is 1 death every 50 minutes. The annual cost of alcohol-related crashes totals more than $44 billion.

The following statistics reveal how big the problem is :

- In 2016, 10,497 people died in alcohol-impaired-driving crashes, accounting for 28 percent of all traffic-related deaths in the United States.

- Of the 1,233 traffic deaths among children ages 0 to 14 years in 2016, 214 (17%) involved an alcohol-impaired driver.

- In 2016, more than 1 million drivers were arrested for driving under the influence of alcohol or narcotics. That's one percent of the 111 million self-reported episodes of alcohol-impaired driving among U.S. adults each year.

- Drugs other than alcohol (legal and illegal) are involved in about 16 percent of motor vehicle crashes.

- Marijuana use is increasing and 13 percent of nighttime, weekend drivers have marijuana in their system.

- Marijuana users were about 25 percent more likely to be involved in a crash than drivers with no evidence of marijuana use; however, other factors—such as age and gender—may account for the increased crash risk among marijuana users.

Why Is Drugged Driving Dangerous?

The effects of specific drugs differ depending on how they act in the brain. For example, marijuana can slow reaction time, impair judgment of time and distance, and decrease coordination. Drivers who have used cocaine or methamphetamine can be aggressive and reckless when driving. Certain kinds of sedatives, called "benzodiazepines," can cause dizziness and drowsiness. All of these impairments can lead to vehicle crashes.

Research studies have shown negative effects of marijuana on drivers, including an increase in lane weaving, poor reaction time, and altered attention to the road. Use of alcohol with marijuana made drivers more impaired, causing even more lane weaving.

It is difficult to determine how specific drugs affect driving because people tend to mix various substances, including alcohol. But we do know that even small amounts of some drugs can have a measurable effect. As a result, some states have zero-tolerance laws for drugged driving. This means a person can face charges for driving under the influence (DUI) if there is any amount of drug in the blood or urine. It's important to note that many states are waiting for research to better define blood levels that indicate impairment, such as those they use with alcohol.

How Many People Take Drugs and Drive?

According to the 2016 National Survey on Drug Use and Health (NSDUH), in 2016, 20.7 million people age 16 or older drove under the influence of alcohol in the past year and 11.8 million drove under the influence of illicit drugs.

369

NSDUH findings also show that men are more likely than women to drive under the influence of drugs or alcohol. And a higher percentage of young adults age 18 to 25 drive after taking drugs or drinking than do adults 26 or older.

Which Drugs Are Linked to Drugged Driving?

After alcohol, marijuana is the drug most often found in the blood of drivers involved in crashes. Tests for detecting marijuana in drivers measure the level of delta-9- tetrahydrocannabinol (THC), marijuana mind-altering ingredient, in the blood. But the role that marijuana plays in crashes is often unclear. THC can be detected in body fluids for days or even weeks after use, and it is often combined with alcohol. The risk associated with marijuana in combination with alcohol, cocaine, or benzodiazepines appears to be greater than that for either drug by itself.

Several studies have shown that drivers with THC in their blood were roughly twice as likely to be responsible for a deadly crash or be killed than drivers who hadn't used drugs or alcohol. However, a large National Highway Traffic Safety Administration (NHTSA) study found no significant increased crash risk traceable to marijuana after controlling for drivers' age, gender, race, and presence of alcohol.

Along with marijuana, prescription drugs are also commonly linked to drugged driving crashes. A 2010 nationwide study of deadly crashes found that about 47 percent of drivers who tested positive for drugs had used a prescription drug, compared to 37 percent of those had used marijuana and about 10 percent of those who had used cocaine. The most common prescription drugs found were pain relievers. However, the study didn't distinguish between medically supervised and illicit use of prescription drugs.

How Often Does Drugged Driving Cause Crashes?

It's hard to measure how many crashes are caused by drugged driving. This is because:

- A good roadside test for drug levels in the body doesn't yet exist

- Police don't usually test for drugs if drivers have reached an illegal blood alcohol level because there's already enough evidence for a DUI charge

- Many drivers who cause crashes are found to have both drugs and alcohol or more than one drug in their system, making it hard to know which substance had the greater effect

One NHTSA study found that in 2009, 18 percent of drivers killed in a crash tested positive for at least one drug. A 2010 study showed that 11 percent of deadly crashes involved a drugged driver.

Why Is Drugged Driving a Problem in Teens and Young Adults?

Teen drivers are less experienced and are more likely than older drivers to underestimate or not recognize dangerous situations. They are also more likely to speed and allow less distance between vehicles. When lack of driving experience is combined with drug use, the results can be tragic. Car crashes are the leading cause of death among young people age 16 to 19 years.

A 2011 survey of middle- and high-school students showed that, in the 2 weeks before the survey, 12 percent of high-school seniors had driven after using marijuana, compared to around 9 percent who had driven after drinking alcohol.

A study of college students with access to a car found that 1 in 6 had driven under the influence of a drug other than alcohol at least once in the past year. Marijuana was the most common drug used, followed by cocaine and prescription pain relievers.

What Steps Can People Take to Prevent Drugged Driving?

Because drugged driving puts people at a higher risk for crashes, public-health experts urge people who use drugs and alcohol to develop social strategies to prevent them from getting behind the wheel of a car while impaired. Steps people can take include:

- Offering to be a designated driver

- Appointing a designated driver to take all car keys

- Getting a ride to and from parties where there are drugs and alcohol

- Discussing the risks of drugged driving with friends in advance

Drugs include illicit substances and prescription and over-the-counter (OTC) medicines. The study excluded nicotine, aspirin, alcohol, and drugs given after the crash.

Chapter 35

Health Consequences of Drug Addiction

Chapter Contents

Section 35.1

Poor Health Outcomes of Commonly Abused Drugs

This section includes text excerpted from "Drugs, Brains, and Behavior: The Science of Addiction," National Institute on Drug Abuse (NIDA), July 2018.

People with addiction often have one or more associated health issues, which could include lung or heart disease, stroke, cancer, or mental-health conditions. Imaging scans, chest X-rays*, and blood tests can show the damaging effects of long-term drug use throughout the body.

* In low doses, X-rays are used to diagnose diseases by making pictures of the inside of the body.

For example, it is now well-known that tobacco smoke can cause many cancers; methamphetamine can cause severe dental problems, known as "meth mouth;" and that opioids can lead to overdose and death. In addition, some drugs, such as inhalants, may damage or destroy nerve cells, either in the brain or the peripheral nervous system (PNS) (the nervous system outside the brain and spinal cord).

Drug use can also increase the risk of contracting infections. Human immunodeficiency virus (HIV) and hepatitis C (a serious liver disease) infection can occur from sharing injection equipment and from impaired judgment leading to unsafe sexual activity. Infection of the heart and its valves (endocarditis) and skin infection (cellulitis) can occur after exposure to bacteria by injection-drug use.

Does Drug Use Cause Mental Disorders, or Vice Versa?

Drug use and mental illness often coexist. In some cases, mental disorders such as anxiety, depression, or schizophrenia may come before addiction; in other cases, drug use may trigger or worsen those mental-health conditions, particularly in people with specific vulnerabilities.

Some people with disorders such as anxiety or depression may use drugs in an attempt to alleviate psychiatric symptoms, which may exacerbate their mental disorder in the long run, as well as increase the risk of developing the addiction. Treatment for all conditions should happen concurrently.

The Impact of Addiction Can Be Far-Reaching

Addiction can lead to health risks such as:

- Cardiovascular disease (CVD)

- Stroke

- Cancer

- Human immunodeficiency virus (HIV)/acquired immunodeficiency syndrome (AIDS)

- Hepatitis B and C

- Lung disease

- Mental disorders

How Can Addiction Harm Other People?

Beyond the harmful consequences for the person with the addiction, drug use can cause serious health problems for others. Some of the more severe consequences of addiction are:

- **Negative effects of drug use while pregnant or breastfeeding.** A mother's substance or medication use during pregnancy can cause her baby to go into withdrawal after it's born, which is called neonatal abstinence syndrome (NAS). Symptoms will differ depending on the substance used but may include tremors, problems with sleeping and feeding, and even seizures. Some drug-exposed children will have developmental problems involving behavior, attention, and thinking. Ongoing research is exploring if these effects on the brain and behavior extend into the teen years, causing continued developmental problems. In addition, some substances can make their way into a mother's breast milk. Scientists are still learning about long-term effects on a child who is exposed to drugs through breastfeeding.

- **Negative effects of secondhand smoke.** Secondhand tobacco smoke exposes bystanders to at least 250 chemicals that are known to be harmful, particularly to children. Involuntary exposure to secondhand smoke increases the risks of heart disease and lung cancer in people who have never smoked. Additionally, the known health risks of secondhand exposure to tobacco smoke raise questions about whether secondhand exposure to marijuana smoke poses similar risks. At this point, little research on this question has been conducted. However, a study found that some nonsmoking participants exposed for an hour to high-THC marijuana in an unventilated room reported mild effects of the drug, and another study showed positive urine tests in the hours directly following exposure. If you inhale secondhand marijuana smoke, it's unlikely you would fail a drug test, but it is possible.

- **Increased spread of infectious diseases.** Injection of drugs accounts for one in ten cases of HIV. Injection drug use is also a major factor in the spread of hepatitis C and can be the cause of endocarditis and cellulitis. Injection drug use is not the only way that drug use contributes to the spread of infectious diseases. Drugs that are misused can cause intoxication, which hinders judgment and increases the chance of risky sexual behaviors.

- **Increased risk of motor vehicle accidents.** Use of illicit drugs or misuse of prescription drugs can make driving a car unsafe—just like driving after drinking alcohol. Drugged driving puts the driver, passengers, and others who share the road at risk. In 2016, almost 12 million people ages 16 or older reported driving under the influence of illicit drugs, including marijuana. After alcohol, marijuana is the drug most often linked to impaired driving. Research studies have shown negative effects of marijuana on drivers, including an increase in lane weaving, poor reaction time, and altered attention to the road.

Section 35.2

Substance Abuse and Medical Complications

This section includes text excerpted from "Health Consequences of Drug Misuse," National Institute on Drug Abuse (NIDA), March 2017.

Drug use can have a wide range of short- and long-term, direct and indirect effects. These effects often depend on the specific drug or drugs used, how they are taken, how much is taken, the person's health, and other factors. Short-term effects can range from changes in appetite, wakefulness, heart rate, blood pressure, and/or mood to heart attack, stroke, psychosis, overdose, and even death. These health effects may occur after just one use.

Long-term effects can include heart or lung disease, cancer, mental illness, human immunodeficiency virus (HIV)/acquired immune deficiency syndrome (AIDS), hepatitis, and others. Long-term drug use can also lead to addiction. Drug addiction is a brain disorder. Not everyone who uses drugs will become addicted, but for some, drug use can change how certain brain circuits work. These brain changes interfere with how people experience normal pleasures in life such as food and sex, their ability to control their stress level, their decision-making, their ability to learn and remember, etc. These changes make it much more difficult for someone to stop taking the drug even when it's having negative effects on their lives and they want to quit.

Drug use can also have indirect effects on both the people who are taking drugs and on those around them. This can include affecting a person's nutrition; sleep; decision-making and impulsivity; and risk of trauma, violence, injury, and communicable diseases. Drug use can also affect babies born to women who use drugs while pregnant. Broader negative outcomes may be seen in education level, employment, housing, relationships, and criminal-justice involvement.

How Various Drugs Affect Different Parts of the Body and Disease Risk
Human Immunodeficiency Virus, Hepatitis, and Other Infectious Diseases

Drug use is linked to risky behaviors such as needle sharing and unsafe sex and can also weaken the immune system. This combination greatly increases the likelihood of contracting HIV, hepatitis, and other infectious diseases.

Cancer

Cigarette smoking is the most preventable cause of cancer in the United States. Smoking cigarettes has been linked to cancer of the mouth, neck, stomach, and lungs, among others. Nonsmoking people exposed to secondhand cigarette smoke increase their chances of developing lung cancer in addition to other health problems.

Young adult males who use marijuana and began their use during adolescence are at risk for an aggressive form of testicular cancer.

Cardiovascular Effects

Researchers have found that most drugs can have adverse cardiovascular effects, ranging from abnormal heart rate to heart attack. Injection drug use can also lead to cardiovascular problems such as collapsed veins and bacterial infections of the blood vessels and heart valves.

Respiratory Effects

Drug use can lead to a variety of respiratory problems. Smoking cigarettes, for example, has been shown to cause bronchitis, emphysema, and lung cancer. Marijuana smoke can also cause respiratory problems, including chronic bronchitis. Smoking crack cocaine can also cause lung damage and severe respiratory problems. The use of some drugs, such as opioids, may cause breathing to slow, block air from entering the lungs, or make asthma symptoms worse.

Gastrointestinal Effects

Among other adverse effects, many drugs can cause nausea and vomiting after use. Cocaine use can also cause abdominal pain and bowel tissue decay, and opioid use can cause abdominal pain, acid reflux, and severe constipation.

Musculoskeletal Effects

Steroid use during childhood or adolescence, resulting in artificially high sex hormone levels, can signal the bones to stop growing earlier than they normally would, leading to short stature. Other drugs may also cause severe muscle cramping and overall muscle weakness.

Kidney Damage

Some drugs may cause kidney damage or failure, either directly or indirectly, from dehydration, dangerous increases in body temperature, and muscle breakdown.

Liver Damage

Chronic use of some drugs, such as heroin, inhalants, and steroids (appearance and performance-enhancing drugs), may lead to significant damage to the liver. This damage can be worse when these drugs are combined with alcohol or other drugs.

Neurological Effects

All addictive drugs act in the brain to produce their euphoric effects. However, some can also cause damage due to seizures, stroke, and direct toxic effects on brain cells. Drug use can also lead to addiction, a brain disorder that occurs when repeated drug use leads to changes in the function of multiple brain circuits that control pleasures/reward, stress, decision-making, impulse control, learning and memory, and other functions. These changes make it harder for those with an addiction to experience pleasure in response to natural rewards—such as food, sex, or positive social interactions—or to manage their stress, control their impulses, and make the healthy choice to stop drug-seeking and use.

Hormonal Effects

Appearance and performance-enhancing drugs disrupt the normal production of hormones in the body, causing both reversible and irreversible changes. These changes include infertility and testicle shrinkage in men as well as body hair growth and male- pattern baldness in women.

Prenatal Effects

Studies show that various drugs may result in miscarriage, premature birth, low birth weight, and a variety of behavioral and cognitive problems in the child. A baby can also be born dependent on the drug if the mother uses it regularly—a condition called "neonatal abstinence syndrome."

Other Health Effects

In addition to the effects that various drugs may have on specific organs of the body, many drugs produce global body changes such as dramatic changes in appetite and increases in body temperature, which may impact a variety of health conditions. Withdrawal from drug use also may lead to numerous adverse health effects, including restlessness, mood swings, fatigue, changes in appetite, muscle and bone pain, mental-health problems, insomnia, cold flashes, diarrhea, vomiting, and others.

Section 35.3

Marijuana's Long-Term Effects on the Brain

This section includes text excerpted from "Marijuana,"
National Institute on Drug Abuse (NIDA), June 2018.

Substantial evidence from animal research and a growing number of studies in humans indicate that marijuana exposure during development can cause long-term or possibly permanent adverse changes in the brain. Rats exposed to tetrahydrocannabinol (THC) before birth, soon after birth, or during adolescence show notable problems with specific learning and memory tasks later in life. Cognitive impairments in adult rats exposed to THC during adolescence are associated with structural and functional changes in the hippocampus. Studies in rats also show that adolescent exposure to THC is associated with an altered reward system, increasing the likelihood that an animal will self-administer other drugs (e.g., heroin) when given an opportunity.

Imaging studies of marijuana's impact on brain structure in humans have shown conflicting results. Some studies suggest regular marijuana use in adolescence is associated with altered connectivity and reduced volume of specific brain regions involved in a broad range of executive functions such as memory, learning, and impulse control compared to people who do not use. Other studies have not found significant structural differences between the brains of people who do and do not use the drug.

Several studies, including two large longitudinal studies, suggest that marijuana use can cause functional impairment in cognitive abilities but that the degree and/or duration of the impairment depends on the age when a person began using and how much and how long he or she used.

Among nearly 4,000 young adults in the Coronary Artery Risk Development in Young Adults (CARDIA) study tracked over a 25-year period until mid-adulthood, cumulative lifetime exposure to marijuana was associated with lower scores on a test of verbal memory but did not affect other cognitive abilities such as processing speed or executive function. The effect was sizeable and significant even after eliminating those involved with current use and after adjusting for confounding factors such as demographic factors, other drug and alcohol use, and other psychiatric conditions such as depression.

A large longitudinal study in New Zealand found that persistent marijuana use disorder with frequent use starting in adolescence was associated with a loss of an average of six or up to eight intelligence quotient (IQ) points measured in mid-adulthood. Significantly, in that study, those who used marijuana heavily as teenagers and quit using as adults did not recover the lost IQ points. People who only began using marijuana heavily in adulthood did not lose IQ points. These results suggest that marijuana has its strongest long-term impact on young people whose brains are still busy building new connections and maturing in other ways. The endocannabinoid system is known to play an important role in the proper formation of synapses (the connections between neurons) during early brain development, and a similar role has been proposed for the refinement of neural connections during adolescence. If the long-term effects of marijuana use on cognitive functioning or IQ are upheld by future research, this may be one avenue by which marijuana use during adolescence produces its long-term effects.

However, results from two prospective longitudinal twin studies did not support a causal relationship between marijuana use and IQ loss. Those who used marijuana did show a significant decline in verbal ability (equivalent to 4 IQ points) and in general knowledge between the preteen years (ages 9 to 12, before use) and late adolescence/early adulthood (ages 17 to 20). However, at the start of the study, those who would use in the future already had lower scores on these measures than those who would not use in the future, and no predictable difference was found between twins when one used marijuana and one did not. This suggests that observed IQ declines, at least across adolescence, may be caused by shared familial factors (e.g., genetics, family environment), not by marijuana use itself. It should be noted, though, that these studies were shorter in duration than the New Zealand study and did not explore the impact of the dose of marijuana (i.e., heavy use) or the development of a *Cannabis*-use disorder; this may have masked a dose or diagnosis-dependent effect.

The ability to draw definitive conclusions about marijuana's long-term impact on the human brain from past studies is often limited by the fact that study participants use multiple substances, and there is often limited data about the participants' health or mental functioning prior to the study.

Marijuana, Memory, and the Hippocampus

Distribution of cannabinoid receptors in the rat brain. Brain image reveals high levels (shown in orange and yellow) of cannabinoid receptors in many areas, including the cortex, hippocampus, cerebellum, and nucleus accumbens (ventral striatum).

Memory impairment from marijuana use occurs because THC alters how the hippocampus, a brain area responsible for memory formation, processes information. Most of the evidence supporting this assertion comes from animal studies. For example, rats exposed to THC in utero, soon after birth, or during adolescence, show notable problems with specific learning/memory tasks later in life. Moreover, cognitive impairment in adult rats is associated with structural and functional changes in the hippocampus from THC exposure during adolescence.

As people age, they lose neurons in the hippocampus, which decreases their ability to learn new information. Chronic THC exposure may hasten age-related loss of hippocampal neurons. In one study, rats exposed to THC every day for 8 months (approximately 30% of their lifespan) showed a level of nerve cell loss at 11 to 12 months of age that equaled that of unexposed animals twice their age.

Section 35.4

Opioid Overdose

This section includes text excerpted from "Opioid Overdose," MedlinePlus, National Institutes of Health (NIH), August 27, 2018.

What Are Opioids?

Opioids, sometimes called narcotics, are a type of drug. They include strong prescription pain relievers, such as oxycodone, hydrocodone, fentanyl, and tramadol. The illegal drug heroin is also an opioid.

A healthcare provider may give you a prescription opioid to reduce pain after you have had a major injury or surgery. You may get them if you have severe pain from health conditions like cancer. Some healthcare providers prescribe them for chronic pain.

Prescription opioids used for pain relief are generally safe when taken for a short time and as prescribed by your healthcare provider. However, people who take opioids are at risk for opioid dependence and addiction, as well as an overdose. These risks increase when opioids are misused. Misuse means you are not taking the medicines according to your provider's instructions, you are using them to get high, or you are taking someone else's opioids.

What Is an Opioid Overdose?

Opioids affect the part of the brain that regulates breathing. When people take high doses of opioids, it can lead to an overdose, with the slowing or stopping of breathing and sometimes death.

What Causes an Opioid Overdose

An opioid overdose can happen for a variety of reasons, including if you:

- Take an opioid to get high
- Take an extra dose of a prescription opioid or take it too often (either accidentally or on purpose)
- Mix an opioid with other medicines, illegal drugs, or alcohol. An overdose can be fatal when mixing an opioid and certain anxiety treatment medicines, such as Xanax or Valium.
- Take an opioid medicine that was prescribed for someone else. Children are especially at risk of an accidental overdose if they take medicine not intended for them.

There is also a risk of overdose if you are getting medication-assisted treatment (MAT). MAT is a treatment for opioid abuse and addiction. Many of the medicines used for MAT are controlled substances that can be misused.

Who Is at Risk for an Opioid Overdose?

Anyone who takes an opioid can be at risk of an overdose, but you are at higher risk if you

- Take illegal opioids
- Take more opioid medicine than you are prescribed
- Combine opioids with other medicines and/or alcohol
- Have certain medical conditions, such as sleep apnea, or reduced kidney or liver function
- Are over 65 years old

What Are the Signs of an Opioid Overdose?

Signs of an opioid overdose include:

- Face is extremely pale and/or feeling clammy to the touch
- Limp body
- Fingernails or lips that have a purple or blue color
- Vomiting or making gurgling noises
- Cannot be awakened or are unable to speak
- Their breathing or heartbeat slows or stops

What Should You Do If You Think That Someone Is Having an Opioid Overdose?

If you think someone is having an opioid overdose,

- Call 9-1-1 immediately.
- Administer naloxone, if it is available. Naloxone is a safe medication that can quickly stop an opioid overdose. It can be injected into the muscle or sprayed into the nose to rapidly block the effects of the opioid on the body.
- Try to keep the person awake and breathing.
- Lay the person on their side to prevent choking.
- Stay with the person until emergency workers arrive.

How Can You Prevent an Opioid Overdose?

There are steps you can take to help prevent an overdose:

- Take your medicine exactly as prescribed by your healthcare provider. Do not take more medicine at once or take medicine more often than you are supposed to.
- Never mix pain medicines with alcohol, sleeping pills, or illegal substances.
- Store medicine safely where children or pets can't reach it. Consider using a medicine lockbox. Besides keeping children safe, it also prevents someone who lives with you or visits your house from stealing your medicines.

- Dispose of unused medicine promptly.

- If you take an opioid, it is also important to teach your family and friends how to respond to an overdose. If you are at high risk for an overdose, ask your healthcare provider about whether you need a prescription for naloxone.

Chapter 36

Preventing Disease in Drug-Abusing Populations

Chapter Contents

Section 36.1

Drug Abuse and Infectious Diseases

This section includes text excerpted from "Drug Use and
Viral Infections (HIV, Hepatitis)," National Institute on
Drug Abuse (NIDA), April 2018.

What's the Relationship between Drug Use and Viral Infections?

People who engage in drug use or high-risk behaviors associated
with drug use put themselves at risk for contracting or transmitting
viral infections such as human immunodeficiency virus (HIV)/acquired
immunodeficiency syndrome (AIDS) or hepatitis. This is because
viruses spread through blood or body fluids. It happens primarily in
two ways: when people inject drugs and share needles or other drug
equipment and when drugs impair judgment and people have unprotected sex with an infected partner. This can happen with both men
and women. Women who become infected with a virus can pass it to
their baby during pregnancy, whether or not they use drugs. They can
also pass HIV to the baby through breastmilk. Drug use can also affect
the symptoms a person has from a viral infection.

The viral infections of greatest concern related to drug use are HIV
and hepatitis.

What Is Human Immunodeficiency Virus/Acquired Immunodeficiency Syndrome?

HIV stands for "human immunodeficiency virus." This virus infects
the body's immune cells, called "CD4 cells" (T cells), which are needed to
fight infections. HIV lowers the number of these T cells in the immune
system, making it harder for the body to fight off infections and disease.

Acquired immune deficiency syndrome, or AIDS, is the final stage
of an HIV infection when the body is unable to fend off disease. A
healthcare provider diagnoses a patient with AIDS when that person
has one or more infections and a T cell count of less than 200. A person
with a healthy immune system has a T cell count between 500 and
1,600. Being infected with HIV doesn't automatically mean that it will
progress to AIDS.

More than 1.1 million people in the United States live with an
HIV infection, with an estimated 162,500 who are unaware of their

condition. While there are medicines that help prevent the transmission and spread of HIV and its progression to AIDS, there is no vaccine for the virus, and there is no cure. Drug use and addiction have been inseparably linked with HIV/AIDS since the beginning of the HIV/AIDS epidemic. People who inject drugs accounted for about six percent of HIV diagnoses in 2015.

What Is Hepatitis

Hepatitis is an inflammation (painful swelling and irritation) of the liver, most often caused by a family of viruses: A, B, C, D, and E. Each has its own way of spreading to other people and its own treatment. Hepatitis B virus (HBV) and hepatitis C virus (HCV) can spread through sharing needles and other drug equipment. Infections can also be transmitted through risky sexual behaviors linked to drug use, though this is not common with HCV.

Hepatitis can lead to cirrhosis—scarring of the liver—resulting in loss of liver function. It can also lead to liver cancer. In fact, HBV and HCV infections are the major risk factors for liver cancer in the United States.

There is a vaccine to prevent HBV infection and medicines to treat it. There are also medicines to treat HCV infection, but no vaccine for prevention. Some people recover from infection without treatment. Other people need to take medicine for the rest of their lives and be monitored for liver failure and cancer.

How Does Drug Use Affect Symptoms and Outcomes of a Viral Infection?

Drug use can worsen HIV symptoms, making it easier for HIV to enter the brain and causing greater nerve-cell injury and problems with thinking, learning, and memory. Drug and alcohol use can also directly damage the liver, increasing the risk for chronic liver disease and cancer among those infected with HBV or HCV.

How Can People Lessen the Spread of Viral Infections?

People can reduce the risk of getting or passing on a viral infection by:

- **Not using drugs.** This decreases the chance of engaging in unsafe behavior, such as sharing drug-use equipment and having unprotected sex, which can lead to these infections.

389

- **Pre-exposure prophylaxis (PrEP).** PrEP is when people who are at significant risk for contracting HIV take a daily dose of HIV medications to prevent them from getting the infection. Research has shown that PrEP has been effective in reducing the risk of HIV infection in people who inject drugs.

- **Getting treatment.** People in treatment for drug use should receive counseling to learn how to stop or reduce their drug use and related risky behaviors. Healthcare providers can use the Seek, Test, Treat, and Retain model of care to seek out and test hard-to-reach people who use drugs and offer them treatment.

- **Post-exposure prophylaxis (PEP).** PEP is when people take antiretroviral medicines to prevent becoming infected after being potentially exposed to HIV. According to the Centers for Disease Control and Prevention (CDC), PEP should be used within 72 hours after a recent possible exposure and only be used in emergency situations. If you think you've recently been exposed to HIV during sex, through sharing needles, or sexual assault, talk to your healthcare provider or an emergency room doctor about PEP right away.

- **Getting tested.** People who use drugs should get tested for HIV, HBV, and HCV. Those who are infected may look and feel fine for years and may not even be aware of the infection. Therefore, testing is needed to help prevent the spread of disease—among those most at risk and in the general population.

- **Practicing safer sex every time.** People can reduce their chances of transmitting or getting HIV, HBV, and HCV by using a condom every time they have sex. This is true for those who use drugs and those in the general population.

Section 36.2

The Connection between HIV/AIDS and Drug Abuse

This section includes text excerpted from "Substance
Use and HIV Risk," HIV.gov, U.S. Department of Health
and Human Services (HHS), August 27, 2018.

How Can Using Drugs Put You at Risk for Getting or Transmitting Human Immunodeficiency Virus?

Using drugs affects your brain, alters your judgment, and lowers your inhibitions. When you're high, you may be more likely to make poor decisions that put you at risk for getting or transmitting human immunodeficiency virus (HIV), such as having sex without a condom, have a hard time using a condom the right way every time you have sex, have more sexual partners, or use other drugs. These behaviors can increase your risk of exposure to HIV and other sexually transmitted diseases (STDs). Or, if you have HIV, they can increase your risk of spreading HIV to others. Using drugs affects your brain, alters your judgment, and lowers your inhibitions.

And if you inject drugs, you are at risk for getting or transmitting HIV and hepatitis B and C if you share needles or equipment (or "works") used to prepare drugs, like cotton, cookers, and water. This is because the needles or works may have blood in them, and blood can carry HIV. You should not share needles or works for injecting silicone, hormones, or steroids for the same reason.

Here are some commonly used substances and their link to HIV risk:

- **Alcohol.** Excessive alcohol consumption, notably binge drinking, can be an important risk factor for HIV because it is linked to risky sexual behaviors and, among people living with HIV, can hurt treatment outcomes.

- **Opioids.** Opioids, a class of drugs that reduce pain, include both prescription drugs and heroin. They are associated with HIV-risk behaviors such as needle sharing when infected and risky sexual behaviors and have been linked to outbreaks of HIV and viral hepatitis. People who are addicted to opioids are also at risk of turning to other ways to get the drug, including trading sex for drugs or money, which increases HIV risk.

- **Methamphetamine.** "Meth" is linked to risky sexual behaviors, such as having more sexual partners or sex without a condom, that place people at greater risk for HIV and other STDs. Meth can be injected, which also increases HIV risk if people share needles and other injection equipment.

- **Crack cocaine.** Crack cocaine is a stimulant that can create a cycle in which people quickly exhaust their resources and may engage in behaviors to obtain the drug that increases their HIV risk.

- **Inhalants.** Use of amyl nitrite ("poppers") has long been linked to risky sexual behaviors, illegal-drug use, and STDs among gay and bisexual men.

Therapy, medicines, and other methods are available to help you stop or cut down on drinking or using drugs. Talk with a counselor, doctor, or other healthcare providers about options that might be right for you. To find a substance-abuse treatment center near you, visit Substance Abuse and Mental Health Services Administration's (SAMHSA) treatment locator or call 800-662-4357.

How Can You Prevent Getting or Transmitting HIV from Injection-Drug Use?

Your risk is high for getting or transmitting HIV and hepatitis B and C if you share needles or equipment (or "works") used to prepare drugs, like cotton, cookers, and water. This is because the needles or works may have blood in them, and blood can carry HIV.

If you inject drugs, you are also at risk of getting HIV (and other STDs) because you may be more likely to take risks with sex when you are high.

The best way to lower your chances of getting HIV is to stop injecting drugs. You may need help to stop or cut down using drugs, but there are many resources available to help you.

If you keep injecting drugs, here are some ways to lower your risk for getting HIV and other infections:

- Use only new, sterile needles and works each time you inject. Many communities have needle exchange programs where you can get new needles and works, and some pharmacies may sell needles without a prescription.

- Never share needles or works.

- Clean used needles with bleach only when you can't get new ones. Bleaching a needle may reduce the risk of HIV but doesn't eliminate it.

- Use sterile water to fix drugs.

- Clean your skin with a new alcohol swab before you inject.

- Be careful not to get someone else's blood on your hands or your needle or works.

- Dispose of needles safely after one use. Use a sharps container, or keep used needles away from other people.

- Get tested for HIV at least once a year.

- Ask your doctor about taking daily medicine to prevent HIV called pre-exposure prophylaxis (PrEP).

- If you think you've been exposed to HIV within the last 3 days, ask a healthcare provider about post-exposure prophylaxis (PEP) right away. PEP can prevent HIV, but it must be started within 72 hours.

- Don't have sex if you're high. If you do have sex, make sure to protect yourself and your partner by using a condom the right way every time or by using other effective methods.

Staying Healthy

If you are living with HIV, substance use can be harmful to your brain and body and affect your ability to stick to your HIV treatment regimen. Learn about the health effects of alcohol and other substance use and how to access substance-abuse treatment programs if you need them.

Section 36.3

Hepatitis Infection and Drug Use

This section includes text excerpted from "Viral Hepatitis—A Very
Real Consequence of Substance Use," National Institute on Drug
Abuse (NIDA), May 2018.

What Is Hepatitis?

Hepatitis is an inflammation of the liver. It can be caused by a
variety of toxins (such as drugs or alcohol), autoimmune conditions,
or pathogens (including viruses, bacteria, or parasites). Viral hepatitis
is caused by a family of viruses labeled A, B, C, D, and E. Hepatitis
B (HBV) and hepatitis C (HCV) are the most common viral hepatitis infections transmitted through the sometimes risky behaviors by
people who use drugs—particularly among people who inject drugs
(PWID). Approximately 850,000 to 2.2 million people are living with
HBV and an estimated 3.5 million people are living with HCV in the
United States.

Left untreated, hepatitis can lead to cirrhosis, a progressive deterioration and malfunction of the liver. It can also lead to a type of
liver cancer called "hepatocellular carcinoma." In fact, HBV and

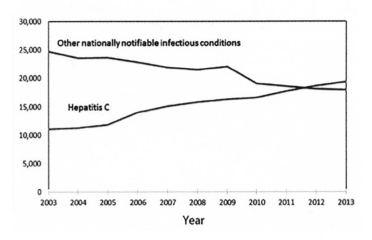

Figure 36.1. *Deaths due to Hepatitis.* (Source: U.S. Department of Health
and Human Services (HHS).)

HCV infections are related to about 65 percent of liver malfunction worldwide. Nearly 50 percent of the cases are caused by HCV alone. During the next 40 to 50 years, one million people with untreated chronic HCV infection will likely die from complications related to their HCV.

Since 2012, there have been more deaths due to hepatitis C than all 60 of the other reportable infectious diseases combined.

In an effort to fight viral hepatitis in the United States, the U.S. Department of Health and Human Services (HHS) developed the National Hepatitis Action Plan for 2017–2020. The plan outlines strategies to achieve the following goals:

1. Prevent new viral hepatitis infections

2. Reduce deaths and improve the health of people living with viral hepatitis

3. Reduce viral health disparities (differences among ethnicities, race, income, and gender, etc.)

4. Coordinate, monitor, and report on implementation of viral hepatitis activities

What Is the Relationship between Drug Use and Viral Hepatitis?

Drug and alcohol use places people at particular risk for contracting viral hepatitis. Engaging in risky sexual behavior that often accompanies drug use increases the risk of contracting HBV and, less frequently, HCV. People who inject drugs (PWID) are at high risk for contracting HBV and HCV from shared needles and other drug-preparation equipment, which exposes them to bodily fluids from other infected people. Because drug use often impairs judgment, PWID repeatedly engages in these unsafe behaviors, which can increase their risk of contracting viral hepatitis. One study reported that each person who injects drugs infected with HCV is likely to infect about 20 others and that this rapid transmission of the disease occurs within the first three years of initial infection. Drug and alcohol use can also directly damage the liver, increasing risk for chronic liver disease and cancer among those infected with hepatitis. This underscores that early detection and treatment of hepatitis infections in PWID and other drug users is paramount to protecting both the health of the person and that of the community.

What Are the Other Health Challenges for People with Hepatitis Who Inject Drugs?

PWID with hepatitis often from several other health conditions at the same time, including mental illness and HIV/AIDS, thus requiring care from multiple healthcare providers. This is sometimes referred to as co-occurring disorders. Substance-use disorder (SUD) treatment is critical for PWID, as it can reduce risky behaviors that increase the chance of transmitting hepatitis. Research has shown that patients with hepatitis receiving medication-assisted treatment for their opioid addiction can be safely treated with antiviral medications.

To enhance HCV care, National Institute on Drug Abuse (NIDA) is examining coordinated care models that utilize case managers to integrate HCV specialty care with primary care, SUD treatment, and mental-health services so that these patients get treatment regimens that address all of their healthcare needs. The Health Resources and Services Administration's (HRSA) Ryan White HIV/AIDS Program developed a free, online curriculum about HIV/hepatitis C for healthcare providers and healthcare staff to increase knowledge about coinfection among people of color in the United States.

What Treatments Are Available for Viral Hepatitis?

Many medications are available for the treatment of chronic HBV and HCV infection. For chronic HBV infection, there are several antiviral drugs. People who are chronically infected with HBV require consistent medical monitoring to ensure that the medications are keeping the virus in check and that the disease is not progressing to liver damage or cancer.

There are also antiviral medications available for HCV treatment and new treatments have been approved over the years. Many antiviral HCV treatments can cure more than 90 percent of people who take them within 8 to 12 weeks. HCV treatment dramatically reduces deaths, and people who are cured are much less likely to develop cirrhosis or liver cancer. However, not everyone infected with HCV needs or can benefit from treatment. NIDA researchers have identified genes that are associated with spontaneous clearance of HCV. These genes also enable people who are unable to clear HCV on their own to respond more favorably to treatment medications. This information can be used to determine which patients can benefit most from HCV treatment. More studies must be done, but this is the first step to personalized medicine for the treatment of HCV.

How Do You Know If You Are Infected with Viral Hepatitis?

The number of new HBV and HCV infections has been declining in recent years, but the number of people living with chronic hepatitis infections is considerable, and deaths associated with untreated, chronic hepatitis infections have been on the rise. This is because most people don't know they are infected until the disease has begun to damage the liver—highlighting why screening for viral hepatitis is so important. People with a history of drug use are generally at higher risk and should discuss their substance use with their healthcare providers.

Initial screening for HBV or HCV involves antibody tests, which show whether you have been exposed to the hepatitis virus, although not necessarily whether you are still infected. A positive antibody test should then be followed up with a test that measures the amount of virus in your blood. If this follow-up test is positive, then you should seek advice from a physician who specializes in viral hepatitis treatment. Because screening for hepatitis is so critical for linking people who test positive to the care they need, NIDA is studying new rapid HCV antibody tests that can be used in drug treatment settings.

The Centers for Disease Control and Prevention (CDC) recommends that people who use or have used drugs be tested for hepatitis B and C as part of routine medical care.

What Do You Do If You Find out You Have Viral Hepatitis?

After learning from your doctor that you have hepatitis, your first step will be to learn more about the virus. Read government resources to find current, scientific information. Adopting a healthy lifestyle is important to prevent the virus from becoming serious. Don't drink or misuse drugs because they are hard on your liver. Get plenty of rest, eat healthy foods, and exercise. Work to protect others by not donating blood or participating in risky behaviors, including sharing needles when using drugs or having unprotected sex.

Section 36.4

Sterile Syringe Programs

This section includes text excerpted from "Syringe Services Programs," Centers for Disease Control and Prevention (CDC), December 13, 2018.

Persons who inject drugs can substantially reduce their risk of getting and transmitting human immunodeficiency virus (HIV), viral hepatitis, and other blood-borne infections by using a sterile needle and syringe for every injection. In many jurisdictions, persons who inject drugs can access sterile needles and syringes through syringe services programs (SSPs) and through pharmacies without a prescription. Though less common, access to sterile needles and syringes may also be possible through a prescription written by a doctor and through other healthcare services.

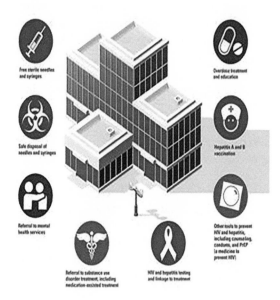

Figure 36.2. *What Is SSP?*

What Are Syringe Services Programs?

SSPs, which have also been referred to as syringe exchange programs (SEPs), needle exchange programs (NEPs), and needle-syringe programs (NSPs) are community-based programs that provide, access to sterile needles and syringes free of cost, facilitate safe disposal of used needles and syringes, and offer safer injection education. Many SSPs also provide linkages to critical services and programs, including substance-use disorder (SUD) treatment programs; overdose prevention education; screening, care, and treatment for HIV and viral hepatitis; HIV pre- and post-exposure prophylaxis (PrEP); prevention of mother-to-child transmission; hepatitis A and hepatitis B vaccination; screening for other sexually transmitted diseases (STDs) and tuberculosis (TB); partner services; and other medical, social, and mental-health services.

What Are the Benefits of Syringe Services Programs?

Based on existing evidence, the U.S. Surgeon General has determined that SSPs, when part of a comprehensive prevention strategy, can play a critical role in preventing HIV among persons who inject drugs (PWID); can facilitate entry into drug treatment and medical services; and do not increase the unsafe illegal injection of drugs. These programs have also been associated with reduced risk for infection with hepatitis C virus (HCV).

Many SSPs offer other infection-prevention materials (e.g., alcohol swabs, vials of sterile water), condoms, and services, such as education on safer injection practices and wound care; overdose prevention; referral to substance-use disorder (SUD) treatment programs including medication-assisted treatment; and counseling and testing for HIV and viral hepatitis. SSPs also provide linkages to other critical services and programs, including screening, care, and treatment for HIV and viral hepatitis, HIV pre- and post-exposure prophylaxis (PrEP), prevention of mother-to-child transmission, hepatitis A and hepatitis B vaccination, screening for other STDs and TB, partner services, and other medical, social, and mental-health services. SSPs also protect the public and first responders by providing safe needle disposal and by reducing the number of people living with HIV and HCV infections who could transmit those infections to others.

Do Syringe Services Programs Increase Drug Use in a Community?

No. Based on existing evidence, the U.S. Surgeon General has determined that SSPs, when part of a comprehensive HIV prevention strategy, do not increase the illegal use of drugs by injection. The opportunity to expand HIV and viral hepatitis prevention services through

SSPs will support communities in their efforts to identify and prevent new infections. SSPs are an effective public-health intervention that can reduce the transmission of HIV and facilitate entry into drug treatment and medical services, without increasing illegal injection of drugs. SSPs often provide other services important to improving the health of persons who inject drugs (PWID), including referrals to SUD and mental-health services, physical healthcare, social services, overdose prevention, and recovery support services. Studies also show that SSPs protect the public and first responders by providing safe needle disposal.

Chapter 37

Mental Illness and Addiction

Chapter Contents

Section 37.1

Addiction and Mental-Health Disorders

This section includes text excerpted from "Comorbidity:
Substance Use Disorders and Other Mental Illnesses,"
National Institute on Drug Abuse (NIDA), August 2018.

What Is Comorbidity?

Comorbidity describes two or more disorders or illnesses occurring
in the same person. They can occur at the same time or one after the
other. Comorbidity also implies interactions between the illnesses that
can worsen the course of both.

Is Drug Addiction a Mental Illness?

Yes. Addiction changes the brain in fundamental ways, changing
a person's normal needs and desires and replacing them with new
priorities connected with seeking and using the drug. This results
in compulsive behaviors that weaken the ability to control impulses,
despite the negative consequences, and are similar to hallmarks of
other mental illnesses.

How Common Are Comorbid Substance-Use Disorders and Other Mental Illnesses?

Many people who have a substance-use disorder (SUD) also develop
other mental illnesses, just as many people who are diagnosed with
mental illness are often diagnosed with a SUD. For example, about
half of people who experience a mental illness will also experience a
SUD at some point in their lives and vice versa. Few studies have been
done on comorbidity in children, but those that have been conducted
suggest that youth with SUDs also have high rates of co-occurring
mental illness, such as depression and anxiety.

Why Do These Disorders Often Co-Occur?

Although SUDs commonly occur with other mental illnesses,
this does not mean that one caused the other, even if one appeared
first. In fact, establishing which came first or why can be difficult.
However, research suggests three possibilities for this common
co-occurrence:

- **Common risk factors can contribute to both mental illness and SUDs.** Research suggests that there are many genes that can contribute to the risk of developing both a SUD and mental illness. For example, some people have a specific gene that can make them at an increased risk of mental illness as an adult, if they frequently used marijuana as a child. A gene can also influence how a person responds to a drug—whether or not using the drug makes them feel good. Environmental factors, such as stress or trauma, can cause genetic changes that are passed down through generations and may contribute to the development of mental illnesses or a SUD.

- **Mental illnesses can contribute to drug use and SUDs.** Some mental-health conditions have been identified as risk factors for developing a SUD. For example, some research suggests that people with mental illness may use drugs or alcohol as a form of self-medication. Although some drugs may help with mental-illness symptoms, sometimes this can also make the symptoms worse. Additionally, when a person develops a mental illness, brain changes may enhance the rewarding effects of substances, predisposing the person to continue using the substance.

- **Substance use and addiction can contribute to the development of mental illness.** Substance use may change the brain in ways that make a person more likely to develop a mental illness.

How Are These Comorbid Conditions Diagnosed and Treated?

The high rate of comorbidity between substance-use disorders and other mental illnesses calls for a comprehensive approach that identifies and evaluates both. Accordingly, anyone seeking help for either substance use, misuse, or addiction or another mental disorder should be evaluated for both and treated accordingly.

Several behavioral therapies have shown promise for treating comorbid conditions. These approaches can be tailored to patients according to age, the specific drug misused, and other factors. They can be used alone or in combinations with medications. Some effective behavioral therapies for treating comorbid conditions include:

- **Cognitive-behavioral therapy (CBT)** helps to change harmful beliefs and behaviors

- **Dialectical behavioral therapy (DBT)** was designed specifically to reduce self-harm behaviors, including suicide attempts, thoughts, or urges; cutting; and drug use

- **Assertive community treatment (ACT)** emphasizes outreach to the community and an individualized approach to treatment

- **Therapeutic communities (TC)** are a common form of long-term residential treatment that focuses on the "resocialization" of the person

- **Contingency management (CM)** gives vouchers or rewards to people who practice healthy behaviors

Effective medications exist for treating opioid, alcohol, and nicotine addiction and for alleviating the symptoms of many other mental disorders, yet most have not been well studied in comorbid populations. Some medications may benefit multiple problems. For example, bupropion is approved for treating both depression (Wellbutrin®) and nicotine dependence (Zyban®).

Section 37.2

Depression and Initiation of Alcohol and Drug Abuse in Teens

This section contains text excerpted from the following sources:
Text in this section begins with excerpts from "Alcohol," National Institute on Drug Abuse (NIDA) for Teens, January 2016; Text under the heading "Research Findings on Depressive Symptoms and Drug Abuse in Adolescents" is excerpted from "Depressive Symptoms and Drug Abuse in Adolescents," National Institute on Drug Abuse (NIDA), January 6, 2015. Reviewed January 2019.

Underage drinking is drinking alcohol before a person turns age 21, which is the minimum legal drinking age in the United States. Underage drinking is a serious problem, as you may have seen from your friends' or your own experiences. Alcohol is the most commonly used substance of abuse among young people in America, and drinking when you're underage puts your health and safety at risk.

Teens drink for a variety of reasons. Some teens want to experience new things. Others feel pressured into drinking by peers. And some are looking for a way to cope with stress or other problems. Unfortunately, drinking will only make any problems a person has already worse, not better.

Research Findings on Depressive Symptoms and Drug Abuse in Adolescents

Research has suggested that depressive symptoms are linked to the initiation of drug-taking in adolescents. A study by researchers at the University of Southern California examined negative urgency—or acting rashly during periods of extreme negative emotion—as the mechanism linking depressive symptoms and substance-abuse initiation.

Ninth-graders in two Los Angeles public high schools completed confidential surveys assessing negative urgency, depression levels, use of a variety of drugs, and other emotional-health behaviors. Students' depressive symptom levels were found to be associated with lifetime use of cigarettes and other forms of tobacco, marijuana, alcohol, inhalants, and prescription painkillers, and negative urgency was linked to the adolescents' depression levels and age of first use and lifetime use of alcohol. These findings suggest that emotional vulnerability increases the likelihood of trying a variety of drugs in early adolescence. Interventions that target emotional coping mechanisms and the reduction of negative urgency may be useful in preventing early drug use, warranting further study.

Chapter 38

Substance Abuse and Suicide Prevention

In 2015, over 33,000 Americans died from opioids—either prescription drugs or heroin or, in many cases, more powerful synthetic opioids like fentanyl. Hidden behind the terrible epidemic of opioid overdose deaths looms the fact that many of these deaths are far from accidental. They are suicides.

In a study of nearly five million veterans published in *Addiction*, scientists reported that presence of a diagnosis of any substance-use disorder (SUD) and specifically, diagnosis of opioid-use disorders (OUDs) led to increased risk of suicide for both males and females. The risk for suicide death was over two-fold for men with OUD. For women, it was more than eight-fold. Interestingly, when the researchers controlled the statistical analyses for other factors, including comorbid psychiatric diagnoses, greater suicide risk for females with OUD remained quite elevated, still more than two times greater than that for unaffected women. For men, it was 30 percent greater. The researchers also calculated that the suicide rate among those with

This chapter contains text excerpted from the following sources: Text in this chapter begins with excerpts from "Opioid Use Disorders and Suicide: A Hidden Tragedy (Guest Blog)," National Institute on Drug Abuse (NIDA), April 20, 2017; Text under the heading "Warning Signs of Suicidal Behavior" is excerpted from "Suicide Prevention," Substance Abuse and Mental Health Services Administration (SAMHSA), September 15, 2017.

OUD was 86.9/100,000. Compare that with an already alarming rate of 14/100,000 in the general U.S. population.

You may be tempted to think that these shocking findings about the effects of OUD on suicide risk are true only for this very special population. But that turns out not to be the case.

Another U.S. study, published in the *Journal of Psychiatric Research*, focused on 41,053 participants from the 2014 National Survey of Drug Use and Health (NSDUH). This survey uses a sample specifically designed to be representative of the entire U.S. population. After controlling for overall health and psychiatric conditions, the researchers found that prescription opioid misuse was associated with anywhere between a 40 and 60 percent increased risk for suicidal ideation (thoughts of suicide). Those reporting at least weekly opioid misuse were at much greater risk for suicide planning and attempts than those who used less often. They were about 75 percent more likely to make plans for suicide and made suicide attempts at a rate 200 percent greater than those unaffected.

Using a different strategy, a review of the literature in the journal *Drug and Alcohol Dependence* estimated standardized mortality ratios for suicide. This is a way of comparing the risk of death in individuals with a given condition compared to individuals from the general population. The researchers found that for people with OUD, the standardized mortality ratio was 1,351 and for injection drug use it was 1,373. This means that compared to the general population, OUD and injection-drug use are both associated with a more than 13-fold increased risk for suicide death.

These are stunning numbers and should be a strong call to action.

Persons who suffer from OUD are highly stigmatized. They often talk about their experience that others view them as "not deserving" treatment or "not deserving" to be rescued if they overdose because they are perceived as a scourge on society. The devastating impact of this brain disorder needs to be addressed. People who could be productive members of society and contribute to their families, their communities, and the general economy deserve treatment and attention.

Warning Signs of Suicidal Behavior

These signs may mean that someone is at risk for suicide. The risk is greater if the behavior is new, or has increased, and if it seems related to a painful event, loss, or change:

- Talking about wanting to die or kill oneself

- Looking for a way to kill oneself
- Talking about feeling hopeless or having no reason to live
- Talking about feeling trapped or being in unbearable pain
- Talking about being a burden to others
- Increasing the use of alcohol or drugs
- Acting anxious or agitated; behaving recklessly
- Sleeping too little or too much
- Withdrawing or feeling isolated
- Showing rage or talking about seeking revenge
- Displaying extreme mood swings

Part Five

Drug-Abuse Treatment
and Recovery

Chapter 39

Recognizing Drug Use

Chapter Contents

Section 39.1

Signs of Drug Use

This section contains text excerpted from the following sources:
Text in this section begins with excerpts from "Substance Abuse,"
U.S. Department of Health and Human Services (HHS), October 4,
2014. Reviewed January 2019; Text under the heading "How Can
You Tell If Your Child Is Using Drugs or Alcohol?" is excerpted
from "Signs of Drug Use," Get Smart About Drugs, U.S. Drug
Enforcement Administration (DEA), April 13, 2017.

Substance abuse has a major impact on individuals, families, and communities. The effects of substance abuse are cumulative, significantly contributing to costly social, physical, mental, and public health problems. These problems include:

- Teenage pregnancy
- Human immunodeficiency virus/acquired immunodeficiency syndrome (HIV/AIDS)
- Other sexually transmitted diseases (STDs)
- Domestic violence
- Child abuse
- Motor vehicle crashes
- Physical fights
- Crime
- Homicide
- Suicide

How Can You Tell If Your Child Is Using Drugs or Alcohol?

Teens are known to have mood swings. However, some behavior may indicate more serious issues, such as abuse of drugs and alcohol. Here are some of the warning signs of drug use.

Problems at School

The warning signs of drug use at school include:

- Frequently forgetting homework

- Missing classes or skipping school

- Disinterest in school or school activities

- A drop in grades

Physical Signs

The physical signs of drug use include:

- Lack of energy and motivation

- Red eyes and cheeks or difficulty focusing—alcohol use

- Red eyes and constricted pupils—marijuana use

- A strange burn on your child's mouth or fingers—smoking something (possibly heroin) through a metal or glass pipe

- Chronic nosebleeds—cocaine abuse

Neglected Appearance

Lack of interest in clothing, grooming, or appearance is not normal. Teenagers are usually very concerned about how they look.

Changes in Behavior

There is a marked change in their behavior.

- Teenagers enjoy privacy, but be aware of excessive attempts to be alone.

- Exaggerated efforts not to allow family members into their rooms

- Not letting you know where they go with friends, or whom they go with

- Breaking curfew without a good excuse

- Changes in relationships with family

Changes in Friends

- No longer is friends with childhood friends

- Seems interested in hanging out with older kids

- Acts secretive about spending time with new friends

Money Issues

- Sudden requests for money without a good reason

- Money stolen from your wallet or from safe places at home

- Items gone from your home and perhaps sold to buy drugs

Specific Smells

- Odor of marijuana, cigarettes, or alcohol on teen's breath, on clothing, in the bedroom, or in the car

Drug Paraphernalia

- Finding items in your child's room, backpack, or car related to drug use

Section 39.2

Am I Drug Addicted?

This section includes text excerpted from "What to Do If You Have a Problem with Drugs: For Teens and Young Adults," National Institute on Drug Abuse (NIDA), January 2016.

How Do You Know If You Have a Drug-Abuse Problem?

Addiction can happen at any age, but it usually starts when a person is young. If you continue to use drugs despite harmful consequences, you could be addicted. It is important to talk to a medical professional about it—your health and future could be at stake.

Have friends or family told you that you are behaving differently for no apparent reason—such as acting withdrawn, frequently tired or depressed, or hostile? You should listen and ask yourself if they are right—and be honest with yourself. These changes could be a sign you are developing a drug-related problem. Parents sometimes overlook such signs, believing them to be a normal part of the teen years. Only you know for sure if you are developing a problem because of your drug use. Here are some other signs:

- Hanging out with different friends
- Not caring about your appearance
- Getting worse grades in school
- Missing classes or skipping school
- Losing interest in your favorite activities
- Getting in trouble in school or with the law
- Having different eating or sleeping habits
- Having more problems with family members and friends

There is no special type of person who becomes addicted. It can happen to anyone.

Thanks to science, it is now known how drugs work in the brain, and that addiction can be successfully treated to help young people stop using drugs and lead productive lives. Asking for help early, when you first suspect you have a problem, is important; don't wait to become addicted before you seek help. If you think you are addicted, there is a treatment that can work. Don't wait another minute to ask for help.

Why Can't You Stop Using Drugs on Your Own?

Repeated drug use changes the brain. Brain imaging studies of drug-addicted people show changes in areas of the brain that are needed to learn and remember, make good decisions, and control yourself. Quitting is difficult, even for those who feel ready.

If You Want to Ask for Help, Where Do You Start?

Asking for help is the first important step. If you have a good relationship with your parents, you should start there. If you do not have a good relationship with your parents (or if they are having some problems of their own and might need help), find an adult you trust and ask him or her for help.

The next step is to go to your doctor. You might want to ask your parents to call your doctor in advance to see if she or he is comfortable discussing drug use. Believe it or not, sometimes doctors are as uncomfortable discussing it as teens are! You will want to find a doctor who has experience with these issues.

Together with your parents and doctor, you can decide if you should enter a treatment program. If you do not have a good relationship with your parents, ask another adult you trust to help you.

It takes a lot of courage to seek help for a possible drug problem because there is a lot of hard work ahead and it might get in the way of school and social activities. But treatment works, and you can recover. It just takes time, patience, and hard work. It is important because you will not be ready to go out into the world on your own until you take care of this issue. Treatment will help you counteract addiction's powerful hold on your brain and behavior so you can regain control of your life.

Keeping It to Yourself

There are privacy laws that prevent your doctor from telling your parents everything. They can't even tell law enforcement about your drug use, in case that worries you. But your parents might ask you to sign a permission form that allows your doctor to discuss your issues with them. If you feel your parents are truly trying to help you, you should consider signing the form, because having accurate information will help them find the right care and treatment for you.

There is one exception to this rule: Doctors can speak to parents and some officials if they think you are in danger of hurting yourself or others.

If you feel you are being abused by your parents or caretakers, you should discuss it with your doctor or contact a school counselor. If you are being abused, you can call the National Child Abuse Hotline for help at 800-422-4453.

What the Doctor Will Ask You

The doctor will ask you a series of questions about your use of alcohol and drugs and other risky behaviors such as driving under the influence or riding with other people who have been using drugs or alcohol. Your doctor can help you best if you tell the truth. The doctor might also give a urine and/or blood test. This will provide important information about your drug use and how it is affecting your health.

If your goal is to truly get better and get your old life back, you should cooperate with your doctor. If you think problems at home are only making it harder to stay clean, share that information with your doctor. If he or she recommends counseling or treatment, you should give it a try. There is a whole network of trained adults out there who want to help you.

What the Treatment Is Like

Treatment for drug problems is tailored to each patient's unique drug-abuse patterns and other medical, psychiatric, and social problems.

Some treatment centers offer outpatient treatment programs, which would allow you to stay in school, at least part-time. Some teens and young adults, though, do better in inpatient (residential) treatment, where you stay overnight for a period of time. An addiction specialist can advise you about your best options.

Do Treatment Centers Force People to Stop Taking Drugs Immediately?

Treatment is always based on the person's needs. However, if you are still using a drug when you are admitted to a treatment program, one of the first things addiction specialists need to do is help you safely remove drugs from your system (called "detox"). This is important because drugs impair the mental abilities you need to make treatment work for you.

When people first stop using drugs, they can experience different physical and emotional withdrawal symptoms, including depression, anxiety, and other mood disorders, as well as restlessness and sleeplessness. Remember that treatment centers are very experienced in helping you get through this process and keeping you safe and comfortable during it. Depending on your situation, you might also be given medications to reduce your withdrawal symptoms, making it easier to stop using.

Who Will Be Helping You in Treatment?

Different kinds of addiction specialists will likely be involved in your care—including doctors, nurses, therapists, social workers, and others. They will work as a team.

Are There Medications That Can Help You Stop Using?

There are medications that help treat addiction to alcohol, nicotine, and opioids (heroin and pain relievers). These are usually prescribed for adults, but sometimes doctors may prescribe them for younger patients. When medication is available, it can be combined with behavioral therapy for added benefit.

Medications are also sometimes prescribed to help with drug withdrawal and to treat possible mental-health conditions (such as depression) that might be contributing to your drug problem.

Your treatment provider will let you know what medications are available for your particular situation. You should be aware that some treatment centers don't believe a drug addiction should be treated with other drugs, so they may not want to prescribe medications. But scientific research shows that medication does help in many cases.

Why You Should Try Rehab If It Failed in Your Previous Attempt

If you have already been in rehab, it means you have already learned many of the skills needed to recover from addiction, and you should try it again. Relapsing (going back to using drugs after getting off them temporarily) does not mean the first treatment failed. People with all kinds of diseases relapse; people with other chronic diseases such as high blood pressure, diabetes, and asthma—which have both physical and behavioral components—relapse about as much as people who have addictions.

Treatment of all chronic diseases, including addiction, involves making tough changes in how you live and act, so setbacks are expected along the way. A return to drug use means treatment needs to be started again or adjusted, or that you might need a different treatment this time.

What Kind of Counseling Should You Get?

Behavioral treatments ("talk therapy") help teens and young adults increase healthy life skills and learn how to be happy without drugs. They can give you some coping skills and will keep you motivated to recover from your drug problem.

Treatment can be one-on-one with a doctor, but some of the most effective treatments for teens are ones that involve one or more of your parents or other family members.

What Are Support Groups Like?

These groups—called peer support groups—aren't the same thing as treatment, but they can help you a lot as you go through treatment and afterward. Self-help groups and other support services offer you an added layer of social support to help you stick with your healthy choices over the course of a lifetime. If you are in treatment, ask your treatment provider about good support groups.

The most well-known self-help groups are those affiliated with Alcoholics Anonymous (AA), Narcotics Anonymous (NA), Cocaine Anonymous (CA), and Teen-Anon, all of which are based on the 12-step approach.

There are other kinds of groups that can provide a lot of support, depending on where you live. To find support groups in your area, contact local hospitals, treatment centers, or faith-based organizations.

Other services available for teens include recovery high schools (in which teens attend school with other students who are also recovering) and peer recovery support services.

How Can You Avoid Fighting with Your Parents While Discussing Your Drug Addiction?

First of all, remember that they were teens once, and they understand teen life more than you think. Second, when you first tell them about your problem, they might get angry out of fear and worry. They might raise their voices because they are very worried about you and your future. Try to remain calm and simply ask for help. Repeat over and over again that you need their help.

Parents do get angry when they find out their kids have been lying to them. You'd do the same! Be honest with them. Let them know you want to change and need their help.

Is Driving A Vehicle Advisable While You Are Seeking Help for Drug Use?

The single most responsible thing you can do is stop driving until you get help for your drug use. This might be inconvenient, but if you do drugs and drive, you could end up not only killing yourself but killing others as well. That could lead to a lifetime in prison. This is no different than drinking and driving.

Taking Drugs Helps You Feel Less Depressed— What's Wrong with That?

The relief you feel is only temporary and can cause more problems down the road as your brain and body start to crave more and more drugs just to feel normal. It is possible you need to find treatment for your depression as well as for your drug use. This is very common. It is called "comorbidity" or "co-occurrence" when you have more than one health problem at the same time.

Be certain to tell your doctor about your depression (or other mental-health problems) as well as your drug use. There are many nonaddictive medicines that can help with depression or other mental-health issues. Sometimes doctors do not talk to each other as much as they should, so you need to be your own best friend and advocate and make sure all of your healthcare providers know about all of the health issues that concern you. You should be treated for all of them at the same time.

If you ever feel so depressed that you think about hurting yourself, there is a hotline you can call: 800-273-8255. This is called the National Suicide Prevention Lifeline (NSPL), and you can share all of your problems with them. A caring, nonjudgmental voice will be on the other end, listening.

Section 39.3

How to Identify Drug Paraphernalia

This section includes text excerpted from "How to Identify Drug Paraphernalia," Get Smart About Drugs, U.S. Drug Enforcement Administration (DEA), June 28, 2017.

A critical part of understanding teen drug use is awareness about drug paraphernalia—the items kids use to hide or consume drugs. You may find these items in your child's bedroom, car, or backpack.

- Plastic baggies or small paper bags

- Cigarette packages

- Electronic cigarettes (also called e-cigarettes)

- Small glass vials

- Pill bottles

- Candy or gum wrappers

- Baseball cap/ski cap

- Belt buckle
- Felt tip marker and lipstick dispensers
- Makeup bags

Drugs and Specific Paraphernalia
Marijuana

- Rolling papers
- Cigars used to fill with marijuana to make a blunt
- Pipes (metal, wooden, acrylic, glass, stone, plastic, or ceramic)
- Bongs (a filtration device used to smoke marijuana)
- Roach clips (a metal holder used to hold a marijuana cigarette)
- E-cigarettes (to smoke marijuana concentrates)

Heroin

- Needles
- Tin foil
- Pipes
- Plastic pen case or cut up drinking straw
- Small spoon

Cocaine

- Pipes
- Small mirrors, small spoons, short plastic straws, and rolled-up paper tubes
- Razor blades
- Lighters

Ecstasy / 3,4-Methylenedioxymethamphetamine / Molly

- Glow sticks, surgical mask/dust mask
- Pacifiers and lollipops (to prevent teeth grinding and jaw clenching)

- Bags of candy to hide pills

Inhalants

- Rags for sniffing
- Tubes of glue
- Balloons
- Nozzles
- Bottles or aerosol cans with hardened glue, sprays, paint, or chemical odors

Items Used to Cover up Drug Use

- Mouthwash, mints, and breathe sprays
- Eye drops for bloodshot eyes
- Sunglasses for red eyes, changes in pupil size, or eye movements

Items or Associations That May Indicate Interest in Illegal Drugs or Drug Use

- Clothing, jewelry, tattoos, and teen slang with drug culture messages
- Websites, music, or publications that glamorize drug use

Where Do Kids Buy Paraphernalia?

- Over the Internet, at tobacco shops, head shops, gift and novelty shops, gas stations, and convenience stores

Legal Consequences

Federal law states it is illegal for any person:

- To sell or offer for sale drug paraphernalia
- To use the mail or any other facility of interstate commerce to transport drug paraphernalia

For more information on possession of drug paraphernalia, check your state's drug paraphernalia laws found in the state's criminal code.

Chapter 40

Drug-Abuse Intervention

Principles of Adolescent Substance-Use Disorder Treatment

Adolescent substance use needs to be identified and addressed as soon as possible. Drugs can have long-lasting effects on the developing brain and may interfere with family, positive peer relationships, and school performance. Most adults who develop a substance-use disorder report having started drug use in adolescence or young adulthood, so it is important to identify and intervene in drug use early.

Adolescents can benefit from a drug-abuse intervention even if they are not addicted to a drug. Substance-use disorders (SUDs) range from problematic use to addiction and can be treated successfully at any stage and at any age. For young people, any drug use (even if it seems like only "experimentation") is cause for concern, as it exposes them to dangers from the drug and associated risky behaviors and may lead to more drug use in the future. Parents and other adults should monitor young people and not underestimate the significance of what may appear as isolated instances of drug taking.

Routine annual medical visits are an opportunity to ask adolescents about drug use. Standardized screening tools are available

This chapter includes text excerpted from "Principles of Adolescent Substance Use Disorder Treatment: A Research-Based Guide," National Institute on Drug Abuse (NIDA), January 2014. Reviewed January 2019.

to help pediatricians, dentists, emergency-room doctors, psychiatrists, and other clinicians determine an adolescent's level of involvement (if any) in tobacco, alcohol, and illicit and nonmedical prescription-drug use. When an adolescent reports substance use, the healthcare provider can assess its severity and either provide an onsite brief intervention or refer the teen to a substance-abuse treatment program.

Legal interventions and sanctions or family pressure may play an important role in getting adolescents to enter, stay in, and complete treatment. Adolescents with SUDs rarely feel they need treatment and almost never seek it on their own. Research shows that treatment can work even if it is mandated or entered into unwillingly.

SUD treatment should be tailored to the unique needs of the adolescent. Treatment planning begins with a comprehensive assessment to identify the person's strengths and weaknesses to be addressed. Appropriate treatment considers an adolescent's level of psychological development, gender, relations with family and peers, how well he or she is doing in school, the larger community, cultural and ethnic factors, and any special physical or behavioral issues.

Treatment should address the needs of the whole person, rather than just focusing on her or his drug use. The best approach to treatment includes supporting the adolescent's larger life needs, such as those related to medical, psychological, and social well-being, as well as housing, school, transportation, and legal services. Failing to address such needs simultaneously could sabotage the adolescent's treatment success.

Behavioral therapies are effective in addressing adolescent drug use. Behavioral therapies, delivered by trained clinicians, help an adolescent stay off drugs by strengthening his or her motivation to change. This can be done by providing incentives for abstinence, building skills to resist and refuse substances and deal with triggers or craving, replacing drug use with constructive and rewarding activities, improving problem-solving skills, and facilitating better interpersonal relationships.

Families and the community are important aspects of treatment. The support of family members is important for an adolescent's recovery. Several evidence-based interventions for adolescent drug abuse seek to strengthen family relationships by improving communication and improving family members' ability to support abstinence from drugs. In addition, members of the community (such as school counselors, parents, peers, and mentors) can encourage young people who need help to get into treatment—and support them along the way.

Effectively treating SUDs in adolescents requires also identifying and treating any other mental-health conditions they may have. Adolescents who abuse drugs frequently also suffer from other conditions including depression, anxiety disorders, attention deficit hyperactivity disorder (ADHD), oppositional defiant disorder (ODD), and conduct problems. Adolescents who abuse drugs, particularly those involved in the juvenile justice system, should be screened for other psychiatric disorders. Treatment for these problems should be integrated with the treatment for a SUD.

Sensitive issues such as violence and child abuse or risk of suicide should be identified and addressed. Many adolescents who abuse drugs have a history of physical, emotional, and/or sexual abuse or other trauma. If abuse is suspected, referrals should be made to social and protective services, following local regulations and reporting requirements.

It is important to monitor drug use during treatment. Adolescents recovering from SUDs may experience relapse or a return to drug use. Triggers associated with relapse vary and can include mental stress and social situations linked with prior drug use. It is important to identify a return to drug use early before an undetected relapse progresses to more serious consequences. A relapse signals the need for more treatment or a need to adjust the individual's current treatment plan to better meet her or his needs.

Staying in treatment for an adequate period of time and continuity of care afterward are important. The minimal length of drug treatment depends on the type and extent of the adolescent's problems, but studies show outcomes are better when a person stays in treatment for three months or more. Because relapses often occur, more than one episode of treatment may be necessary. Many adolescents also benefit from continuing care following treatment, including drug-use monitoring, follow-up visits at home, and linking the family to other needed services.

Testing adolescents for sexually transmitted diseases such as human immunodeficiency virus (HIV) and hepatitis B and C, is an important part of drug treatment. Adolescents who use drugs—whether injecting or noninjecting—are at an increased risk for diseases that are transmitted sexually as well as through the blood, including HIV and hepatitis B and C. All drugs of abuse alter judgment and decision making, increasing the likelihood that an adolescent will engage in unprotected sex and other high-risk behaviors, including sharing contaminated drug-injection equipment and unsafe tattooing and body piercing practices—potential routes of virus transmission. Substance-use treatment can reduce this risk both by reducing adolescents' drug use (and thus keeping them out of situations in which they are not thinking clearly) and by providing risk-reduction counseling to help them modify or change their high-risk behaviors.

Chapter 41

Drug-Abuse Treatment in a Healthcare Setting

Chapter Contents

Section 41.1

Medical Professionals Need to Identify Substance-Use Disorders

This section includes text excerpted from "What Role Can Medical Professionals Play in Addressing Substance Abuse (Including Abuse of Prescription Drugs) among Adolescents?" National Institute on Drug Abuse (NIDA), January 2014. Reviewed January 2019.

Role of Medical Professionals in Addressing Substance Abuse among Adolescents

Medical professionals have an important role to play in screening their adolescent patients for drug use, providing brief interventions, referring them to substance-abuse treatment if necessary, and providing ongoing monitoring and follow-up. Screening and brief interventions do not have to be time-consuming and can be integrated into general medical settings.

- **Screening.** Screening and brief assessment tools administered during annual routine medical checkups can detect drug use before it becomes a serious problem. The purpose of screening is to look for evidence of any use of alcohol, tobacco, or illicit drugs or abuse of prescription drugs and assess how severe the problem is. Results from such screens can indicate whether a more extensive assessment and possible treatment are necessary. Screening as a part of routine care also helps to reduce the stigma associated with being identified as having a drug problem.

- **Brief intervention.** Adolescents who report using drugs can be given a brief intervention to reduce their drug use and other risky behaviors. Specifically, they should be advised how continued drug use may harm their brains, general health, and other areas of their life, including family relationships and education. Adolescents reporting no substance use can be praised for staying away from drugs and rescreened during their next physical.

- **Referral.** Adolescents with substance-use disorders (SUDs) or those that appear to be developing a SUD may need a referral to substance-abuse treatment for more extensive assessment and care.

- **Follow-up.** For patients in treatment, medical professionals can offer ongoing support of treatment participation and abstinence from drugs during follow-up visits. Adolescent patients who relapse or show signs of continuing to use drugs may need to be referred back to treatment.

- **Assessing risk factors.** Before prescribing medications that can potentially be abused, clinicians can assess patients for risk factors such as mental illness or a family history of substance abuse, consider an alternative medication with less abuse potential, more closely monitor patients at high risk, reduce the length of time between visits for refills so fewer pills are on hand, and educate both patients and their parents about appropriate use and potential risks of prescription medications, including the dangers of sharing them with others.

Screening Tools and Brief Assessments Used with Adolescents

Screening tools are available and outlined in the American Academy of Pediatrics (AAP) publications.

In addition, the *Alcohol Screening and Brief Intervention for Youth: A Practitioner's Guide* developed by the National Institute on Alcohol Abuse and Alcoholism (NIAAA) provides information on identifying adolescents at high risk for alcohol abuse.

Section 41.2

Addiction Treatment Neglected in the Healthcare Setting

This section includes text excerpted from "Principles of
Adolescent Substance Use Disorder Treatment: A Research-Based
Guide—Treatment Settings," National Institute on Drug
Abuse (NIDA), January 2014. Reviewed January 2019.

Treatment for substance-use disorders (SUDs) is delivered at varying levels of care in many different settings. Because no single treatment is appropriate for every adolescent, treatments must be tailored for the individual. Based on the consensus of drug-treatment experts, the American Society of Addiction Medicine (ASAM) has developed guidelines for determining the appropriate intensity and length of treatment for adolescents with substance-abuse problems, based on an assessment involving six areas:

- Level of intoxication and potential for withdrawal

- Presence of other medical conditions

- Presence of other emotional, behavioral, or cognitive conditions

- Readiness or motivation to change

- Risk of relapse or continued drug use

- Recovery environment (e.g., family, peers, school, legal system)

With a SUD—as with any other medical condition—treatment must be long enough and strong enough to be effective. Just as an antibiotic must be taken for sufficient time to kill a bacterial infection, even though symptoms may already have subsided, substance-abuse treatment must continue for a sufficient length of time to treat the disease. Undertreating a SUD—providing lower than the recommended level of care or a shorter length of treatment than recommended—will increase the risk of relapse and could cause the patient, his or her family members, or the referring juvenile justice system to lose hope in the treatment because they will see it as ineffective.

Outpatient/Intensive Outpatient

Adolescent drug-abuse treatment is most commonly offered in outpatient settings. When delivered by well-trained clinicians, this can be highly effective. Outpatient treatment is traditionally recommended for adolescents with less severe addictions, few additional mental-health problems, and a supportive living environment, although evidence suggests that more severe cases can be treated in outpatient settings as well. Outpatient treatment varies in the type and intensity of services offered and may be delivered on an individual basis or in a group format (although research suggests group therapy can carry certain risks). Low- or moderate-intensity outpatient care is generally delivered once or twice a week. Intensive outpatient services are delivered more frequently, typically more than twice a week for at least three hours per day. Outpatient programs may offer drug abuse-prevention programming (focused on deterring further drug use) or other behavioral and family interventions.

Partial Hospitalization

Adolescents with more severe SUDs but who can still be safely managed in their home living environment may be referred to a higher level of care called "partial hospitalization" or "day treatment." This setting offers adolescents the opportunity to participate in treatment four to six hours a day at least five days a week while living at home.

Residential/Inpatient Treatment

Residential treatment is a resource-intense high level of care, generally for adolescents with severe levels of addiction whose mental-health and medical needs and addictive behaviors require a 24-hour structured environment to make recovery possible. These adolescents may have complex psychiatric or medical problems or family issues that interfere with their ability to avoid substance use. One well-known long-term residential treatment model is the therapeutic community (TC). TCs use a combination of techniques to "resocialize" the adolescent and enlist all the members of the community, including residents and staff, as active participants in treatment. Treatment focuses on building personal and social responsibility and developing new coping skills. Such programs offer a range of family services and may require family participation if the TC is sufficiently close to where the family lives. Short-term residential programs also exist.

Chapter 42

Detoxification

Few clear definitions of detoxification and related concepts are in general use at this time. Criminal justice, healthcare, substance abuse, mental health, and many other systems all define detoxification differently. This chapter offers a clear and uniform set of definitions for the various components of detoxification and substance-abuse treatment.

What Is Detoxification?

Detoxification is a set of interventions aimed at managing acute intoxication and withdrawal. It denotes a clearing of toxins from the body of the patient who is acutely intoxicated and/or dependent on substances of abuse. Detoxification seeks to minimize the physical harm caused by the abuse of substances.

The Washington Circle Group (WCG), a body of experts organized to improve the quality and effectiveness of substance-abuse prevention and treatment, defines detoxification as "a medical intervention that manages an individual safely through the process of acute withdrawal." The WCG makes an important distinction, however, in noting that "a detoxification program is not designed to resolve the long-standing psychological, social, and behavioral problems associated with alcohol and drug abuse." Detoxification is not substance-abuse treatment and rehabilitation.

This chapter includes text excerpted from "TIP 45 Detoxification and Substance Abuse Treatment," Substance Abuse and Mental Health Services Administration (SAMHSA), October 2015. Reviewed January 2019.

Detoxification as Distinct from Substance-Abuse Treatment

Detoxification is a set of interventions aimed at managing acute intoxication and withdrawal. Supervised detoxification may prevent potentially life-threatening complications that might appear if the patient were left untreated. At the same time, detoxification is a form of palliative care (reducing the intensity of a disorder) for those who want to become abstinent or who must observe mandatory abstinence from drug use as a result of hospitalization or legal involvement. Finally, for some patients, it represents a point of the first contact with the treatment system and the first step to recovery. Treatment/rehabilitation, on the other hand, involves a constellation of ongoing therapeutic services ultimately intended to promote recovery for substance-abuse patients.

Components of Detoxification

Detoxification, as a broad process, has three essential components that may take place concurrently or as a series of steps:

- **Evaluation** entails testing for the presence of substances of abuse in the bloodstream, measuring their concentration, and screening for co-occurring mental and physical conditions. The evaluation also includes a comprehensive assessment of the patient's medical and psychological conditions and social situation to help determine the appropriate level of treatment following detoxification. Essentially, the evaluation serves as the basis for the initial substance-abuse treatment plan once the patient has been withdrawn successfully.

- **Stabilization** includes the medical and psychosocial processes of assisting the patient through acute intoxication and withdrawal to the attainment of a medically stable, fully supported, substance-free state. This often is done with the assistance of medications, though in some approaches to detoxification no medication is used. Stabilization includes familiarizing patients with what to expect in the treatment milieu and their role in treatment and recovery. During this time practitioners also seek the involvement of the patient's family, employers, and other significant people when appropriate and with the release of confidentiality.

- **Fostering** the patient's entry into treatment involves preparing the patient for entry into substance-abuse treatment by stressing the importance of following through with the complete substance-abuse treatment continuum of care. For patients who have demonstrated a pattern of completing detoxification services and then failing to engage in substance-abuse treatment, a written treatment contract may encourage entrance into a continuum of substance-abuse treatment and care. This contract, which is not legally binding, is voluntarily signed by patients when they are stable enough to do so at the beginning of treatment. In it, the patient agrees to participate in a continuing care plan, with details and contacts established prior to the completion of detoxification.

All three components (evaluation, stabilization, and fostering a patient's entry into treatment) involve treating the patient with compassion and understanding. Patients undergoing detoxification need to know that someone cares about them, respects them as individuals, and has hope for their future.

Chapter 43

Treatment for Drug Addiction: An Overview

Can Drug Addiction Be Treated?

Yes, but it's not simple. Because addiction is a chronic disease, people can't simply stop using drugs for a few days and be cured. Most patients need long-term or repeated care to stop using completely and recover their lives.

Addiction treatment must help the person do the following:

- Stop using drugs
- Stay drug-free
- Be productive in the family, at work, and in society

Based on scientific research since the mid-1970s, the following key principles should form the basis of any effective treatment program:

- Addiction is a complex but treatable disease that affects brain function and behavior.
- No single treatment is right for everyone.
- People need to have quick access to treatment.

This chapter includes text excerpted from "Treatment Approaches for Drug Addiction," National Institute on Drug Abuse (NIDA), January 2018.

- Effective treatment addresses all of the patient's needs, not just his or her drug use.

- Staying in treatment long enough is critical.

- Counseling and other behavioral therapies are the most commonly used forms of treatment.

- Medications are often an important part of treatment, especially when combined with behavioral therapies.

- Treatment plans must be reviewed often and modified to fit the patient's changing needs.

- Treatment should address other possible mental disorders.

- Medically assisted detoxification is only the first stage of treatment.

- Treatment doesn't need to be voluntary to be effective.

- Drug use during treatment must be monitored continuously.

- Treatment programs should test patients for human immunodeficiency virus (HIV), acquired immunodeficiency syndrome (AIDS), hepatitis B and C, tuberculosis (TB), and other infectious diseases as well as teach them about steps they can take to reduce their risk of these illnesses.

What Are Treatments for Drug Addiction?

There are many options that have been successful in treating drug addiction, including:

- Behavioral counseling

- Medication

- Medical devices and applications used to treat withdrawal symptoms or deliver skills training

- Evaluation and treatment for co-occurring mental-health issues such as depression and anxiety

- Long-term follow-up to prevent relapse

A range of care with a tailored treatment program and follow-up options can be crucial to success. Treatment should include both medical and mental-health services as needed. Follow-up care may include community- or family-based recovery support systems.

How Are Medications and Devices Used in Drug Addiction Treatment?

Medications and devices can be used to manage withdrawal symptoms, prevent relapse, and treat co-occurring conditions.

Withdrawal. Medications and devices can help suppress withdrawal symptoms during detoxification. Detoxification is not in itself "treatment," but only the first step in the process. Patients who do not receive any further treatment after detoxification usually resume their drug use. One study of treatment facilities found that medications were used in almost 80 percent of detoxifications. In November 2017, the U.S. Food and Drug Administration (FDA) granted a new indication to an electronic stimulation device, NSS-2 Bridge, for use in helping reduce opioid-withdrawal symptoms. This device is placed behind the ear and sends electrical pulses to stimulate certain brain nerves.

Relapse prevention. Patients can use medications to help reestablish normal brain function and decrease cravings. Medications are available for treatment of opioid (heroin, prescription pain relievers), tobacco (nicotine), and alcohol addiction. Scientists are developing other medications to treat stimulant (cocaine, methamphetamine) and *Cannabis* (marijuana) addiction. People who use more than one drug, which is very common, need treatment for all of the substances they use.

- **Opioids.** Methadone (Dolophine®, Methadose®), buprenorphine (Suboxone®, Subutex®, Probuphine ®, Sublocade™), and naltrexone (Vivitrol®) are used to treat opioid addiction. Acting on the same targets in the brain as heroin and morphine, methadone and buprenorphine suppress withdrawal symptoms and relieve cravings. Naltrexone blocks the effects of opioids at their receptor sites in the brain and should be used only in patients who have already been detoxified. All medications help patients reduce drug-seeking and related criminal behavior and help them become more open to behavioral treatments. A National Institute on Drug Abuse (NIDA) study found that, once treatment is initiated, both a buprenorphine/naloxone combination and an extended-release naltrexone formulation are similarly effective in treating opioid addiction. Because full detoxification is necessary for treatment with naloxone, initiating treatment among active users was difficult, but once detoxification was complete, both medications had similar effectiveness.

441

- **Tobacco.** Nicotine-replacement therapies have several forms, including the patch, spray, gum, and lozenges. These products are available over-the-counter (OTC). The FDA has approved two prescription medications for nicotine addiction: bupropion (Zyban®) and varenicline (Chantix®). They work differently in the brain, but both help prevent relapse in people trying to quit. The medications are more effective when combined with behavioral treatments, such as group and individual therapy as well as telephone quitlines.

- **Alcohol.** Three medications have been FDA-approved for treating alcohol addiction and a fourth, topiramate, has shown promise in clinical trials (large-scale studies with people). The three approved medications are as follows:

  - **Naltrexone** blocks opioid receptors that are involved in the rewarding effects of drinking and in the craving for alcohol. It reduces relapse to heavy drinking and is highly effective in some patients. Genetic differences may affect how well the drug works in certain patients.

  - **Acamprosate (Campral®)** may reduce symptoms of long-lasting withdrawal, such as insomnia, anxiety, restlessness, and dysphoria (generally feeling unwell or unhappy). It may be more effective in patients with severe addiction.

  - **Disulfiram (Antabuse®)** interferes with the breakdown of alcohol. Acetaldehyde builds up in the body, leading to unpleasant reactions that include flushing (warmth and redness in the face), nausea, and irregular heartbeat if the patient drinks alcohol. Compliance (taking the drug as prescribed) can be a problem, but it may help patients who are highly motivated to quit drinking.

- **Co-occurring conditions.** Other medications are available to treat possible mental-health conditions, such as depression or anxiety, that may be contributing to the person's addiction.

How Are Behavioral Therapies Used to Treat Drug Addiction?

Behavioral therapies help patients:

- Modify their attitudes and behaviors related to drug use
- Increase healthy life skills

442

- Persist with other forms of treatment, such as medication

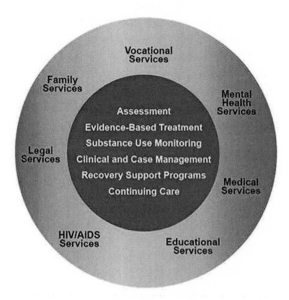

Figure 43.1. *Components of Comprehensive Drug-Addiction Treatment*

Patients can receive treatment in many different settings with various approaches.

Outpatient behavioral treatment includes a wide variety of programs for patients who visit a behavioral-health counselor on a regular schedule. Most of the programs involve individual or group drug counseling, or both. These programs typically offer forms of behavioral therapy such as:

- **Cognitive-behavioral therapy (CBT)**, which helps patients recognize, avoid, and cope with the situations in which they are most likely to use drugs

- **Multidimensional family therapy (MDFT)**—developed for adolescents with drug-abuse problems as well as their families— which addresses a range of influences on their drug-abuse patterns and is designed to improve overall family functioning

- **Motivational interviewing (MI)**, which makes the most of people's readiness to change their behavior and enter treatment

- **Motivational incentives** (contingency management), which uses positive reinforcement to encourage abstinence from drugs

Treatment is sometimes intensive at first, and patients attend multiple outpatient sessions each week. After completing intensive treatment, patients transition to regular outpatient treatment, which meets less often and for fewer hours per week to help sustain their recovery. In September 2017, the FDA permitted marketing of the first mobile application, reSET®, to help treat substance-use disorders (SUDs). This application is intended to be used with outpatient treatment to treat alcohol, cocaine, marijuana, and stimulant substance-use disorders (SUDs).

Inpatient or residential treatment can also be very effective, especially for those with more severe problems (including co-occurring disorders). Licensed residential-treatment facilities offer 24-hour structured and intensive care, including safe housing and medical attention. Residential treatment facilities may use a variety of therapeutic approaches, and they are generally aimed at helping the patient live a drug-free, crime-free lifestyle after treatment. Examples of residential treatment settings include:

- **Therapeutic communities (TCs)**, which are highly structured programs in which patients remain at a residence, typically for 6 to 12 months. The entire community, including treatment staff and those in recovery, act as key agents of change, influencing the patient's attitudes, understanding, and behaviors associated with drug use.

- **Shorter-term residential treatment**, which typically focuses on detoxification as well as providing initial intensive counseling and preparation for treatment in a community-based setting.

- **Recovery housing**, which provides supervised, short-term housing for patients, often following other types of inpatient or residential treatment. Recovery housing can help people make the transition to an independent life—for example, helping them learn how to manage finances or seek employment, as well as connecting them to support services in the community.

How Many People Get Treatment for Drug Addiction?

According to Substance Abuse and Mental Health Services Administration's (SAMHSA) National Survey on Drug Use and Health (NSDUH), 22.5 million people (8.5% of the U.S. population) age 12 or older needed treatment for an illicit-drug or alcohol-use problem in 2014. Only 4.2 million (18.5% of those who needed treatment) received any substance-use treatment in the same year. Of these, about 2.6 million people received treatment at specialty treatment programs (Center for Behavioral Health Statistics and Quality (CBHSQ), 2015).

The term "illicit" refers to the use of illegal drugs, including marijuana, according to federal law, and misuse of prescription medications.

Chapter 44

Medication and Counseling Treatment

Chapter Contents

Section 44.1

What Is Medication and Counseling Treatment?

This section includes text excerpted from "Medication and Counseling Treatment," Substance Abuse and Mental Health Services Administration (SAMHSA), September 28, 2015. Reviewed January 2019.

Medication-assisted treatment (MAT) is the use of medications, in combination with counseling and behavioral therapies, to provide a "whole-patient" approach to the treatment of substance-use disorders (SUDs). Research shows that a combination of medication and therapy can successfully treat these disorders, and for some people struggling with addiction, MAT can help sustain recovery.

MAT is primarily used for the treatment of addiction to opioids such as heroin and prescription pain relievers that contain opiates. The prescribed medication operates to normalize brain chemistry, block the euphoric effects of alcohol and opioids, relieve physiological cravings, and normalize body functions without the negative effects of the abused drug. Medications used in MAT are approved by the U.S. Food and Drug Administration (FDA), and MAT programs are clinically driven and tailored to meet each patient's needs. Combining medications used in MAT with anxiety-treatment medications can be fatal. Types of anxiety treatment medications include derivatives of Benzodiazepine, such as Xanax or valium.

Opioid-Treatment Programs

Opioid-treatment programs (OTPs) provide MAT for individuals diagnosed with an opioid-use disorder (OUD). OTPs also provide a range of services to reduce, eliminate, or prevent the use of illicit drugs, potential criminal activity, and/or the spread of infectious disease. OTPs focus on improving the quality of life of those receiving treatment.

OTPs must be accredited by a Substance Abuse and Mental Health Services Administration (SAMHSA)-approved accrediting body and certified by SAMHSA. The Division of Pharmacologic Therapies (DPT), part of the SAMHSA Center for Substance Abuse Treatment (CSAT), oversees accreditation standards and certification processes for OTPs.

Federal law requires patients who receive treatment in an OTP to receive medical, counseling, vocational, educational, and other assessment and treatment services, in addition to prescribed medication. The law allows MAT professionals to provide treatment and services in a range of settings, including hospitals, correctional facilities, offices, and remote clinics.

As of 2015, OTPs were located in every U.S. state except North Dakota and Wyoming. The District of Columbia (DC) and the territories of Puerto Rico and the Virgin Islands also had OTPs in operation.

Counseling and Behavioral Therapies

Under federal law, MAT patients must receive counseling, which could include different forms of behavioral therapy. These services are required along with medical, vocational, educational, and other assessment and treatment services.

Medication-Assisted Treatment Effectiveness

In 2013, an estimated 1.8 million people had an opioid-use disorder (OUD) related to prescription pain relievers, and about 517,000 had an opioid-use disorder related to heroin use. MAT has proved to be clinically effective and to significantly reduce the need for inpatient detoxification services for these individuals. MAT provides a more comprehensive, individually tailored program of medication and behavioral therapy. MAT also includes support services that address the needs of most patients.

The ultimate goal of MAT is a full recovery, including the ability to live a self-directed life. This treatment approach has been shown to:

- Improve patient survival

- Increase retention in treatment

- Decrease illicit opiate use and other criminal activity among people with SUDs

- Increase patients' ability to gain and maintain employment

- Improve birth outcomes among women who have SUDs and are pregnant

Research also shows that these medications and therapies can contribute to lowering a person's risk of contracting human immunodeficiency virus (HIV) or hepatitis C by reducing the potential for relapse.

Unfortunately, medication-assisted treatment (MAT) is greatly underused. For instance, according to SAMHSA's Treatment Episode Data Set (TEDS) 2002–2010, the proportion of heroin admissions with treatment plans that included receiving medication-assisted opioid therapy fell from 35 percent in 2002 to 28 percent in 2010. The slow adoption of these evidence-based treatment options for alcohol and opioid dependence is partly due to misconceptions about substituting one drug for another. Discrimination against MAT patients is also a factor, despite state and federal laws clearly prohibiting it. Other factors include lack of training for physicians and negative opinions toward MAT in communities and among healthcare professionals.

Medication-Assisted Treatment and Patient Rights

SAMHSA's Partners for Recovery Initiative produced a brochure designed to assist MAT patients and to educate and inform others. This Medication-Assisted Treatment (MAT) Know Your Rights Brochure—2009 presents and explains the federal laws that prohibit discrimination against individuals with disabilities and how they protect people receiving MAT for opioid addiction.

Under the Confidentiality Regulation, 42 Code of Federal Regulations (CFR) 2, personally identifiable health information relating to substance-use and alcohol treatment must be handled with a higher degree of confidentiality than other medical information.

Medications Used in Medication-Assisted Treatment

The FDA has approved several different medications to treat opioid addiction and alcohol dependence.

A common misconception associated with MAT is that it substitutes one drug for another. Instead, these medications relieve the withdrawal symptoms and psychological cravings that cause chemical imbalances in the body. MAT programs provide a safe and controlled level of medication to overcome the use of an abused opioid. And research has shown that when provided at the proper dose, medications used in MAT have no adverse effects on a person's intelligence, mental capability, physical functioning, or employability.

Medications used in MAT for opioid treatment can only be dispensed through a SAMHSA-certified OTP. Some of the medications used in MAT are controlled substances due to their potential for misuse. Drugs, substances, and certain chemicals used to make drugs are classified by the U.S. Drug Enforcement Administration (DEA) into five distinct categories, or schedules, depending upon a drug's acceptable medical use and potential for misuse.

Medication-Assisted Treatment Medications and Child Safety

It's important to remember that if medications are allowed to be kept at home, they must be locked in a safe place away from children. Methadone in its liquid form is colored and is sometimes mistaken for a soft drink. Children who take medications used in MAT may overdose and die.

Section 44.2

Medication and Counseling Treatment—Buprenorphine

This section includes text excerpted from "Buprenorphine,"
Substance Abuse and Mental Health Services
Administration (SAMHSA), May 31, 2016.

Buprenorphine is used in medication-assisted treatment (MAT) to help people reduce or quit their use of heroin or other opiates, such as pain relievers like morphine.

Approved for clinical use in October 2002 by the U.S. Food and Drug Administration (FDA), buprenorphine represents the advancement in medication-assisted treatment (MAT). Medications such as buprenorphine, in combination with counseling and behavioral therapies, provide a whole-patient approach to the treatment of opioid dependency. When taken as prescribed, buprenorphine is safe and effective.

Unlike methadone treatment, which must be performed in a highly structured clinic, buprenorphine is the first medication to treat opioid dependency that is permitted to be prescribed or dispensed in physician offices, significantly increasing treatment access. Under the Drug

Addiction Treatment Act (DATA) of 2000 (DATA 2000), qualified U.S. physicians can offer buprenorphine for opioid dependency in various settings, including in an office, community hospital, health department, or correctional facility.

Substance Abuse and Mental Health Services Administration (SAMHSA)-certified opioid treatment programs (OTPs) also are allowed to offer buprenorphine, but only are permitted to dispense treatment.

As with all medications used in MAT, buprenorphine is prescribed as part of a comprehensive treatment plan that includes counseling and participation in social-support programs.

Buprenorphine offers several benefits to those with opioid dependency and to others for whom treatment in a methadone clinic is not preferred or is less convenient. The FDA has approved the following buprenorphine products:

- Bunavail (buprenorphine and naloxone) buccal film

- Suboxone (buprenorphine and naloxone) film

- Zubsolv (buprenorphine and naloxone) sublingual tablets

- Buprenorphine-containing transmucosal products for opioid dependency

How Buprenorphine Works

Buprenorphine has unique pharmacological properties that help:

- Lower the potential for misuse

- Diminish the effects of physical dependency to opioids, such as withdrawal symptoms and cravings

- Increase safety in cases of overdose

Buprenorphine is an opioid partial agonist. This means that, like opioids, it produces effects such as euphoria or respiratory depression (hypoventilation). With buprenorphine, however, these effects are weaker than those of full drugs such as heroin and methadone.

Buprenorphine's opioid effects increase with each dose until at moderate doses they level off, even with further dose increases. This "ceiling effect" lowers the risk of misuse, dependency, and side effects. Also, because of buprenorphine's long-acting agent, many patients may not have to take it every day.

Side Effects of Buprenorphine

Buprenorphine's side effects are similar to those of opioids and can include:

- Nausea, vomiting, and constipation
- Muscle aches and cramps
- Cravings
- Inability to sleep
- Distress and irritability
- Fever

Buprenorphine Misuse Potential

Because of buprenorphine's opioid effects, it can be misused, particularly by people who do not have an opioid dependency. Naloxone is added to buprenorphine to decrease the likelihood of diversion and misuse of the combination drug product. When these products are taken as sublingual tablets, buprenorphine's opioid effects dominate and naloxone blocks opioid withdrawals. If the sublingual tablets are crushed and injected, however, the naloxone effect dominates and can bring on opioid withdrawals.

Buprenorphine Safety

People should use the following precautions when taking buprenorphine:

- Do not take other medications without first consulting your doctor.
- Do not use illegal drugs, drink alcohol, or take sedatives, tranquilizers, or other drugs that slow breathing. Mixing large amounts of other medications with buprenorphine can lead to overdose or death.
- Do ensure that a physician monitors any liver-related health issues that you may have

Treatment with Buprenorphine

The ideal candidates for opioid dependency treatment with buprenorphine:

- Have been objectively diagnosed with an opioid dependency

- Are willing to follow safety precautions for the treatment

- Have been cleared of any health conflicts with using
  buprenorphine

- Have reviewed other treatment options before agreeing to
  buprenorphine treatment

Before buprenorphine treatment begins, policies and procedures should be in place to guarantee patient privacy and the confidentiality of personally identifiable health information. Under the Confidentiality Regulation, 42 Code of Federal Regulations (CFR) 2, information relating to substance use and alcohol treatment must be handled with a higher degree of confidentiality than other medical information.

Buprenorphine treatment happens in three phases:

- **The Induction Phase** is the medically monitored startup
  of buprenorphine treatment performed in a qualified
  physician's office or certified opioid-treatment programs (OTP)
  using approved buprenorphine products. The medication is
  administered when a person with an opioid dependency has
  abstained from using opioids for 12 to 24 hours and is in the
  early stages of opioid withdrawal. It is important to note that
  buprenorphine can bring on acute withdrawal for patents, who
  are not in the early stages of withdrawal and who have other
  opioids in their bloodstream.

- **The Stabilization Phase** begins after a patient has
  discontinued or greatly reduced their misuse of the problem
  drug, no longer has cravings, and experiences few, if any, side
  effects. The buprenorphine dose may need to be adjusted during
  this phase. Because of the long-acting agent of buprenorphine,
  once patients have been stabilized, they can sometimes switch to
  alternate-day dosing instead of dosing every day.

- **The Maintenance Phase** occurs when a patient is doing
  well on a steady dose of buprenorphine. The length of time
  of the maintenance phase is tailored to each patient and
  could be indefinite. Once an individual is stabilized, an
  alternative approach would be to go into a medically supervised
  withdrawal, which makes the transition from a physically
  dependent state smoother. People then can engage in further

rehabilitation—with or without medication-assisted treatment (MAT)—to prevent a possible relapse.

Treatment of opioid dependency with buprenorphine is most effective in combination with counseling services, which can include different forms of behavioral therapy and self-help programs.

Section 44.3

Medication and Counseling Treatment—Methadone

This section includes text excerpted from "Methadone," Substance Abuse and Mental Health Services Administration (SAMHSA), September 28, 2015. Reviewed January 2019.

What Is Methadone?

Methadone is a medication used in medication-assisted treatment (MAT) to help people reduce or quit their use of heroin or other opiates.

Methadone has been used for decades to treat people who are addicted to heroin and narcotic pain medicines. When taken as prescribed, it is safe and effective. It allows people to recover from their addiction and to reclaim active and meaningful lives. For optimal results, patients should also participate in a comprehensive medication-assisted treatment (MAT) program that includes counseling and social support.

How Does Methadone Work?

Methadone works by changing how the brain and nervous system respond to pain. It lessens the painful symptoms of opiate withdrawal and blocks the euphoric effects of opiate drugs such as heroin, morphine, and codeine, as well as semi-synthetic opioids such as oxycodone and hydrocodone.

Methadone is offered in pill, liquid, and wafer forms and is taken once a day. Pain relief from a dose of methadone lasts about four to eight hours. Substance Abuse and Mental Health Services Administration (SAMHSA's) TIP 43: Medication-Assisted Treatment for Opioid Addiction in Opioid Treatment Programs (OTP)–2008 shows that methadone is effective in higher doses, particularly for heroin users, helping them stay in treatment programs longer.

As with all medications used in medication-assisted treatment (MAT), methadone is to be prescribed as part of a comprehensive treatment plan that includes counseling and participation in social support programs.

How Can a Patient Receive Methadone?

Patients taking methadone to treat opioid addiction must receive the medication under the supervision of a physician. After a period of stability (based on progress and proven, consistent compliance with the medication dosage), patients may be allowed to take methadone at home between program visits. By law, methadone can only be dispensed through an opioid-treatment program (OTP) certified by SAMHSA.

The length of time in methadone treatment varies from person to person. According to the National Institute on Drug Abuse (NIDA) publication *Principles of Drug Addiction Treatment: A Research-Based Guide—2012*, the length of methadone treatment should be a minimum of 12 months. Some patients may require treatment for years. Even if a patient feels that they are ready to stop methadone treatment, it must be stopped gradually to prevent withdrawal. Such a decision should be supervised by a doctor.

Patients who develop a problem with methadone or have questions can access information through SAMHSA's Find Help.

Methadone Safety

Methadone can be addictive, so it must be used exactly as prescribed. This is particularly important for patients who are allowed to take methadone at home and aren't required to take medication under supervision at an OTP. Methadone medication is specifically tailored for the individual patient (as doses are often adjusted and readjusted) and is never to be shared with or given to others. Patients should share their complete health history with health providers to ensure the safe use of the medication.

Other medications may interact with methadone and cause heart conditions. Even after the effects of methadone wear off, the medication's active ingredients remain in the body for much longer. Taking more methadone can cause unintentional overdose.

The following tips can help achieve the best treatment results:

- Never use more than the amount prescribed, and always take at the times prescribed. If a dose is missed, or if it feels like it's not working, do not take an extra dose of methadone.

- Do not consume alcohol while taking methadone.

- Be careful driving or operating machinery on methadone.

- **Call 911** if too much methadone is taken or if an overdose is suspected.

- Take steps to prevent children from accidentally taking methadone.

- Store methadone at room temperature and away from light.

- Dispose of unused methadone by flushing it down the toilet.

Side Effects of Methadone

Side effects should be taken seriously, as some of them may indicate an emergency. Patients should stop taking methadone and contact a doctor or emergency services right away if they:

- Experience difficulty breathing or shallow breathing

- Feel lightheaded or faint

- Experience hives or a rash, or swelling of the face, lips, tongue, or throat

- Feel chest pain

- Experience a fast or pounding heartbeat

- Experience hallucinations or confusion

Pregnant or Breastfeeding Women and Methadone

Women who are pregnant or breastfeeding can safely take methadone. When withdrawal from an abused drug happens to a pregnant woman, it causes the uterus to contract and may bring on miscarriage or premature birth. Methadone's ability to prevent withdrawal symptoms helps pregnant women better manage their addiction while avoiding health risks to both mother and baby.

Undergoing methadone maintenance treatment while pregnant will not cause birth defects, but some babies may go through withdrawal after birth. This does not mean that the baby is addicted. Infant withdrawal usually begins a few days after birth but may begin two to four weeks after birth.

Mothers taking methadone can still breastfeed. Research has shown that the benefits of breastfeeding outweigh the effect of the small amount of methadone that enters the breast milk. A woman who is thinking of stopping methadone treatment due to breastfeeding or pregnancy concerns should speak with her doctor first.

Section 44.4

Medication and Counseling Treatment—Naltrexone

This section includes text excerpted from "Naltrexone,"
Substance Abuse and Mental Health Services
Administration (SAMHSA), September 12, 2016.

What Is Naltrexone?

Naltrexone is a medication approved by the U.S. Food and Drug Administration (FDA) to treat opioid-use disorders (OUD) and alcohol-use disorders (AUD). It comes in a pill form or as an injectable. The pill form of naltrexone (ReVia, Depade) can be taken at 50 mg once per day. The injectable extended-release form of the drug (Vivitrol) is administered at 380 mg intramuscular once a month. Naltrexone can be prescribed by any healthcare provider who is licensed to prescribe medications. To reduce the risk of precipitated withdrawal, patients are warned to abstain from illegal opioids and opioid medication for a minimum of 7 to 10 days before starting naltrexone. If switching from methadone to naltrexone, the patient has to be completely withdrawn from the opioids.

How Naltrexone Works

Naltrexone blocks the euphoric and sedative effects of drugs such as heroin, morphine, and codeine. It works differently in the body than buprenorphine and methadone, which activate opioid receptors in the body that suppress cravings. Naltrexone binds and blocks opioid receptors, and is reported to reduce opioid cravings. There is no abuse and diversion potential with naltrexone.

If a person relapses and uses the problem drug, naltrexone prevents the feeling of getting high. People using naltrexone should not use any other opioids or illicit drugs; drink alcohol; or take sedatives, tranquilizers, or other drugs.

Patients on naltrexone may have reduced tolerance to opioids and may be unaware of their potential sensitivity to the same, or lower, doses of opioids that they used to take. If patients who are treated with naltrexone relapse after a period of abstinence, it is possible that the dosage of opioid that was previously used may have life-threatening consequences, including respiratory arrest and circulatory collapse.

As with all medications used in medication-assisted treatment (MAT), naltrexone is to be prescribed as part of a comprehensive treatment plan that includes counseling and participation in social-support programs.

Naltrexone for Opioid-Use Disorders

Extended-release injectable naltrexone is approved for treatment of people with opioid-use disorder (OUD). It can be prescribed by any healthcare provider who is licensed to prescribe medications; special training is not required. It is important that medical-managed withdrawal (detoxification) from opioids be completed at least seven to ten days before extended-release injectable naltrexone is initiated or resumed. Research has shown that naltrexone decreases reactivity to drug-conditioned cues and decreases craving. Patients who have been treated with extended-release injectable naltrexone may have reduced tolerance to opioids and may be unaware of their potential sensitivity to the same, or lower, doses of opioids that they used to take. Extended-release naltrexone should be part of a comprehensive management program that includes psychosocial support.

Naltrexone for Alcohol Dependence

When used as a treatment for alcohol dependency, naltrexone blocks the euphoric effects and feelings of intoxication. This allows people with alcohol addiction to reduce their drinking behaviors enough to remain motivated to stay in treatment and avoid relapses. Naltrexone is not addictive nor does it react adversely with alcohol.

Long-term naltrexone therapy extending beyond three months is considered most effective by researchers, and therapy may also be used indefinitely.

Side Effects of Naltrexone

People taking naltrexone may experience side effects, but they should not stop taking the medication. Instead, they should consult their healthcare provider or substance-misuse treatment practitioner to adjust the dose or change the medication. Some side effects include:

- Upset stomach or vomiting

- Diarrhea

- Headache

- Nervousness

- Sleep problems/tiredness

- Joint or muscle pain

Seek a healthcare provider right away for:

- **Liver injury.** Naltrexone may cause liver injury. Seek evaluation if there are symptoms and or signs of liver disease.

- **Injection site reactions.** This may occur from the injectable naltrexone. Seek evaluation for worsening skin reactions.

- **Allergic pneumonia.** It may cause allergic pneumonia. Seek evaluation for signs and symptoms of pneumonia.

Section 44.5

Medication and Counseling Treatment—Naloxone

This section includes text excerpted from "Naloxone,"
Substance Abuse and Mental Health Services
Administration (SAMHSA), March 3, 2016.

What Is Naloxone?

Naloxone is a medication approved by the U.S. Food and Drug Administration (FDA) to prevent overdose by opioids such as heroin, morphine, and oxycodone. It blocks opioid receptor sites, reversing the toxic effects of the overdose. Naloxone is administered when a patient is showing signs of opioid overdose. The medication can be given by intranasal spray, intramuscular (into the muscle), subcutaneous (under the skin), or intravenous injection.

Naloxone is also added to buprenorphine to decrease the likelihood of diversion and misuse of the combination drug product.

A doctor can prescribe naloxone to patients who are in medication-assisted treatment (MAT), especially if the patient is taking medications used in MAT or considered a risk for opioid overdose. Candidates for naloxone are those who:

- Take high doses of opioids for long-term management of chronic pain

- Receive rotating opioid-medication regimens

- Have been discharged from emergency medical care following opioid poisoning or intoxication

- Take certain extended-release or long-acting opioid medications

- Are completing mandatory opioid detoxification or drug abstinence programs

Pregnant women can be safely given naloxone in limited doses under the supervision of a doctor.

A doctor or pharmacist can show patients, their family members, or caregivers how to administer naloxone. Intravenous injection every two to three minutes is recommended in emergencies.

Patients given an automatic injection device or nasal spray should keep the item available at all times. Medication should be replaced when the expiration date passes.

Naloxone is effective if opioids are misused in combination with other sedatives or stimulants. It is not effective in treating overdoses of benzodiazepines or stimulant overdoses involving cocaine and amphetamines.

Side Effects of Naloxone

Patients who experience an allergic reaction from naloxone, such as hives or swelling in the face, lips, or throat, should seek medical help immediately. They should not drive or perform other potentially unsafe tasks.

Use of naloxone may cause symptoms of opioid withdrawal, including:

- Feeling nervous, restless, or irritable

- Body aches

- Dizziness or weakness

- Diarrhea, stomach pain, or nausea

- Fever, chills, or goosebumps

- Sneezing or a runny nose in the absence of a cold

Opioid Overdose

Opioid overdose can happen:

- When a patient misunderstands the directions for use, accidentally takes an extra dose, or deliberately misuses a prescription opioid or an illicit drug like heroin

- If a person takes opioid medications prescribed for someone else

- If a person mixes opioids with other medications, alcohol, or over-the-counter (OTC) drugs

Opioid overdose is life-threatening and requires immediate emergency attention. Recognizing the signs of opioid overdose is essential to saving lives.

Section 44.6

Medication and Counseling Treatment—Opioid Overdose

This section includes text excerpted from "Opioid Overdose," Substance Abuse and Mental Health Services Administration (SAMHSA), March 10, 2016.

Substance-use disorders (SUDs) impact the lives of millions of Americans. According to the Substance Abuse and Mental Health Services Administration (SAMHSA) Opioid Overdose Prevention Toolkit—2016, there were almost 17,000 prescription drug overdose deaths in 2010, which was almost double the number of similar deaths in 2001. Also, according to SAMHSA's CBHSQ Report—2015, the number of people age 12 and older who received treatment for heroin use during their most recent treatment in the past year has risen from 277,000 people in 2002 to 526,000 people in 2013.

An opioid overdose can occur for a variety of reasons, including:

- When a person overdoses on an illicit opioid drug such as heroin or morphine

- When a person overdoses on a medication used in medication-assisted treatment (MAT), many of which are controlled substances that have the potential for misuse. This can occur when someone accidentally takes an extra dose, deliberately misuses a prescription opioid, or mixes opioids with other medications, alcohol, or over-the-counter medications. An overdose can be fatal when mixing an opioid and anxiety treatment medications, including derivatives of Benzodiazepine, such as Xanax or valium.

- When a person takes an opioid medication prescribed for someone else. Children are particularly vulnerable to accidental overdoses if they take medication not intended for them.

Opioid overdose is life-threatening and requires immediate emergency attention. Recognizing the signs of opioid overdose is essential to saving lives.

Call 911 immediately if a person exhibits any of these symptoms:

- Their face is extremely pale and/or feels clammy to the touch

- Their body goes limp

- Their fingernails or lips have a purple or blue color

- They start vomiting or making gurgling noises

- They cannot be awakened or are unable to speak

- Their breathing or heartbeat slows or stops

Treating Opioid Overdose

Opioid overdose can be fatal and requires immediate medical attention. Consider the following actions:

- Call 911 if you suspect that an overdose has occurred.

- If the person has stopped breathing or if breathing is very weak, begin cardiopulmonary resuscitation (CPR).

- Make sure that your family members, caregivers, or the people who spend time with you know how to tell if you are experiencing an overdose and what to do until emergency medical help arrives. You will probably be unable to treat yourself if you experience an opioid overdose.

Naloxone is a medication used in treating opioid overdose.

Preventing Opioid Overdose

Overdose can occur even with prescription opioid pain relievers and medications used in medication-assisted treatment MAT. Always follow the instructions you receive with your medication. Ask your doctor or pharmacist if you have questions or are unsure of how to take your medication.

The following tips can help you or a loved one avoid opioid overdose:

- Take medicine as prescribed by your doctor

- Do not take more medication or take it more often than instructed

- Never mix pain medicines with alcohol, sleeping pills, or illicit substances

- Store medicine safely where children or pets can't reach it

- Dispose of unused medication promptly

Chapter 45

Treatment for Methamphetamine Addiction

Methamphetamine—meth for short—is a very addictive stimulant drug. It is a powder that can be made into a pill or a shiny rock (called a crystal). The powder can be eaten or snorted up the nose. It can also be mixed with liquid and injected into your body with a needle. Crystal meth is smoked in a small glass pipe.

Meth at first causes a rush of good feelings, but then users feel edgy, overly excited, angry, or afraid. Meth use can quickly lead to addiction. It causes medical problems including:

- Making your body temperature so high that you pass out

- Severe itching

- "Meth mouth"—broken teeth and dry mouth

- Thinking and emotional problems

This chapter contains text excerpted from the following sources: Text in this chapter begins with excerpts from "Methamphetamine," MedlinePlus, National Institutes of Health (NIH), May 6, 2016; Text under the heading "What Treatments Are Effective for People Who Abuse Methamphetamine?" is excerpted from "Methamphetamine," National Institute on Drug Abuse (NIDA), September 2013, Reviewed January 2019.

What Treatments Are Effective for People Who Abuse Methamphetamine?

The most effective treatments for methamphetamine addiction at this point are behavioral therapies, such as cognitive behavioral intervention (CBI) and contingency-management (CM) interventions. For example, the Matrix Model, a 16-week comprehensive behavioral-treatment approach that combines behavioral therapy, family education, individual counseling, 12-step support, drug testing, and encouragement for nondrug-related activities, has been shown to be effective in reducing methamphetamine abuse. CM interventions, which provide tangible incentives in exchange for engaging in treatment and maintaining drug abstinence, have also been shown to be effective. Motivational Incentives for Enhancing Drug Abuse Recovery (MIEDAR), an incentive-based method for promoting cocaine and methamphetamine abstinence, has demonstrated efficacy in methamphetamine abusers through National Institute on Drug Abuse's (NIDA) National Drug Abuse Clinical Trials Network (CTN).

Although medications have proven effective in treating some substance-use disorders, as of now there are no medications that counteract the specific effects of methamphetamine or that prolong abstinence from and reduce the abuse of methamphetamine by an individual addicted to the drug. NIDA has made research in the development of medications to treat addiction to stimulants and other drugs a priority, however. One approach being tried is to target the activity of glial cells. A drug called AV411 (ibudilast) that suppresses the neuroinflammatory actions of glial cells has been shown to inhibit methamphetamine self-administration in rats and is now being fast-tracked in clinical trials to establish its safety and effectiveness in humans with methamphetamine addiction. Also under study are approaches that use the body's immune system to neutralize the drug in the bloodstream before it reaches the brain. These approaches include injecting a user with anti methamphetamine antibodies or with vaccines that would stimulate the body to produce its own such antibodies. Researchers have begun a clinical study to establish the safety of an antimethamphetamine monoclonal antibody known as mAb7F9 in human methamphetamine users.

Chapter 46

Supporting Substance-Abuse Recovery

Chapter Contents

Section 46.1

What Is Recovery?

This section includes text excerpted from "Recovery and Recovery Support," Substance Abuse and Mental Health Services Administration (SAMHSA), October 12, 2018.

The adoption of recovery by behavioral health systems in recent years has signaled a dramatic shift in the expectation for positive outcomes for individuals who experience mental and/or substance-use conditions. Now, when individuals with mental and/or substance-use disorders (SUDs) seek help, they are met with the knowledge and belief that anyone can recover and/or manage their conditions successfully. The value of recovery and recovery-oriented behavioral-health systems is widely accepted by states, communities, healthcare providers, peers, families, researchers, and advocates including the U.S. Surgeon General, the Institute of Medicine (IOM), and others.

Substance Abuse and Mental Health Services Administration (SAMHSA) has established a working definition of recovery that defines "recovery" as a process of change through which individuals improve their health and wellness, live self-directed lives, and strive to reach their full potential. Recovery is built on access to evidence-based clinical treatment and recovery-support services for all populations.

SAMHSA has delineated four major dimensions that support a life in recovery:

- **Health**—overcoming or managing one's diseases or symptoms—for example, abstaining from the use of alcohol, illicit drugs, and nonprescribed medications if one has an addiction problem—and, for everyone in recovery, making informed, healthy choices that support physical and emotional well-being

- **Home**—having a stable and safe place to live

- **Purpose**—conducting meaningful daily activities, such as a job, school volunteerism, family caretaking, or creative endeavors, and the independence, income, and resources to participate in society

- **Community**—having relationships and social networks that provide support, friendship, love, and hope

Hope, the belief that these challenges and conditions can be overcome, is the foundation of recovery. A person's recovery is built on his or her strengths, talents, coping abilities, resources, and inherent values. It is holistic, addresses the whole person and their community, and is supported by peers, friends, and family members.

The process of recovery is highly personal and occurs via many pathways. It may include clinical treatment, medications, faith-based approaches, peer support, family support, self-care, and other approaches. Recovery is characterized by continual growth and improvement in one's health and wellness that may involve setbacks. Because setbacks are a natural part of life, resilience becomes a key component of recovery.

Resilience refers to an individual's ability to cope with adversity and adapt to challenges or change. Resilience develops over time and gives an individual the capacity not only to cope with life's challenges but also to be better prepared for the next stressful situation. Optimism and the ability to remain hopeful are essential to resilience and the process of recovery.

Because recovery is a highly individualized process, recovery services and supports must be flexible to ensure cultural relevancy. What may work for adults in recovery may be very different for youth or older adults in recovery. For example, the promotion of resiliency in young people, and the nature of social supports, peer mentors, and recovery coaching for adolescents and transitional age youth are different than recovery support services for adults and older adults.

The process of recovery is supported through relationships and social networks. This often involves family members who become the champions of their loved one's recovery. They provide essential support to their family member's journey of recovery and similarly experience the moments of positive healing as well as the difficult challenges. Families of people in recovery may experience adversities in their social, occupational, and financial lives, as well as in their overall quality of family life. These experiences can lead to increased family stress, guilt, shame, anger, fear, anxiety, loss, grief, and isolation. The concept of resilience in recovery is also vital for family members who need access to intentional supports that promote their health and well-being. The support of peers and friends is also crucial in engaging and supporting individuals in recovery.

Recovery Support

SAMHSA established recovery-support systems to promote partnering with people in recovery from mental and substance-use disorders and their family members to guide the behavioral-health system and promote individual, program, and system-level approaches that foster health and resilience (including helping individuals with behavioral-health needs be well, manage symptoms, and achieve and maintain abstinence); increase housing to support recovery; reduce barriers to employment, education, and other life goals; and secure necessary social supports in their chosen community.

Recovery support is provided through treatment, services, and community-based programs by behavioral healthcare providers, peer providers, family members, friends and social networks, the faith community, and people with experience in recovery. Recovery-support services help people enter into and navigate systems of care, remove barriers to recovery, stay engaged in the recovery process, and live full lives in communities of their choice.

Recovery-support services include culturally and linguistically appropriate services that assist individuals and families working toward recovery from mental and/or substance-use problems. They incorporate a full range of social, legal, and other services that facilitate recovery, wellness, and linkage to and coordination among service providers, and other supports shown to improve quality of life for people in and seeking recovery and their families.

Recovery-support services also include access to evidence-based practices (EBPs) such as supported employment, education, and housing; assertive community treatment; illness management; and peer-operated services. Recovery-support services may be provided before, during, or after clinical treatment or may be provided to individuals who are not in treatment but seek support services. These services, provided by professionals and peers, are delivered through a variety of community- and faith-based groups, treatment providers, schools, and other specialized services. For example, in the United States, there are 22 recovery high schools that help reduce the risk environment for youth with substance-use disorders. These schools typically have high retention rates and low relapse rates. The broad range of service-delivery options ensures the life experiences of all people are valued and represented.

Cultural Awareness and Competency

Supporting recovery requires that mental-health and addiction services:

- Be responsive and respectful to the health beliefs, practices, and cultural and linguistic needs of diverse people and groups

- Actively address diversity in the delivery of services

- Seek to reduce health disparities in access and outcomes

Cultural competence describes the ability of an individual or organization to interact effectively with people of different cultures. To produce positive change, practitioners must understand the cultural context of the community they serve and have the willingness and skills to work within this context. This means drawing on community-based values, traditions, and customs, and working with knowledgeable people from the community to plan, implement, and evaluate prevention activities.

Individuals, families, and communities that have experienced social and economic disadvantages are more likely to face greater obstacles to overall health. Characteristics such as race or ethnicity, religion, low socioeconomic status, gender, age, mental health, disability, sexual orientation or gender identity, geographic location, or other characteristics historically linked to exclusion or discrimination are known to influence health status.

SAMHSA is committed to addressing these health disparities by providing culturally and linguistically appropriate prevention, treatment, and recovery support programs. This commitment is reinforced through the agency's disparity impact strategy that monitors programs and activities to ensure that access, use, and outcomes are equitable across racial and ethnic minority groups.

The SAMHSA Office of Behavioral Health Equity (OBHE) works to reduce mental-health and substance-use disparities among diverse racial and ethnic populations, as well as lesbian, gay, bisexual, and transgender (LGBT) populations. OBHE was established to improve access to quality care and in accordance with Section 10334(b) of the Affordable Care Act (ACA) of 2010, which requires six agencies under the U.S. Department of Health and Human Services (HHS) to establish an office of minority affairs.

Through the State Peer and Family Network Grant Programs, the Recovery Community Services Program, the National Consumer Supporter Technical Assistance Center and the Targeted Capacity Expansion Peer-to-Peer grant program, SAMHSA is gathering data to assess the effectiveness of recovery supports delivered by peers with specific populations, and to identify program models that best address the needs of individuals in recovery.

A recovery focus is also a preventive approach that simultaneously supports building resiliency, wellness, measurable recovery, and quality of life (QOL).

471

Section 46.2

Recovery Support Services

This section includes text excerpted from "Principles of Adolescent
Substance Use Disorder Treatment: A Research-Based Guide,"
National Institute on Drug Abuse (NIDA), January 2014.
Reviewed January 2019.

To reinforce gains made in treatment and to improve their quality
of life (QOL) more generally, recovering adolescents may benefit from
recovery-support services, which include continuing care, mutual help
groups (such as 12-step programs), peer recovery-support services, and
recovery high schools. Such programs provide a community setting
where fellow recovering persons can share their experiences, provide
mutual support to each other's struggles with drug or alcohol problems, and in other ways support a substance-free lifestyle. Note that
recovery-support services are not substitutes for treatment. Also, the
existing research evidence for these approaches (with the exception
of Assertive Continuing Care (ACC)) is preliminary; anecdotal evidence supports the effectiveness of peer recovery-support services
and recovery high schools, for example, but their efficacy has not been
established through controlled trials.

Assertive Continuing Care

ACC is a home-based continuing-care approach delivered by trained
clinicians to prevent relapse and is typically used after an adolescent
completes therapy utilizing the Adolescent Community Reinforcement
Approach (A-CRA). Using positive and negative reinforcement to shape
behaviors, along with training in problem-solving and communication
skills, ACC combines A-CRA and assertive case-management services
(e.g., use of a multidisciplinary team of professionals, round-the-clock
coverage, assertive outreach) to help adolescents and their caregivers
acquire the skills to engage in positive social activities.

Mutual Help Groups

Mutual help groups such as the 12-step programs Alcoholics Anonymous (AA) and Narcotics Anonymous (NA) provide ongoing support
for people with addictions to alcohol or drugs, respectively, free of
charge and in a community setting. Participants meet in a group with
others in recovery, once a week or more, sharing their experiences

and offering mutual encouragement. Twelve-step groups are guided by a set of fundamental principles that participants are encouraged to adopt—including acknowledging that willpower alone cannot achieve sustained sobriety, that surrender to the group conscience must replace self-centeredness, and that long-term recovery involves a process of spiritual renewal.

Peer Recovery Support Services

Peer recovery-support services, such as recovery community centers, help individuals remain engaged in treatment and/or the recovery process by linking them together both in groups and in one-on-one relationships with peer leaders who have direct experience with addiction and recovery. Depending on the needs of the adolescent, peer leaders may provide mentorship and coaching and help connect individuals to treatment, 12-step groups, or other resources. Peer leaders may also facilitate or lead community-building activities, helping recovering adolescents build alternative social networks and have drug- and alcohol-free social options.

Recovery High Schools

Recovery high schools are schools specifically designed for students recovering from substance-abuse issues. They are typically part of another school or set of alternative school programs within the public school system, but recovery school students are generally separated from other students by means of scheduling and physical barriers. Such programs allow adolescents newly in recovery to be surrounded by a peer group supportive of recovery efforts and attitudes. Recovery schools can serve as an adjunct to formal substance-abuse treatment, with students often referred by treatment providers and enrolled in concurrent treatment for other mental-health problems.

Chapter 47

Know Your Rights: Parity for Mental-Health and Substance-Use Disorder Benefits

Mental-Health Parity and Addiction Equity Act of 2008

Health benefits are physical-health, mental-health, and substance-use disorder (SUD) services paid for by health plans, often called "health insurance." Generally, the Mental Health Parity and Addiction Equity Act (MHPAEA or "parity") requires most health plans to apply similar rules to mental-health and substance-use disorder (MH/SUD) benefits as they do for medical/surgical benefits—referred to here as "physical health" benefits.

Health Plans and Parity

Most health plans are required by law to offer parity for MH/SUD benefits. Generally, these plans include most employer-sponsored

This chapter includes text excerpted from "Know Your Rights: Parity for Mental Health and Substance Use Disorder Benefits," Substance Abuse and Mental Health Services Administration (SAMHSA), June 2016.

group health plans and individual health-insurance coverage, including coverage sold in the health-insurance marketplaces.

What Parity Means to You

Parity means that financial requirements, such as copayments, and treatment limits, such as how many visits your insurance will pay for, must be comparable for physical-health, mental-health, and substance-use disorder services. Parity also applies to rules related to how mental-health and substance-abuse disorder treatment is accessed and under what conditions treatment is covered (such as whether you need permission from your health plan before starting treatment).

Here are some examples of common limits placed on physical-health, mental-health, and substance-abuse disorder benefits and services that are subject to parity:

- Copayments (or simply copays)

- Deductibles

- Yearly visit limits

- Need for prior authorization

- Proof of medical necessity

Although benefits may differ across plans, parity requires that the processes related to plan benefit determinations be comparable.

Parity Protections

Here are examples of how the protections from this law may benefit you:

- Plans must apply comparable copays for mental-health and substance-abuse disorder care and physical healthcare.

- There can be no limit on the number of visits for outpatient mental-health and substance-abuse disorder care if there is no visit limit for outpatient physical healthcare.

- Prior authorization requirements for mental-health and substance-abuse disorder services must be comparable to or less restrictive than those for physical-health services.

Ways to Find Out More

Call your health-plan administrator or human-resources (HR) representative for the "summary plan description" and the "summary of benefits and coverage." You can usually find this number online or on the back of your health-insurance card. You may also be able to check your health-plan benefits online to see what mental-health and substance-abuse disorder services. See if they are comparable to the benefits for physical health.

Your Right to Information

With respect to parity, your health plan must provide information about the mental-health and substance-abuse disorder benefits it offers. You have the right to request this information from your health plan. This includes criteria the plan uses to decide if a service or treatment is medically necessary. If your plan denies payment for mental-health and substance-abuse disorder services, your plan must give you a written explanation of the reason for the denial and must provide more information upon request.

Your Right to Appeal a Claim

If your health plan denies a claim, you have the right to appeal a denied claim. This means you can ask your health plan to look again at its decision, and perhaps reverse the decision and pay the claim. Call your health plan to ask how to submit a request to appeal a claim.

Parity Resources

For more about the federal parity law, go to the U.S. Department of Labor (DOL) Mental Health Parity page or call toll-free at 866-444-3272 to speak to a DOL benefits advisor.

For assistance with parity issues from your state's Department of Insurance, contact information can be found on the National Association of Insurance Commissioners website.

Chapter 48

Employee-Assistance Programs for Substance Abuse

Providing support through an employee-assistance program (EAP) or other means will help your drug-free workplace program succeed.

Employees' work may suffer not only from substance-misuse or substance-use disorders (SUDs), but from marital and family turmoil; medical, financial, or legal problems; or psychological stressors. Providing employees with support for issues that affect their well-being will enhance the effectiveness of your drug-free workplace program.

Local drug-free workplace coalitions or other community-based groups may be able to provide assistance. Contact your state or country office for alcohol and drug misuse services and ask if these resources are available in your area. You can also use Substance Abuse and Mental Health Services Administration's (SAMHSA) Drug-Free Workplace Helpline, 800-967-5752, as a resource.

This chapter includes text excerpted from "Drug-Free Workplace Program—Provide Support," Substance Abuse and Mental Health Services Administration (SAMHSA), January 20, 2017.

Employee-Assistance Programs (EAPs)

Employee-assistance programs (EAPs) can help employees with personal problems that affect their job performance. EAPs can identify and address a wide range of health, financial, and social issues, including mental- and substance-use disorders. Some EAPs concentrate primarily on alcohol, prescription drug, and other drug issues.

To address such issues, EAPs usually offer services, such as employee education, individual assessments, organizational assessments, management consultation, referrals to treatment, and short-term counseling. Counseling services help employees deal with personal problems such as grief, balancing work and family life, and stress management. Some EAPs offer services for the promotion of health and wellness. Some offer legal, financial, and retirement assistance. And some provide specialized trauma-intervention services for dealing with critical incidents in the workplace. Inquire whether your health insurance carriers provide EAP services or can help identify local, regional, national, and international EAP providers.

Types of Employee-Assistance Programs
In-House/Internal Programs

In an in-house or internal program, the EAP professionals are onsite within the workplace to deliver their services. This kind of program is most often found in companies with large numbers of employees in concentrated locations. These professionals may be direct employees of the company, or they may be employees of an EAP vendor that has been contracted to provide onsite services in the workplace.

External Programs

An external program provides employees and their family members with access to a toll-free number for service intake. The EAP intake specialist verifies benefit eligibility and then refers the caller to its specialized network of EAP providers that are geographically convenient to the employee or to the employee's family member.

Blended Programs

Large corporations with dense pockets of employee concentrations, along with smaller concentrations in multiple locations, may want to consider a blended EAP. Under this structure, an employee can meet with an in-house employee-assistance professional, if the location is convenient. Otherwise, the employee can use the vendor EAP network to access EAP counseling services near home.

Management-Sponsored Programs

A management-sponsored program is, as the name indicates, sponsored exclusively by management, as opposed to being sponsored by a union or by both management and a union. Such programs can vary widely in design and scope. Some deal only with substance misuse. Some include proactive prevention and health and wellness activities, as well as problem identification and referral. Some are actively linked to the employee health-benefit structure.

Member-Assistance Programs

A member-assistance program (MAP) is provided by a union. Like EAPs, MAPs can vary widely in design and scope. Unions have a long history of addressing member, family, health, welfare, and working-condition concerns. MAPs support a wide range of prevention, problem identification, referral, and counseling services and activities for workers and their dependents.

Peer-Based Programs

Less common than conventional EAPs, peer-based or coworker-based EAPs offer education, training, assistance, and referrals—all through peers and coworkers. This type of program requires extensive education and training for employees.

Selecting an Employee-Assistance Programs

Not every EAP will be right for every organization. To determine whether a particular EAP will meet your specific needs, ask the EAP provider the following questions:

- Do members of your staff belong to a professional EAP association, such as the Employee Assistance Trade Association (EASNA) or the International Employee Assistance Professionals Association (EAPA)?

- Do the staff who will be assigned to my organization hold the Certified Employee Assistance Professional (CEAP) credential?

- What is the education level of each member of your professional staff?

- Do you have references we may contact?

- Do you provide on-site employee-education and supervisor-training services?

- What fee programs do you offer?

- Will you do on-site visits? Are you able to conduct a needs assessment of our organization?

- What types of counseling services are available to employees? How many sessions?

- How easy will it be for employees to use the EAP? Where and how often is the EAP available to employees?

- To which programs and services do you make referrals, and why?

- Does the EAP have a system for evaluating the effectiveness of the program?

When seeking EAP services, be sure to provide prospective EAPs with information about your health-benefits structure, your drug-free-workplace policy, and a description of the service that you want the EAP program to provide. If you have a preferred budget range, share that information as well. You also might want to share the characteristics of your workplace and employees, such as worksites, job categories, and the numbers and demographics of employees, supervisors, and covered family members.

Costs and Benefits of Employee-Assistance Programs

Numerous studies have supported the business case for the purchase of EAPs and other workplace services, with many employers receiving positive returns on their EAP investments. Research on the prevalence, cost, and characteristics of EAPs suggests that EAPs are worthwhile and can also provide a valuable way for workers with personal problems to access appropriate healthcare.

External EAPs are typically priced on a fixed-fee basis. Under this pricing structure, an employer pays a fixed rate per employee per month, multiplied by the total number of employees across each contract year. The pricing is based on the total package of services that the employer ultimately selects, such as the total number of short-term counseling sessions available per employee or family member, per problem, and per year.

Sometimes an employer may be able to engage in a fee-for-service contract with EAPs. This pricing arrangement is typically available for EAP add-on services such as substance-use professional evaluations, mental-health debriefings, and crisis intervention.

For small employers, securing EAP services through a small-business EAP consortium can prove financially beneficial. The pricing is based on the services available through the consortium, but the total number of covered employees in the consortium drives down the per-employee cost.

Assessing Costs and Services

Be clear about what you want and can afford. Be specific if you are seeking EAP services for policy development, policy critique or legal review, or implementation planning. Let the EAP know if you would like them to develop educational materials, such as written materials for employees or supervisor-training sessions. Also, communicate whether or not you want customized reports on EAP service utilization.

If the costs seem too high, ask what work could be done within your budget, or if payment plans are available. The work could also be done in phases. You may also want to approach other EAPs for bids to see if their fees are closer to your budget.

Be sure to ask questions about:

- Fees and how they are calculated

- What work will be done

- Who will do the work and what qualifications they have

- When work will be completed

- What results can be anticipated

- Who to call for references

Chapter 49

Drug Courts

Drug courts are specialized court docket programs that target criminal defendants and offenders, juvenile offenders, and parents with pending child-welfare cases who have alcohol- and other drug dependency problems.

As of June 2015, the estimated number of drug courts operating in the United States is over 3,000. The majority target adults, including driving while intoxicated (DWI) offenders and a growing number of veterans; others address juvenile, child welfare, and different case types.

Table 49.1. Types of Drug Courts (Number and Types of Drug Courts (As of June 2015))

Type of Drug Court	Number
Adult	1,558
Juvenile	409
Family	312
Veterans	306
DWI	284
Tribal	138
Co-occurring	70

This chapter includes text excerpted from "Drug Courts," National Institute of Justice (NIJ), U.S. Department of Justice (DOJ), August 23, 2018.

Table 49.1. Continued

Type of Drug Court	Number
Re-entry	29
Federal District	27
Federal Veterans	6
Campus	3
Total	3,142

The Drug Court Model

Although drug courts vary in the target population, program design, and service resources, they are generally based on a comprehensive model involving:

- Offender screening and assessment of risks, needs, and responsivity

- Judicial interaction

- Monitoring (e.g., drug testing) and supervision

- Graduated sanctions and incentives

- Treatment and rehabilitation services

Drug courts are usually managed by a nonadversarial and multidisciplinary team including judges, prosecutors, defense attorneys, community corrections, social workers, and treatment-service professionals. Support from stakeholders representing law enforcement, the family, and the community is encouraged through participation in hearings, programming, and events such as graduation.

Impact of Drug Courts on Recidivism and Cost

Lower recidivism. Using retrospective data, researchers in several studies found that drug courts reduced recidivism among program participants in contrast to comparable probationers. For example, one study found that, within a two-year follow-up period, the felony rearrest rate decreased from 40 percent before the drug court to 12 percent after the drug court started in one county, and the felony re-arrest rate decreased from 50 to 35 percent in another county.

In an unprecedented longitudinal study that accumulated recidivism and cost analyses of drug court cohorts over 10 years, National Institute of Justice (NIJ) researchers found that drug courts may lower recidivism rates (rearrests) and significantly lower costs. They used data from a primarily pre-plea adult drug court in Portland, Oregon, to track 6,500 offenders who participated in the Multnomah County Drug Court between 1991 and 2001. Rearrests were lower five years or more later compared to rearrests for similar drug offenders within the same county.

The researchers also found, however, that the drug courts' impact on recidivism varied by year as a result of changes in programming and judge assignments over time. Reductions in recidivism ranged from 17 to 26 percent.

Lower costs. Compared to traditional criminal-justice system processing, treatment, and other investment costs averaged $1,392 lower per drug court participant. Reduced recidivism and other long-term program outcomes resulted in public savings of $6,744 on average per participant (or $12,218 if victimization costs are included).

Factors for success. Although general research findings are that drug-courts can reduce recidivism and promote other positive outcomes such as cost savings, several factors affect a drug court program's success:

- Proper assessment and treatment
- The role assumed by the judge and the nature of offender interactions with the judge
- Other variable influences such as drug-use trends, staff turnover, and resource allocation

Through NIJ's Multisite Adult Drug Court Evaluation (MADCE) program, researchers examined the underlying processes to identify what practices are effective, for whom, and under what conditions.

Part Six

Drug-Abuse Testing and Prevention

Chapter 50

Drug-Abuse Prevention Begins at Home

Chapter Contents

Section 50.1

Talking to Your Child about Tobacco, Alcohol, and Drugs

This section includes text excerpted from "Talk to Your Kids about Tobacco, Alcohol, and Drugs," Office of Disease Prevention and Health Promotion (ODPHP), U.S. Department of Health and Human Services (HHS), July 24, 2018.

The Basics

Talk to your child about the dangers of tobacco, alcohol, and drugs. Knowing the facts will help your child make healthy choices.

What Do You Need to Say?

When you talk about tobacco, alcohol, and drugs:

- Find out what your child already knows.

- Teach your child the facts.

- Give your child clear rules.

- Be prepared to answer your child's questions.

- Talk with your child about how to say "no."

When Should You Start Talking with Your Child?

Start early. By preschool, most children have seen adults smoking cigarettes or drinking alcohol, either in real life, on television (TV), or online.

Make sure your child knows right from the start that you think it's important to stay safe and avoid drugs.

Here are more reasons to start the conversation early:

- Almost 9 out of 10 smokers start smoking before they turn 18.

- By the time they are in eighth grade, most children think that using alcohol is okay.

- At age 12 or 13, some kids are already using drugs such as marijuana or prescription pain relievers.

What If Your Child Is Older?

It's never too late to start the conversation about avoiding drugs. Even if your teen may have tried tobacco, alcohol, or drugs, you can still talk about making healthy choices and how to say "no" next time.

What You Need to Know about Prescription and Other Medicines

When you talk to your child about the dangers of drugs, don't forget about drugs that may already be in your home, such as prescription or over-the-counter (OTC) drugs. These drugs are the third most commonly abused substances by teens age 14 and older (after marijuana and alcohol).

Prescription or OTC drug abuse is when a person uses a drug to get high. People might abuse drugs by:

- Taking too much of a prescription or OTC drug

- Taking a prescription drug prescribed to someone else

When not taken safely, prescription and OTC medicines can be just as addictive and dangerous as other drugs.

Commonly abused prescription or OTC drugs include:

- Opioid painkillers, such as Vicodin, OxyContin®, or codeine

- Medicines used for anxiety or sleep problems, such as Valium or Xanax

- Medicines that treat ADHD (attention deficit hyperactivity disorder), such as Adderall or Ritalin

Make sure to talk to your kids about the dangers of prescription-drug abuse.

Set a good example for your kids:

- Never take someone else's prescription medicine or give yours to anyone else.

- Keep track of the medicines in your home and store them in a locked cabinet.

- Get rid of unused medicines safely.

493

Why You Need to Talk to Your Child

Research shows that kids do listen to their parents. Children who learn about drug risks from their parents are less likely to start using drugs.

When kids choose not to use alcohol or drugs, they are also less likely to:

- Have serious trouble in school
- Get hurt in a car accident
- Be a victim of crime
- Have addiction problems as an adult

If you don't talk about it, your child may think it's okay to use alcohol and other drugs.

Take Action!

Talk with your child about tobacco, alcohol, and drugs—and keep the conversation going.

Talk with Your Child Early and Often

Start conversations about your values and expectations while your child is young. Your child will get used to sharing information and opinions with you. This will make it easier for you to continue talking as your child gets older.

Here are some tips:

- **Use everyday events to start a conversation.** For example, if you see a group of kids smoking, talk about how tobacco harms the body.
- **Give your child your full attention.** Turn off your TV, radio, cell phone, and computer, and really listen.
- **Try not to "talk at" your child.** Encourage your child to ask questions. If you don't know the answer to a question, look it up together.
- **Find age-appropriate ways** to talk to your child about drugs.

Teach Your Child the Facts

Your child needs to know how drugs can harm the brain, affect the body, and cause problems at home and in school. Kids who know the facts are more likely to make good choices.

- If your child likes sports, focus on how smoking can affect athletic performance. Or you can say that tobacco causes bad breath and yellow teeth.

- Remind your child that alcohol is a powerful drug that slows down the body and brain.

- Tell your child how other drugs—such as steroids, marijuana, and prescription medicines—affect the brain and body.

Set Clear Rules for Your Child

Not wanting to upset their parents is the number one reason kids give for not using drugs. Your child will be less tempted to use tobacco, alcohol, and drugs if you explain your rules clearly.

Here are some things to keep in mind when you talk to your child:

- Explain that you set rules to keep your child safe.

- Tell your child you expect your children not to use tobacco, alcohol, or drugs.

- Let your child know what will happen if this rule is broken—and follow through if this happens.

- Praise your child for good behavior.

Help Your Child Learn How to Say "No"

Kids say that they use alcohol and other drugs to "fit in and belong" with other kids. That's why it's important for parents to help children build the confidence to make a healthy choice when someone offers tobacco, drugs, or alcohol.

Check out these strategies to help you talk with your kids about staying healthy and drug-free.

Set a Good Example

Things you can do:

- If you smoke, try to quit.

- If you drink alcohol, don't drink too much or too often.

- If you have a drug problem, find a treatment program near you.

- Use prescription and OTC medicines safely.

- Never drink or use drugs and drive.

What If You Have Used Drugs in the Past?

Be honest with your child, but don't give a lot of details.

Get Help If You Need It

If you think your child may have a drug or alcohol problem, get help. Don't wait. Getting treatment early can make a difference.

What about Cost?

Drug and alcohol assessments for teens are covered under the Affordable Care Act (ACA), the healthcare reform law passed in 2010. Depending on your insurance plan, your child may be able to get an assessment at no cost to you.

Section 50.2

What to Do If Your Teen or Young Adult Has a Problem with Drugs

This section includes text excerpted from "What to Do If Your Teen or Young Adult Has a Problem with Drugs," National Institute on Drug Abuse (NIDA), January 2016.

How Do You Know If Your Teen or Young Adult Has a Substance-Use Disorder?

Addiction can happen at any age, but it usually starts when a person is young. If your teen continues to use drugs despite harmful consequences, she or he may be addicted.

If an adolescent starts behaving differently for no apparent reason—such as acting withdrawn, frequently tired or depressed, or hostile—it could be a sign that he or she is developing a drug-related problem. Parents and others may overlook such signs, believing them to be a normal part of puberty. Other signs include:

- A change in peer group

- Carelessness with grooming

- Decline in academic performance

- Missing classes or skipping school

- Loss of interest in favorite activities

- Trouble in school or with the law

- Changes in eating or sleeping habits

- Deteriorating relationships with family members and friends

Intervening early when you first spot signs of drug use in your teen are critical; don't wait for your teen to become addicted before you seek help. However, if a teen is addicted, treatment is the next step.

Why Can't Some Teens Stop Using Drugs on Their Own?

Repeated drug use changes the brain. Brain imaging studies of people with drug addictions show changes in areas of the brain that are critical to judgment, decision-making, learning and memory, and behavior control. Quitting is difficult, even for those who feel ready.

If You Want to Help Your Teen or Young Adult, Where Do You Start?

Asking for help from professionals is the first important step. You can start by bringing your child to a doctor who can screen for signs of drug use and other related health conditions. You might want to ask in advance if she or he is comfortable screening for drug use with standard assessment tools and making a referral to an appropriate treatment provider. If not, ask for a referral to another provider skilled in these issues.

You can also contact an addiction specialist directly. There are 3,500 board-certified physicians who specialize in addiction in the United States. The American Society of Addiction Medicine (ASAM) website (www.asam.org) has a find-a-physician feature on its homepage, and the American Academy of Child and Adolescent Psychiatry (AACAP) website (www.aacap.org) has a child and adolescent psychiatrist finder on its website. You and the physician can decide if your teen or young adult should be referred to treatment.

It takes a lot of courage to seek help for a child with a possible drug problem because there is a lot of hard work ahead for both of you, and the treatment may interrupt academic, personal, and possibly athletic milestones expected during the teen years. However, treatment works, and teens can recover from addiction, although it may take time and patience. Treatment enables young people to counteract addiction's powerful disruptive effects on their brain and behavior so they can regain control of their lives. You want to be sure your teen is healthy before venturing into the world with more independence, and where drugs are more easily available.

What Kind of Screening Will the Doctor Do?

The doctor will ask your child a series of questions about the use of alcohol and drugs, and associated risk behaviors (such as driving under the influence or riding with other drivers who have been using drugs or alcohol). The doctor might also give a urine and/or blood test to identify drugs that are being abused. This assessment will help determine the extent of a teen's drug use (if any) and whether a referral to a treatment program is necessary.

If Your Child Refuses to Cooperate, Should the Family Conduct an Intervention?

Most teens, and many young adults still being supported by their family, only enter treatment when they are compelled to do so by the pressure of their family, the juvenile-justice system, or other court systems. However, there is no evidence that confrontational "interventions" such as those familiar from TV programs are effective. It is even possible for such confrontational encounters to escalate into violence or backfire in other ways. Instead, parents should focus on creating incentives to get the teen to a doctor. Often, young people will listen to professionals rather than family members, as the latter encounters can sometimes be driven by fear, accusations, and emotions.

People of all ages with substance-use disorders (SUDs) live in fear of what will happen if their drugs are taken away. You can ensure your teen that professional treatment centers will keep her or him safe and as comfortable as possible if a detoxification process is needed. Be sure to let your teen know that family members and loved ones will stand by them and offer loving support.

How Do You Find the Right Treatment Center?

If you or your medical specialist decides your teen can benefit from substance-abuse treatment, there are many options available. You can start by contacting the government's Treatment Locator service at 800-662-4357 and findtreatment.samhsa.gov. (This service is supported by the Substance Abuse and Mental Health Services Administration (SAMHSA) in the U.S. Department of Health and Human Services (HHS).) This Treatment Locator service lets you search for a provider in your area; it will also provide information about the treatment center and if it works with teens.

You can also search the following directories to find board-certified addiction specialists near you. It's recommended to search both directories.

The American Board of Addiction Medicine (ABAM) directory lists physicians who are board-certified in addiction medicine. Many of these physicians are primary-care doctors.

The American Board of Psychiatry and Neurology (ABPN) directory lists psychiatrists who are board-certified in addiction psychiatry. These physicians specialize in mental health.

What Do You Look for in a Treatment Center for This Age Group?

Treatment approaches must be tailored to address each patient's unique substance-abuse patterns and related medical, psychiatric, and social problems. Some treatment centers offer outpatient-treatment programs, which would allow your teen to stay in school on an at least part-time basis. However, some adolescents do better in inpatient (residential) treatment. An addiction specialist can advise you about your best options.

The National Institute on Drug Abuse (NIDA) has dedicated 30 years of research into determining the drug-addiction treatments that are most effective. NIDA offers an online publication that outlines the best treatment practices for this age group. You might want to have these materials handy when you talk to treatment centers to aid you in asking the right questions.

Who Will Provide Treatment to Your Child?

Different kinds of addiction specialists will work together in your teen's care, including doctors, nurses, therapists, social workers, and others.

Is There Medication That Can Help?

There are medications available to treat addictions to alcohol, nicotine, and opioids (heroin and pain relievers). These are generally prescribed for adults but, in some circumstances, doctors may prescribe them for younger patients. When medication is available, it can be combined with behavioral therapy to ensure success for most patients. In addition, nonaddictive medication is sometimes prescribed to help with withdrawal.

Your treatment provider will advise you about what medications are available for your particular situation. Some treatment centers follow the philosophy that they should not treat drug addiction with other drugs, but research shows that medication can help in many cases.

If Your Teen or Young Adult Confides in a Doctor, Will You Be Able to Find out What's Going On?

If your child talks to a doctor or other medical expert, privacy laws might prevent that expert from sharing the information with you. However, you can speak to the doctor before your child's appointment and express your concerns, so the doctor knows the importance of a drug-use screening in your child's situation. In addition, most healthcare providers that specialize in addiction treatment can't share your information with anyone (even other providers) without your written permission.

If health professionals believe your child might be a danger to her- or himself or to others, then the provider may be able to share relevant information with family members.

What If Your Teen or Young Adult Has Been in Rehab Before?

This means your child has already learned many of the skills needed to recover from addiction, and will only benefit from further treatment. Relapse does not mean the first treatment failed. Relapse rates with are similar to rates for other chronic diseases, such as hypertension, diabetes, and asthma. Treatment of chronic diseases involves changing deeply imbedded behaviors, so setbacks are to be expected along the way. A return to substance abuse indicates that treatment needs to be reinstated or adjusted, or that a different approach might be called for.

How Will You Pay for Treatment?

If your child has health insurance, it may cover substance-abuse treatment services. Many insurance plans cover inpatient stays. When setting up appointments with treatment centers, you can ask about payment options and what insurance plans they take. They can also advise you on low-cost options.

The Behavioral Health Treatment Services Locator provided by the SAMHSA provides payment information for each of the treatment services listed, including information on sliding-fee scales and payment assistance. Its "Frequently Asked Questions" feature addresses the cost of treatment. In addition, you can also call the treatment help-line at 800-662-4357 or TTY: 800-487-4889 to ask about treatment centers that offer low- or no-cost treatment. You can contact your state substance-abuse agency. Many states offer help with payment for substance-abuse treatment.

Note that The Mental Health Parity and Addiction Equity Act (MHPAEA) ensures that copays, deductibles, and visit limits are generally not more restrictive for mental health and SUD benefits than they are for medical and surgical benefits. The Affordable Care Act (ACA) builds on this law and requires coverage of mental health and SUD services as one of its ten essential health benefits categories. Under the essential health-benefits rule, individual and small-group health plans are required to comply with these parity regulations.

When you research payment options, be sure you are speaking with people familiar with these new rules.

A note on health insurance for veterans: If the person needing treatment is a veteran or is covered by health benefits for veterans, the U.S. Department of Veterans Affairs (VA) can help you find VA services near you.

What Kind of Counseling Is Best for a Teen or Young Adult?

Your child's treatment provider will probably recommend counseling. Behavioral treatment (also known as "talk therapy") can help patients engage in the treatment process, change their attitudes and behaviors related to substance abuse, and increase healthy life skills. These treatments can also enhance the effectiveness of medications and help people stay in treatment longer.

Treatment for substance abuse and addiction can be delivered in many different settings using a variety of behavioral approaches. With adults, both individual-therapy and group-counseling settings with peers are used. However, studies suggest group therapy can be risky with younger age groups, as some participants in a group may have a negative influence over the others or even steer the conversation toward stories about having fun with drugs. Some research suggests that the most effective treatments for teens are those that involve one or more family members being present.

Will a Support Group Help Your Teen?

While group counseling is sometimes discouraged for teens, peer-support groups for teens can be a useful companion to treatment. Self-help groups and other support services can extend the effects of professional treatment for a teen recovering from an addiction. Such groups can be particularly helpful during recovery, offering an added layer of community-level social support to help teens maintain healthy behaviors over the course of a lifetime. If your teen is in treatment, your treatment provider will likely be able to tell you about good support groups.

The most well-known self-help groups are those affiliated with Alcoholics Anonymous (AA), Narcotics Anonymous (NA), Cocaine Anonymous (CA), and Teen-Anon. All of these are based on the 12-step model. Support groups for family members of people with addictions, like Alateen, can also be helpful. You can check the websites of any of these groups for information about teen programs or meetings in your area. To find other meetings in your area, contact local hospitals, treatment centers, or faith-based organizations.

Other services available for teens include recovery high schools (where teens attend school with others in recovery and apart from potentially harmful peer influences) and peer-recovery support services. There are other groups in the private sector that can provide a lot of support.

How Do You Keep Things Stable in Your Home until Your Teen Is in Treatment?

First, talk to your teen. There are ways to have a conversation about drugs or other sensitive issues that will prevent escalation into an argument.

Acknowledge your child's opinions but know that many people with substance-abuse problems are afraid and ashamed and might not always tell the truth. This is why it is important to involve medical professionals who have experience working with people struggling with substance-abuse issues.

Second, if your teen has a driver's license, and you suspect drug use, you should take away your child's driving privileges. This could cause an inconvenience for the family, but could prevent a tragic accident. This could also be used as an incentive to get your child to agree to be evaluated by a medical professional.

Handling Teens Who Are Depressed and Use Drugs

It is possible your child needs to find treatment for both depression and addiction. This is very common. It is called "comorbidity" or "co-occurrence" when you have more than one health problem at the same time. Parents should encourage their children to tell all of their healthcare providers about all of their symptoms and behaviors. There are many nonaddictive drugs that can help with depression or other mental-health issues. Sometimes healthcare providers do not communicate with each other as well as they should, so you can be your child's advocate and make sure all relevant healthcare providers know about all of your child's health issues. Your child should be treated for all health issues at the same time.

If your child ever feels so depressed that you think he or she will self-harm, there is a hotline you or your child can call. The National Suicide Prevention Lifeline's (NSPL) number is 800-273-8255. You are also welcome to call it to discuss your child's symptoms and get advice on how to best handle the situation.

Section 50.3

How to Minimize Prescription-Drug Misuse and Abuse among Teens

This section includes text excerpted from "Rise in Prescription Drug Misuse and Abuse Impacting Teens," Substance Abuse and Mental Health Services Administration (SAMHSA), April 19, 2016.

The fastest-growing drug problem in the United States isn't cocaine, heroin, or methamphetamines. It is misuse of prescription drugs, and this problem is profoundly affecting the lives of teenagers.

According to the National Institute on Drug Abuse (NIDA) Drug-Facts, prescription-drug misuse and abuse are when someone takes a medication inappropriately (for example, without a prescription). Sadly, prescription-drug misuse and abuse among young people is not an insignificant problem. According to National Survey on Drug Use and Health (NSDUH) data on youth and young adults, more than 5,700 youth in 2014 reported using prescription pain relievers without a doctor's guidance for the first time.

A common misperception is that prescription drugs are safer or less harmful to one's body than other kinds of drugs. However, there is a range of short- and long-term health consequences for each type of prescription drug used inappropriately:

- **Stimulants** have side effects in common with cocaine and may include paranoia, dangerously high body temperatures, and an irregular heartbeat, especially if stimulants are taken in large doses or in ways other than swallowing a pill.

- **Opioids**, which act on the same parts of the brain as heroin, can cause drowsiness, nausea, constipation, and, depending on the amount taken, slowed breathing.

- **Depressants** can cause slurred speech, shallow breathing, fatigue, disorientation, lack of coordination, and seizures upon withdrawal from chronic use.

These impacts can be particularly harmful to a developing adolescent brain and body. Our brains continue to develop until we reach our early- to mid-twenties. During adolescence, the prefrontal cortex (PFC) further develops to enable us to set priorities, formulate strategies, allocate attention, and control impulses. The outer mantle of the brain also experiences a burst of development, helping us to become more sophisticated at processing abstract information and understanding rules, laws, and codes of social conduct. Drug use impacts perception—a skill adolescent brains are actively trying to cultivate—and can fracture developing neural pathways. Additionally, as our brains are becoming hardwired during adolescence, the pathways being reinforced are the ones that stick. If those pathways include addiction, the impact may lead to lifelong challenges.

As with any type of mind-altering drug, prescription-drug misuse and abuse can affect judgment and inhibition, putting adolescents at heightened risk for human immunodeficiency virus (HIV) and other sexually transmitted infections, misusing other kinds of drugs, and engaging in additional risky behaviors.

Solutions to Minimize Prescription-Drug Misuse and Abuse among Teens

Here are several ways to minimize prescription-drug misuse and abuse among young people:

- **Education.** One in four teenagers believe that prescription drugs can be used as a study aid and nearly one-third of parents say that they believe that attention deficit hyperactivity disorder (ADHD) medication can improve a child's academic or testing performance, even if that child does not have ADHD. Parents, children, and prescribers must be educated on the impact of prescription drugs on the developing brain.

- **Safe medication storage and disposal.** Two-thirds of teens who misused pain relievers in the past year say that they got them from family members and friends, including their home's medicine cabinets. Hence, it is important to safeguard medicine in the home, according to the Partnership for Drug-Free Kids. Safe disposal of medications diminishes such opportunities for easy access.

- **Prescription-drug monitoring.** Many people are calling on doctors and pharmacies to better monitor how (and how often) drugs are prescribed. Doctors more readily hand out prescription painkillers than they did ten years ago, and, according to some sources, pharmacists do not habitually check prescription-drug registries, which would help to identify potential over-prescribing and misuse.

In addition, educating adolescents and their parents about the risks of drug misuse and abuse can play a role in combating the problem.

The National Institute on Drug Abuse (NIDA), a component of the National Institutes of Health (NIH), created the website NIDA for Teens (www. teens.drugabuse.gov) to educate teens, their parents, and teachers on the science behind prescription-drug misuse and abuse. Developed with the help of teens to ensure relevance, NIDA scientists created a site that delivers science-based facts about how drugs affect the brain and body so that young people will be armed with better information to make healthy decisions.

Section 50.4

Tips for Parents: The Truth about Club Drugs

This section includes text excerpted from "About Protecting Your Kids," Federal Bureau of Investigation (FBI), February 1, 2002. Reviewed January 2019.

What Are Raves?

Raves are high-energy, all-night dances that feature hard pounding techno-music and flashing laser lights. Raves are found in most metropolitan areas and, increasingly, in rural areas throughout the country. The parties are held in permanent dance clubs, abandoned warehouses, open fields, or empty buildings.

Raves are frequently advertised as "alcohol-free" parties with hired security personnel. Internet sites often advertise these events as "safe" and "drug-free." However, they are dangerously overcrowded parties where your child can be exposed to rampant drug use in a high-crime environment. Numerous overdoses are documented at these events.

Raves are one of the most popular venues in which club drugs are distributed. Club drugs include methylenedioxymethamphetamine (MDMA), more commonly known as "ecstasy," Gamma-hydroxybutyrate (GHB), and rohypnol (also known as the "date rape" drugs), ketamine, methamphetamine (also known as "Meth"), and lysergic acid diethylamide (LSD).

Because some club drugs are colorless, odorless, and tasteless, they can be added without detection to beverages by individuals who want to intoxicate or sedate others in order to commit sexual assaults.

Rave promoters capitalize on the effects of club drugs. Bottled water and sports drinks are sold at raves, often at inflated prices, to manage hyperthermia and dehydration. Also found are pacifiers to prevent involuntary teeth clenching, menthol nasal inhalers, surgical masks, chemical lights, and neon glow sticks to increase sensory perception and enhance the rave experience.

Cool-down rooms are provided, usually at a cost, as a place to cool off due to the increased body temperature of a drug user or dancer dancing in such an overcrowded space.

Don't risk your child's health and safety. Ask questions about where she or he is going and see it for yourself.

What Are Club Drugs?
Methylenedioxymethamphetamine

Street names: ecstasy, E, X, XTC, Adam, Clarity, Lover's Speed
MDMA is an amphetamine-based, hallucinogenic type drug that is taken orally, usually in a tablet or capsule form.
Effects:

- Lasts three to six hours

- Enables dancers to dance for long periods of time

- Increases the chances of dehydration, hypertension, heart or kidney failure, and increased body temperature, which can lead to death

- Long-term effects include confusion, depression, sleep problems, anxiety, paranoia, and loss of memory

Gamma-hydroxybutyrate

Street names: Grievous Bodily Harm, G, Liquid Ecstasy, Georgia Home Boy
GHB is a central-nervous-system (CNS) depressant that is usually ingested in liquid, powder, tablet, and capsule forms.
Effects:

- May last up to 4 hours, depending on the dose used

- Slows breathing and heart rates at dangerous levels

- Also has sedative and euphoric effects that begin up to 10 to 20 minutes after ingestion

- Use in connection with alcohol increases its potential for harm

- Overdose can occur quickly—sometimes death occurs

Methamphetamine

Street names: Speed, Ice, Chalk, Meth, Crystal, Crank, Fire, Glass
Methamphetamine is a CNS stimulant, often found in pill, capsule, or powder form, that can be snorted, injected, or smoked.
Effects:

- Displays signs of agitation

- Excited speech

- Lack of appetite and increased physical activity

- Often results in drastic weight loss

- Violence

- Psychotic behavior

- Paranoia

- Sometimes damage to the heart or nervous system

Ketamin

Street names: Special K, K, Vitamin K, Cat Valium
Ketamine is an injectable anesthetic used primarily by veterinarians, found either in liquid form or as a white powder that can be snorted or smoked, sometimes with marijuana.
Effects:

- Causes reactions similar to those of phencyclidine (PCP), a hallucinatory drug

- Results in impaired attention, learning, and memory function

- In larger doses, it may cause delirium, amnesia, impaired motor function, high blood pressure, and depression

Rohypnol

Street names: Roofies, Rophies, Roche, Forget-me Pill
Rohypnol is a tasteless and odorless sedative, easily soluble in carbonated beverages, with toxic effects that are aggravated by concurrent use of alcohol.

Effects:

- Can cause anterograde amnesia, which contributes to rohypnol's popularity as a "date rape" drug

- Can cause decreased blood pressure, drowsiness, visual disturbances, dizziness, and confusion

Lysergic Acid Diethylamide (LSD)

Street names: Acid, Boomers, Yellow Sunshines

LSDs are hallucinogen that causes distortions in sensory perception, usually taken orally either in tablet or capsule form. Often sold on blotter paper that has been saturated with the drug.

Effects:

- Are often unpredictable and may vary depending on dose, environment, and the user

- Causes dilated pupils, higher body temperature, increased heart rate and blood pressure, sweating, dry mouth, and tremors

- Can cause numbness, weakness, and nausea

- Long-term effects may include persistent psychosis and hallucinogenic-persisting perception disorder, commonly known as "flashbacks"

Know the Signs

Effects of stimulant club drugs, such as MDMA and methamphetamine:

- Increased heart rate

- Convulsions

- Extreme rise in body temperature

- Uncontrollable movements

- Insomnia

- Impaired speech

- Dehydration

- High blood pressure

- Grinding teeth

Effects of sedative/hallucinogenic club drugs, such as GHB, ketamine, LSD, and rohypnol:

- Slow breathing

- Decreased heart rate (Except LSD)

- Respiratory problems

- Intoxication

- Drowsiness

- Confusion

- Tremors

- Nausea

Effects common to all club drugs can include anxiety, panic, depression, euphoria, loss of memory, hallucinations, and psychotic behavior. Drugs, traces of drugs, and drug paraphernalia are direct evidence of drug abuse. Pacifiers, menthol inhalers, surgical masks, and other such items could also be considered indicators.

Where Do You Go for Help?

If you suspect your child is abusing drugs, monitor behavior carefully. Confirm with a trustworthy adult where your child is going and what he or she is doing. Enforce strict curfews. If you have evidence of club drug use, approach your child when he or she is sober, and if necessary, call on other family members and friends to support you in the confrontation.

Once the problem is confirmed, seek the help of professionals. If your child is under the influence of drugs and immediate intervention is necessary, consider medical assistance. Doctors, hospital substance programs, school counselors, the county mental-health society, members of the clergy, organizations such as Narcotics Anonymous (NA), and rape-counseling centers stand ready and waiting to provide information and intervention assistance.

Chapter 51

Drug-Abuse Testing and Prevention in Schools

Chapter Contents

Section 51.1

Drug Testing in Schools

This section includes text excerpted from "Frequently Asked
Questions about Drug Testing in Schools," National
Institute on Drug Abuse (NIDA), May 2017.

About Drug Testing in Schools
How Do Some Schools Conduct Drug Testing?

Following models established in the workplace, some schools conduct random drug testing and/or reasonable suspicion/cause testing.
This usually involves collecting urine samples to test for drugs such as
marijuana, cocaine, amphetamines, phencyclidine (PCP), and opioids
(both heroin and prescription pain relievers).

In random testing, students are selected regardless of their drug-
use history and may include students required to do a drug test as a
condition of participation in an extracurricular activity. In reasonable
suspicion/cause testing, a student can be asked to provide a urine
sample if the school suspects or has evidence that she or he is using
drugs, such as:

- School officials making direct observations

- The student presents with the physical symptoms of being under
  the influence or behaves abnormally or erratically

Why Do Some Schools Conduct Random Drug Tests?

Schools adopt random student drug testing to decrease drug misuse
and illicit-drug use among students. First, they hope random testing
will serve as a deterrent and give students a reason to resist peer pressure to take drugs. Second, drug testing can identify teens who have
started using illicit drugs and would benefit from early intervention,
as well as identify those who already have drug problems and need
a referral to treatment. Using illicit drugs not only interferes with a
student's ability to learn, but can also disrupt the teaching environment, affecting other students as well.

Is Random Drug Testing of Students Legal?

In June 2002, the U.S. Supreme Court broadened the authority
of public schools to test students for illegal drugs. The court ruled to

allow random drug tests for all middle- and high-school students participating in competitive extracurricular activities. The ruling greatly expanded the scope of school drug testing, which previously had been allowed only for student-athletes.

Just Because the U.S. Supreme Court Said Student Drug Testing for Adolescents in Competitive Extracurricular Activities Is Constitutional, Does That Mean It Is Legal in Your City or State?

A school or school district that is interested in adopting a student drug-testing program should seek legal expertise so that it complies with all federal, state, and local laws. Individual state constitutions may dictate different legal thresholds for allowing student drug testing. Communities interested in starting student drug testing programs should become familiar with the law in their respective states to ensure proper compliance.

If a Student Tests Positive for Drugs, Should That Student Face Disciplinary Consequences?

The primary purpose of drug testing is not to punish students who use illicit drugs but to prevent future illicit-drug use and to help students already using become drug-free. If a student tests positive for drugs, schools can respond to the individual situation. If a student tests positive for drug use but has not yet progressed to addiction, the school can require counseling and follow-up testing. For students diagnosed with addiction, parents and a school administrator can refer them to effective drug-treatment programs to begin the recovery process.

Why Test Teenagers at All?

Teens' brains and bodies are still developing, and this makes them especially vulnerable to the harmful effects of drug use. Most teens do not use illicit drugs, but for those who do, it can lead to a wide range of adverse effects on their behavior and health.

Short term. Even a single use of an intoxicating drug can affect a person's judgment and decision-making, resulting in accidents, poor performance in school or sports activities, unplanned risky behavior, and overdose.

Long term. Repeated drug use can lead to serious problems, such as poor academic outcomes, mood changes (depending on the drug:

depression, anxiety, paranoia, psychosis), and social or family problems caused or worsened by drugs.

Repeated drug use can also lead to addiction. Studies show that the earlier a teen begins using drugs, the more likely it is that she or he will develop a substance-use disorder (SUD). A SUD develops when continued drug use causes issues, such as health problems and failure to meet responsibilities at home, work, or school. A SUD can range from mild to severe, with the most severe form being addiction. Conversely, if teens stay away from drugs while in high school, they are less likely to develop a SUD later in life.

How Many Students Actually Use Drugs?

Findings from the 2016 Monitoring the Future (MTF) survey of eighth, tenth, and twelfth graders showed that past-year use of illicit drugs other than marijuana is down from recent peaks in all three grades.

Twenty-one percent of twelfth graders say that they've used any illicit drug other than marijuana at least once in their lifetime, and about 36 percent reported using marijuana in the last year. Misuse of prescription drugs is also a concern—for example, in 2016, more than 6 percent of high-school seniors reported nonmedical use of the prescription stimulant Adderall® in the past year.

What Testing Methods Are Available?

There are several testing methods available that use urine, hair, oral fluids, and sweat. These methods vary in cost, reliability, drugs detected, and detection period. Schools can determine their needs and choose the method that best suits their requirements, as long as the testing kits are from a reliable source.

Which Drugs Can Be Tested For?

Various testing methods normally test for a "panel" of five to ten different drugs. A typical drug panel tests for marijuana, cocaine, opioids (including the prescription pain relievers OxyContin® and Vicodin®), amphetamines, and PCP. If a school has a particular problem with other drugs, such as 3,4-methylenedioxymethamphetamine (MDMA), gamma-hydroxybutyrate (GHB), or appearance- and performance-enhancing drugs (steroids), they can include testing for these drugs as well. It is also possible to screen for synthetic cannabinoids, commonly known as Spice and K2.

What about Alcohol

Alcohol is a drug, and its use is a serious problem among young people. However, alcohol does not remain in the blood long enough for most tests to detect most recent use. Breathalyzers, oral fluid tests, and urine tests can only detect use within the past few hours. The cutoff is usually detection of the presence of alcohol for the equivalent of a blood alcohol content greater than 0.02 percent (20mg/1dL). Teens with substance-use problems often engage in polydrug use (they use more than one drug), so identifying a problem with an illicit or prescription drug may also suggest an alcohol problem.

How Accurate Are Drug Tests? Is There a Possibility a Test Could Give a False Positive?

The accuracy of drug tests from a certified lab is very high, and confirmation tests can help to rule out any false positives. Usually, samples are divided so that, if an initial test is positive, a confirmation test can be conducted. Federal guidelines are in place to ensure accuracy and fairness in drug-testing programs.

Can Students "Beat" the Tests?

Many drug-using students are aware of techniques that supposedly detoxify their systems or mask their drug use. Internet sites give advice on how to dilute urine samples, and there are even companies that sell clean urine or products designed to distort test results. A number of techniques and products are focused on urine tests for marijuana, but masking products are becoming more available for tests on hair, oral fluids, and multiple drugs.

Most of these products do not work, are very costly, and are easily identified in the testing process. Moreover, even if the specific drug is successfully masked, the product itself can be detected, in which case the student using it would become an obvious candidate for additional screening and attention. In fact, some testing programs label a test positive if a masking product is detected.

What Has Research Determined about the Utility of Random Drug Tests in Schools?

Study findings in this area show mixed results, but researchers generally agree that student drug testing should not be a stand-alone strategy for reducing substance use in students and that school climate (the quality and character of school life) is an important factor for achieving success in drug-prevention programs. Because there is not a clear benefit to drug testing in schools, the American Academy of Pediatrics (AAP) "opposes widespread implementation of drug testing as a means of achieving substance-abuse intervention. Relevant studies include the following:

A National Institute on Drug Abuse (NIDA)-funded study published in 2013 found evidence of lower marijuana use in the presence of school drug testing and evidence of higher use of illicit drugs other than marijuana. Otherwise, the study found no causal relationships between school drug testing and patterns of substance use.

A study published in 2013 found that positive school climate was associated with reduced likelihood of marijuana and cigarette initiation and cigarette escalation and that student drug testing was not associated with changes in the initiation or escalation of substance use. The authors conclude that improving school climates is a promising strategy for preventing student substance use, while testing is a relatively ineffective drug-prevention policy.

A study published in 2012 found that students subject to mandatory random student drug testing reported less substance use than comparable students in high schools without such testing. The study found no impact of random drug testing reported by students not participating in testing on the intention to use substances, the perceived consequences of substance use, participation in activities subject to drug testing, or school connectedness.

Results from a study published in 2012 indicate that drug testing is primarily effective at deterring substance use for female students in schools with positive climates. The authors conclude that drug testing should not be implemented as a stand-alone strategy for reducing substance use and that school climate should be considered before implementing drug testing.

A NIDA-funded study published in 2007 found that random drug and alcohol testing had no deterrent effects on student-athletes for past-month use during any of four follow-up periods. However, in two of four follow-up self-reports, student-athletes reduced past-year drug use, and two assessments showed a reduction of drug and alcohol use as well. Because the conflicting findings between the past-month and past-year substance use, more research is needed.

Section 51.2

Drug-Use Prevention Education in Schools

This section includes text excerpted from "Information for Educators, Students, Parents, and Families," Substance Abuse and Mental Health Services Administration (SAMHSA), August 27, 2018.

Federal Commission on School Safety

On March 12, 2018, President Trump established the Federal Commission on School Safety (FCSS) (the Commission), chaired by Secretary of Education (DoED) Betsy DeVos, to address school safety and the culture of school violence. The Commission will recommend policy and best practices for school violence prevention. The Commission is comprised of cabinet members whose agencies have jurisdiction over key school safety issues: the Attorney General, Secretary of Education, Secretary of Homeland Security, and Secretary of the U.S. Department of Health and Human Services (HHS). Within HHS, the Assistant Secretary for Mental Health and Substance Use also works with the Commission.

Ensuring the safety, health, and well-being of children is a top priority for HHS. Studies have shown that approximately one in ten children and youth in the United States experience a serious emotional disturbance, yet only 20 percent of those receive the help they need. Many of these children perform poorly in school and have difficulties at home and in the community. Furthermore, trauma, social isolation, and bullying are highly correlated with the development of serious emotional disturbance and the rates of youth depression, anxiety, self-harm, and most tragically, suicide are climbing.

Schools are on the front lines of addressing mental-health conditions and are vital in identifying and supporting students with these conditions in order to improve student skill and functioning, promote healthy relationships, and reduce challenging behaviors and youth violence.

Role of Educators in Preventing Drug Use

While schools provide a number of programs and activities to promote emotional health and prevent substance use among students, they face unprecedented behavioral-health challenges. The Substance

Abuse and Mental Health Services Administration (SAMHSA) provides helpful information and resources for a variety of educational settings:

- **The Safe Schools/Healthy Students Initiative Road to Success** tours four grant sites across the country and provides success stories about creating sustainable positive and healthy changes among children, youth, and families.

- **Preventing Suicide: A Toolkit for High Schools—2012** assists high-school districts in designing and implementing strategies to prevent suicide and promote behavioral health.

MentalHealth.gov provides information for educators about mental health and student behavior as well as suggestions on how to support students and families.

Role of Students in Preventing Drug Use

Young adults seeking (or in) recovery from a behavioral-health issue can benefit from peer support services that promote individual well-being. Most young people ages 12 to 20 do not drink. Get the facts about alcohol use and the reasons why children and adolescents should be too smart to start. MentalHealth.gov offers resources for children and youth who are looking for information about mental-health problems and how to seek help.

Role of Parents and Families in Preventing Drug Use

By the time most children enter preschool, they may have seen adults drink alcohol and smoke cigarettes in real life, in the media, or both. Even elementary-school children may hear about or see illegal drug use.

Visit SAMHSA's Building Blocks (www.samhsa.gov/building-blocks) for tips on talking about underage drinking, tobacco, drugs, and other sensitive issues with children.

Parents and caregivers are the leading influence in their child's decision not to drink. Check out the parent resources on SAMHSA's "Talk. They Hear You." website to start—and keep up—the conversation about the dangers of drinking alcohol at a young age.

MentalHealth.gov offers parents and caregivers information about what to look for in their children's behavior, how to talk about mental health, and how to seek help if needed.

Chapter 52

Drug Testing

Chapter Contents

Section 52.1

Drug Testing

This section includes text excerpted from "Drug
Testing," MedlinePlus, National Institutes of
Health (NIH), October 11, 2017.

What Is a Drug Test?

A drug test looks for the presence of one or more illegal or prescription drugs in your urine, blood, saliva, hair, or sweat. Urine testing is the most common type of drug screening. The drugs most often tested for include:

- Marijuana

- Opioids, such as heroin, codeine, oxycodone, morphine, hydrocodone, and fentanyl

- Amphetamines, including methamphetamine

- Cocaine

- Steroids

- Barbiturates, such as phenobarbital and secobarbital

- Phencyclidine (PCP)

Other names: Drug screen, drug test, drugs-of-abuse testing, substance-abuse testing, toxicology screen, tox screen, and sports doping tests.

What Is a Drug Test Used For?

Drug screening is used to find out whether or not a person has taken a certain drug or drugs. It may be used for:

- **Employment.** Employers may test you before hiring and/or after hiring to check for on-the-job drug use.

- **Sports organizations.** Professional and collegiate athletes usually need to take a test for performance-enhancing drugs or other substances.

- **Legal or forensic purposes.** Testing may be part of a criminal or motor-vehicle-accident investigation. Drug screening may also be ordered as part of a court case.

- **Monitoring opioid use.** If you've been prescribed an opioid for chronic pain, your healthcare provider may order a drug test to make sure you are taking the right amount of your medicine.

Why Do You Need a Drug Test?

You may have to take a drug test as a condition of your employment, in order to participate in organized sports, or as part of a police investigation or court case. Your healthcare provider may order drug screening if you have symptoms of drug abuse. These symptoms include:

- Slowed or slurred speech
- Dilated or small pupils
- Agitation
- Panic
- Paranoia
- Delirium
- Difficulty breathing
- Nausea
- Changes in blood pressure or heart rhythm

What Happens during a Drug Test

A drug test generally requires that you give a urine sample in a lab. You will be given instructions to provide a "clean catch" sample. The clean-catch method includes the following steps:

Step 1. Wash your hands.

Step 2. Clean your genital area with a cleansing pad given to you by your provider. Men should wipe the tip of their penis. Women should open their labia and clean from front to back.

Step 3. Start to urinate into the toilet.

Step 4. Move the collection container under your urine stream.

Step 5. Collect at least an ounce or two of urine into the container, which should have markings to indicate the amounts.

Step 6. Finish urinating into the toilet.

Step 7. Return the sample container to the lab technician or health-care provider.

In certain instances, a medical technician or other staff members may need to be present while you provide your sample.

For a blood test for drugs, you will go to a lab to provide your sample. During the test, a healthcare professional will take a blood sample from a vein in your arm, using a small needle. After the needle is inserted, a small amount of blood will be collected into a test tube or vial. You may feel a little sting when the needle goes in or comes out. This usually takes less than five minutes.

Will You Need to Do Anything to Prepare for the Drug Test?

Be sure to tell the testing provider or your healthcare provider if you are taking any prescription drugs, over-the-counter (OTC) medicines, or supplements because they may give you a positive result for certain illegal drugs. Also, you should avoid foods with poppy seeds, which can cause a positive result for opioids.

Are There Any Risks to the Drug Test?

There are no known physical risks to having a drug test, but a positive result may affect other aspects of your life, including your job, your eligibility to play sports, and the outcome of a court case.

What Do the Drug Test Results Mean?

If your results are negative, it means no drugs were found in your body, or the level of drugs was below an established level, which differs depending on the drug. If your results are positive, it means one or more drugs were found in your body above an established level. However, false positives can happen. So if your first test shows that you have drugs in your system, you will have further testing to figure out whether or not you are actually taking a certain drug or drugs.

Is There Anything Else You Need to Know about a Drug Test?

Before you take a drug test, you should be told what you are being tested for, why you are being tested, and how the results will be used. If you have questions or concerns about your test, talk to your healthcare provider or contact the individual or organization that ordered the test.

Section 52.2

Home-Use Drug Testing

This section includes text excerpted from "Drugs of Abuse
Home Use Test," U.S. Food and Drug Administration (FDA),
September 27, 2018.

Frequently Asked Questions on Drugs of Abuse Home Use Test
What Do These Tests Do?

These tests indicate if one or more prescription or illegal drugs
are present in urine. These tests detect the presence of drugs such as
marijuana, cocaine, opiates, methamphetamine, amphetamines, phencyclidine (PCP), benzodiazepine, barbiturates, methadone, tricyclic
antidepressants (TCAs), ecstasy, and oxycodone.

The testing is done in two steps. First, you do a quick at-home test.
Second, if the test suggests that drugs may be present, you send the
sample to a laboratory for additional testing.

What Are Drugs of Abuse?

Drugs of abuse are illegal or prescription medicines (for example, Oxycodone or Valium) that are taken for a nonmedical purpose. Nonmedical purposes for a prescription drug include taking
the medication for longer than your doctor prescribed it for or for a
purpose other than what the doctor prescribed it for. Medications
are not drugs of abuse if they are taken according to your doctor's
instructions.

What Type of Test Are These?

They are qualitative tests—you find out if a particular drug may
be in the urine, but not how much is present.

When Should You Do These Tests?

You should use these tests when you think someone might be abusing prescription or illegal drugs. If you are worried about a specific
drug, make sure to check the label to confirm that this test is designed
to detect the drug you are looking for.

523

How Accurate Are These Tests?

The at-home testing part of this test is fairly sensitive to the presence of drugs in the urine. This means that if drugs are present, you will usually get a preliminary (or presumptive) positive test result. If you get a preliminary positive result, you should send the urine sample to the laboratory for a second test.

It is very important to send the urine sample to the laboratory to confirm a positive at-home result because certain foods, food supplements, beverages, or medicines can affect the results of at-home tests. Laboratory tests are the most reliable way to confirm drugs of abuse.

Many things can affect the accuracy of these tests, including (but not limited to):

- The way the person completed the test

- The way the person stored the test or urine

- What the person ate or drank before taking the test

- Any other prescription or over-the-counter (OTC) drugs the person may have taken before the test

Note that a result showing the presence of an amphetamine should be considered carefully, even when this result is confirmed in the laboratory testing. Some OTC medications will produce the same test results as illegally abused amphetamines.

Does a Positive Test Mean That Drugs-of-Abuse Were Found?

Take no serious actions until you get the laboratory's result. Remember that many factors may cause a false positive result in the home test.

Remember that a positive test for a prescription drug does not mean that a person is abusing the drug, because there is no way for the test to indicate acceptable levels compared to abusive levels of prescribed drugs.

If the Test Results Are Negative, Can You Be Sure That the Person You Tested Did Not Abuse Drugs?

No drug test of this type is 100 percent accurate. There are several factors that can make the test results negative even though the person is abusing drugs. First, you may have been tested for the wrong drugs.

Or, you may not have tested the urine when it contained drugs. It takes time for drugs to appear in the urine after a person takes them, and they do not stay in the urine indefinitely; you may have collected the urine too late or too soon. It is also possible that the chemicals in the test went bad because they were stored incorrectly or they passed their expiration date.

If you get a negative test result, but still suspect that someone is abusing drugs, you can test again at a later time. Talk to your doctor if you need more help deciding what steps to take next.

How Soon after a Person Takes Drugs Will They Show up in a Drug Test? and How Long after a Person Takes Drugs Will They Continue to Show up in a Drug Test?

The drug clearance rate tells how soon a person may have a positive test after taking a particular drug. It also tells how long the person may continue to test positive after the last time she or he took the drug. Clearance rates for common drugs of abuse are given below. These are only guidelines, however, and the times can vary significantly from these estimates based on how long the person has been taking the drug, the amount of drug they use, or the person's metabolism.

Table 52.1. Clearance Rates for Common Drugs of Abuse

Drug	How Soon after Taking Drug Will There Be a Positive Drug Test?	How Long after Taking Drug Will There Continue to Be a Positive Drug Test?
Marijuana/Pot	1–3 hours	1–7 days
Crack (Cocaine)	2–6 hours	2–3 days
Heroin (Opiates)	2–6 hours	1–3 days
Speed/Uppers (Amphetamine, methamphetamine)	4–6 hours	2–3 days
Angel Dust/PCP	4–6 hours	7–14 days
Ecstasy	2–7 hours	2–4 days
Benzodiazepine	2–7 hours	1–4 days
Barbiturates	2–4 hours	1–3 weeks
Methadone	3–8 hours	1–3 days
Tricyclic Antidepressants	8–12 hours	2–7 days
Oxycodone	1–3 hours	1–2 days

How Is a Drugs-of-Abuse Test Performed?

These tests usually contain a sample collection cup, the drug test (it may be test strips, a test card, a test cassette, or other methods for testing the urine), and an instruction leaflet or booklet. It is very important that the person doing the test reads and understands the instructions first, before even collecting the sample. This is important because, with most test kits, the result must be visually read within a certain number of minutes after the test is started.

You collect urine in the sample collection cup and test it according to the instructions. If the test indicates the preliminary presence of one or more drugs, the sample should be sent to a laboratory where a more specific chemical test will be used in order to obtain a final result. Some home-use kits have a shipping container and preaddressed mailer in them. If you have questions about using these tests or the results that you are getting, you should contact your healthcare provider.

Chapter 53

Preventing Drug Abuse in the Workplace

Chapter Contents

Section 53.1

Drug-Free Workplace Policies

This section includes text excerpted from "Develop a Policy," Substance Abuse and Mental Health Services Administration (SAMHSA), January 20, 2017.

Creating a written drug-free policy that reflects the needs of your workplace and applicable laws is a key part of a successful drug-free workplace program.

After assessing your workplace's needs, your drug-free workplace team members should develop a policy that is customized to your organization. Organizations in safety- and security-sensitive industries are subject to additional rules and regulations.

There are many reasons to put the drug-free workplace policy in writing:

- A written policy may be required by law or by the organization's insurance carriers.

- A written policy makes legal review possible.

- A written policy provides a record of the organization's efforts and a reference if the policy is challenged. It might protect the employer from certain kinds of claims by employees.

- A written policy is easier to explain to employees, supervisors, and others.

- Putting the policy in writing helps employers and employees concentrate on important policy information.

When developing a policy, take into account:

- Legal requirements such as drug-free workplace laws and regulations that may apply

- Characteristics of the workplace and employees

- The values and priorities of the organization

Basic Elements of an Effective Policy

A drug-free workplace policy can include a statement of purpose and a discussion of implementation approaches. The other main elements of an effective policy are:

- Goals

- Definitions, expectations, and prohibitions

- Dissemination strategies

- Benefits and assurances

- Consequences and appeals

Policy Approaches

Policy approaches can range from meeting the minimum requirements mandated by law to broader policies that address other issues that might be related to drug use, such as employee absenteeism.

Option 1. Meeting the Requirements of the Law

To meet legal requirements, you must know exactly what those requirements are. If necessary, seek the advice of an appropriate legal expert.

In general, an organization's leadership should be familiar with the three types of federal laws and regulations that cover

- Federal grantees and contractors in general

- Safety-sensitive industries

- Security-sensitive industries working with the U.S. Department of Defense

Organizations not covered by these requirements may still decide to meet some or all of these requirements in their drug-free workplace policies.

At a minimum, the organization must:

- **Prepare and distribute a formal drug-free workplace policy statement.** This statement should clearly prohibit the manufacture, use, and distribution of controlled substances in the workplace and spell out the specific consequences of violating this policy.

- **Establish a drug-free awareness program.** The program should inform employees of the dangers of workplace substance use; review the requirements of the organization's drug-free workplace policy; and offer information about any counseling, rehabilitation, or employee assistance plans that may be available.

- **Ensure that all employees working on the federal contract understand their personal reporting obligations.** Under the terms of the Drug-Free Workplace Act, an employee must notify the employer within five calendar days if she or he is convicted of a criminal drug violation in the workplace.

- **Notify the federal contracting agency of any covered violation.** Under the terms of the Drug-Free Workplace Act, the employer has 10 days to report that a covered employee has been convicted of a criminal drug violation in the workplace.

- **Take direct action against an employee convicted of a workplace drug violation.** This action may involve imposing a penalty or requiring that the employee participate in an appropriate rehabilitation or counseling program.

- **Maintain an ongoing good-faith effort to meet all the requirements of the Drug-Free Workplace Act throughout the life of the contract.**

Covered organizations that fail to comply with terms of the Drug-Free Workplace Act may be subject to a variety of penalties, including suspension or termination of their federal grants or contracts and prohibition from applying for federal funds in the future.

Option 2. Addressing Other Substances

In addition, you may want your drug-free workplace policy to cover one or more types of legally obtainable substances, as well as illegal drugs. Under certain circumstances, alcohol, tobacco, legalized marijuana, and prescription drugs can adversely affect workplace health, safety, and productivity.

Options for addressing these substances include:

- **Alcohol.** Working under the influence of alcohol can be dangerous, especially in safety-sensitive positions. You may want your drug-free workplace policy to make clear that working under the influence of alcohol will not be tolerated.

- **The presence and use of alcohol in the workplace.** The mere presence of alcohol in the workplace can compromise safety and productivity because it makes workplace alcohol use more likely. You may want your policies to prohibit the presence and consumption of alcohol in the workplace.

- **Alcoholic and nonalcoholic beverages at work-related parties.** You may want to restrict the use of alcohol at work-related parties and other events. At minimum, your policy could require that nonalcoholic beverages be available at work-related events.

- **Tobacco.** You may choose to maintain a smoke-free workplace. Or you may designate certain areas as smoke-free and prohibit the sale of tobacco products at worksites.

- **Prescription drugs.** The Substance Abuse and Mental Health Services Administration (SAMHSA) has identified prescription-drug misuse and abuse as a growing national problem. You may decide to establish guidelines for employees using particular prescription medications and medical marijuana, especially if the medications could affect job performance.

Option 3. Addressing Other Problems That May Be Related to Drug Use

Drug-free workplace policies can also mention other problem behaviors that may be related to drug use. These may include damaging inventory, repeatedly missing production schedules, and repeatedly being absent after holidays and weekends. In addition, some organizations may want to frame the issue of drug-related workplace behaviors in the larger context of employee health and productivity.

You may want to emphasize:

- **The policy's immediate objectives**, which are to comply with drug-free workplace laws and regulations (if applicable) and to prevent drug-related workplace accidents, illnesses, absenteeism, and performance problems

- **The policy's long-term goals** of protecting and improving worker health, safety, and productivity more broadly, in part by addressing workplace alcohol and drug misuse

Statement of Purpose

The statement of purpose should contain the organization's goals for the workplace policy, the organization's definition of "substance use," and a description of how the policy was developed. For example, was it developed in meetings with union representatives or employees representing different and diverse segments of the workforce? Or in collaboration with the organization's legal counsel? Some organizations may want the policy to have a very narrow goal, such as meeting the minimum requirements of law. Other organizations may prefer broader goals.

Organizations that are covered by drug-free workplace laws and regulations may want to use or adapt one of the sample statements of purpose below. Even if drug-free workplace laws and regulations do not apply to your organization, you still can adopt one of the sample statements of purpose below by simply omitting the words "to meet the requirements of applicable laws and regulations."

Example Statements of Purpose

Meeting the requirements of the law. The purpose of this policy is to meet the requirements of applicable laws and regulations to ensure that the workplace is free of illegal drugs.

Addressing other substances as well. The purpose of this policy is:

- To meet the requirements of applicable laws and regulations to ensure that the workplace is free of illegal drugs

- To establish restrictions on the workplace-related use of legal substances, such as alcohol, cigarettes, legalized marijuana, and prescription drugs

- **Addressing other problems that can be related to drug use.** The purpose of this policy is to meet the requirements of applicable laws and regulations to ensure that the workplace is free of illegal drugs

- To establish restrictions on the workplace-related use of legal substances, such as alcohol, cigarettes, legalized marijuana, and prescription drugs

- To address fitness-for-duty behaviors (such as repeatedly calling in sick or being absent directly before and after holidays and weekends, repeatedly damaging inventory or failing to meet reasonable production schedules, and being involved in frequent accidents that can be related to the use of drugs and other substances)

- To explain the steps that will be taken to protect employees, identify problems, and provide assistance

Goals

Questions that you may want to consider in defining your policy goals include:

- What are the drug-free workplace laws and regulations (federal, state, or local) with which your organization must comply, if applicable?

- What other goals does your organization expect to achieve? For example, does your organization hope to reduce or eliminate drug-related workplace accidents, illnesses, and absenteeism?

- Does your organization want to address the issue of preventing and treating workplace drug use and misuse in the context of accomplishing a broader goal? These broader goals may include promoting employee health and safety.

Definitions, Expectations, and Prohibitions

For this part of the policy, you may want to address the following:

- How does your organization define substance use?

- What employee behaviors are expected?

- Exactly what substances and behaviors are prohibited?

- Who is covered by the policy?

- When will the policy apply? For example, will it apply during work hours only, or also during organization-sponsored events after normal business hours?

- Where will the policy apply? For example, will it apply in the workplace while workers are on duty, outside the workplace while they are on duty, or in the workplace and in organization-owned vehicles while they are off duty?

- Who is responsible for carrying out and enforcing the policy?

- Will the policy include any form of testing for alcohol, prescription drugs, or other drugs?

- Are any employees covered by the terms of a collective bargaining agreement, and, if so, how do the terms affect the way the policy will be implemented and enforced for those employees?

Dissemination Strategies

How will your organization educate employees about the policy? For example, you can train supervisors, discuss the policy during orientation sessions for new employees, and inform all employees about the policy using a variety of formats. The employee handbook, posters in gathering places at worksites, information on the organization intranet, and mobile applications or other types of technological approaches can all approach for disseminating the policy.

Benefits and Assurances

Think about how your organization will help:

- Employees comply with the policy
- Protect employees' confidentiality
- Employees find help for drug-related problems
- Employees who are in treatment or recovery
- Ensure that all aspects of the policy are implemented fairly and consistently for all employees

Consequences and Appeals

Consider addressing the consequences of violating the policy, and the procedures for determining whether an employee has violated the policy. Your policy should also outline the procedures for appealing a determination that an employee may have violated the policy.

Section 53.2

Drug Testing in the Workplace

This section includes text excerpted from "Drug Testing," Substance Abuse and Mental Health Services Administration (SAMHSA), November 2, 2015. Reviewed January 2019.

Workplace drug-testing programs are designed to detect the presence of alcohol, illicit drugs, or certain prescription drugs. Drug testing is a prevention and deterrent method that is often part of a comprehensive drug-free workplace program. Both federal and nonfederal workplaces may have drug testing programs in place.

Any workplace drug-testing program should comply with applicable local, state, and federal laws.

Conducting Drug Tests

Federal agencies must use certified labs and follow other guidelines for drug testing.

Before beginning drug testing, ask the following questions and consider how they will affect your testing program. Be sure to address each question in your drug-free workplace policy.

- Who receives testing?

- When are the drug tests given?

- Who conducts the testing?

- What substances are tested for?

- Who pays for the drug testing?

- What steps are taken to ensure the accuracy of the drug tests?

- What are the legal rights of employees who receive a positive test result?

Tests may be performed by a trained collector who visits your workplace to collect specimens, or employees may go to a certified laboratory. To ensure accuracy, the specimen's chain of custody must be continuous from receipt until disposal.

Develop a system to protect the confidentiality of employee drug-testing records. Select a person within your organization who will be responsible for receiving employee drug-test results, and make sure that the person is aware of confidentiality protocols. Explain the relationship of the drug-testing program to your organization's employee assistance plan (EAP), if one is offered. Let employees know how drug-testing results can be used to inform their treatment, rehabilitation, and re-integration into the workplace.

Types of Drug Tests

Drug tests vary, depending on what types of drugs are being tested for and what types of specimens are being collected. Urine, hair, saliva (oral fluid), or sweat samples can be used as test specimens.

In federally regulated programs, only urine samples are collected, although the Secretary of the U.S. Department of Health and Human Service (HHS) has released proposed guidelines for the inclusion of oral fluid specimens.

Tests are commonly used for five categories of drugs:

- Amphetamines

- Cocaine

- Marijuana

- Opiates

- Phencyclidine (PCP)

Additional categories may include barbiturates, benzodiazepines, ethanol (alcohol), hydrocodone, 3,4-methylenedioxymethamphetamine (MDMA), methadone, methaqualone, or propoxyphene.

Random tests are the most effective for deterring illicit-drug use. Employers conduct random tests using an unpredictable selection process.

Drug testing may also be used in the following set times or circumstances:

Pre-Employment Tests

You can make passing a drug test a condition of employment. With this approach, all job candidates will receive drug testing prior to being hired.

Annual Physical Tests

You can test your employees for alcohol and other drug use as part of an annual physical examination. Be sure to inform employees that drug-testing will be part of the exam. Failure to provide prior notification is a violation of the employee's constitutional rights.

For-Cause and Reasonable Suspicion Tests

You may decide to test employees who show discernible signs of being unfit for duty (for-case testing), or who have a documented pattern of unsafe work behavior (reasonable suspicion testing). These kinds of tests help to protect the safety and well-being of the employee and other coworkers.

Post-Accident Tests

Testing employees who were involved in a workplace accident or unsafe practices can help determine whether alcohol or other drug use were contributing factors to the incident.

Post-Treatment Tests

Testing employees who return to work after completing a rehabilitation program can encourage them to remain drug-free.

Test Results of Drug Tests

Ensuring the accuracy of drug-testing results is critical. Using an HHS-certified laboratory to test the specimens and a Medical Review Officer (MRO) to interpret the test results will help prevent inaccurate testing. MROs are licensed physicians who receive laboratory results and have knowledge of substance-use disorders (SUDs) and federal drug-testing regulations. MROs are trained to interpret and evaluate test results together with the employee's medical history and other relevant information.

A negative test result does not indicate that an employee has never used alcohol or illicit drugs, nor is it a guarantee against future use.

Federal employees or employees in safety- and security-sensitive industries regulated by the Department of Defense (DoD) or the Department of Transportation (DOT) who show positive test results have the right to have the specimen tested by a second HHS-certified laboratory. Although a second test is not required, all employers should include this right in their drug-testing programs.

Depending on the workplace and the circumstances, employees who test positive may be referred to EAPs, into treatment, or for disciplinary action.

Chapter 54

Substance-Misuse-Prevention Media Campaigns

Substance-Misuse-Prevention Media Campaigns

The following are examples of media campaigns developed by states, jurisdictions, and national organizations. The examples fall into the following focus areas: alcohol use, prescription-drug misuse and abuse, public health, and underage drinking.

Most are social-marketing campaigns, developed to promote specific prevention or health-promotion messages. Inclusion in this list does not reflect message endorsement.

State and Jurisdiction Campaigns
Alcohol Use

- **One Nation Guam**, Guam's alcohol-free movement, aims to promote healthy lifestyles free of alcohol, tobacco, and other drugs. The campaign works to reduce the social acceptability of alcohol use and to challenge the notion that alcohol is part

This chapter includes text excerpted from "Substance Misuse Prevention Media Campaigns," Substance Abuse and Mental Health Services Administration (SAMHSA), August 6, 2015. Reviewed January 2019.

of Guam culture by featuring local people who live healthy alcohol-free lifestyles. One Nation Guam's target demographic includes youth, parents, and Chamorro and other Micronesian ethnicities.

Prescription-Drug Misuse and Abuse

- **Georgia's Generation Rx Project** is a three- year, Substance Abuse and Mental Health Services Administration (SAMHSA)-funded project to prevent the misuse of prescription drugs among young people ages 12 to 25 years in three Georgia counties. The campaign encourages the safe disposal of unused and expired prescription medications by providing secure drop boxes to facilitate proper disposal. Generation Rx also trains youth as advocates for preventing prescription-drug misuse and abuse, supplying them with skills to serve as leaders in the effort.

- **New Mexico's Dose of Reality Campaign** is a SAMHSA-funded statewide prevention campaign designed to educate teens and their parents about the risks associated with prescription-painkiller misuse. The campaign uses multifaceted communication strategies, comprising television (TV), radio, online, print, and outdoor messaging. Resources are tailored to various populations (medical providers, students, parents, businesses, educators, and coaches) and include advertisements that promote the safe storage and proper disposal of prescription drugs, commercials aimed at teens, and a parent resource toolkit.

- **The North Dakota Prescription-Drug Abuse Campaign**, developed by the Substance Abuse Prevention Division of North Dakota's Department of Human Services, provides posters, flyers, factsheets, and media toolkits designed to educate the public about prescription-drug misuse and abuse. The campaign offers suggestions for safeguarding medications in the home and information about the state's safe prescription-drug-disposal program. As part of the campaign, the North Dakota Department of Human Services, Office of the Attorney General, and Association of Realtors collaborated to create a set of resources for realtors to share with their clients about the risk of prescription-drug theft during open houses.

- **Ohio's Prescription for Prevention: Stop the Epidemic** campaign launched by the Ohio Department of Health (ODH), is an education and awareness campaign designed to prevent prescription-drug misuse and abuse. The campaign includes public-service announcements, drug-disposal guidelines, and factsheets that include both country-specific and statewide data.

- **Wisconsin's Good Drugs Gone Bad**, a program and toolkit originally created in 2009 by the Northeast Wisconsin Coalition, undergoes regular revisions to provide the most up-to-date information about substance misuse. After producing successful public-service announcements, the campaign collaborated with filmmakers to create a film for teens about the dangers of prescription-drug misuse and abuse. Other materials include customizable posters that community organizations can use to support their substance-misuse prevention efforts, Powerpoint presentations, handouts for prevention practitioners, and a nonfiction book about a former police officer's struggle with prescription-drug abuse.

Public Health

- **Montana's Most of Us** campaign, developed by Montana's Center for Health and Safety Culture (CHSC), uses social norms marketing techniques to address public-health issues such as tobacco use and substance misuse. The Montana Model of Social Norms comprises a seven-step process that involves planning, assessment, pilot testing, implementation, and evaluation. Campaign topics include methamphetamine education and prevention, drinking and driving prevention, and underage drinking reduction.

Underage Drinking

- **Colorado's SpeakNow!** campaign was developed under the state's Partnerships for Success (PFS) grant. The campaign encourages parents and caregivers to talk to their children about the dangers of alcohol misuse. It provides an action plan for engaging in open discussions about the challenges associated with underage drinking and healthy alternatives. The SpeakNow! website also enables parents to text their teenagers as a way to informally begin these conversations. In addition, the campaign provides information on Colorado's underage-drinking laws and associated legal consequences.

- **Hawaii's Be a Jerk** campaign encourages adults to "be a jerk" by saying no to underage drinking. Rather than targeting individuals, Be a Jerk focuses on creating an environment where alcohol is less available to youth, and changing community attitudes toward underage drinking. To achieve these goals, Be a Jerk works with community members to:
  - Limit the number of alcohol advertisements aimed at youth
  - Ask local stores and bars to implement more stringent ID checks
  - Change community norms related to the acceptability of underage drinking

- **Maine's Parent Media Campaign** aims to raise awareness of underage alcohol use. Campaign materials include brochures for parents that contain state-specific data on teenage drinking, adolescent brain development, perception vs. fact, and signs of teen alcohol use. In addition to brochures, the campaign uses radio advertisements, posters, and parent contact cards to increase awareness of teenage alcohol use.

- **Massachusetts' Reality Check** campaign supplies parents with information about laws related to underage drinking, local data, and tips for starting conversations with youth and with other parents. The campaign also describes different ways that youth procure alcohol and offers tips for preventing access. The campaign is run by the Cambridge Prevention Coalition, an innovative community-based coalition that engages youth and adults to reduce underage drinking.

National Campaigns
Prescription-Drug Misuse and Abuse

- **The AWARxE Prescription-Drug Safety Program** is designed to spread awareness about prescription-drug misuse and abuse. It offers tips for understanding prescription information, safely acquiring and administering medications, and properly disposing of unused medications. The campaign also encourages people to share their personal stories about prescription-drug misuse and connects website users with prescription-drug awareness events happening across the United States.

- **Up and Away and Out of Sight** is an educational program to remind families of the importance of safe medicine storage. It is an initiative of PROTECT, in partnership with the Centers for Disease Control and Prevention (CDC) and the Consumer Healthcare Products Association Educational Foundation, among others. The campaign encourages adults to keep medicine out of the reach of small children and to teach children about medicine safety. Other tips include never telling a child that medicine is candy (even if having trouble administering medicine) and instructing guests to keep purses, bags, and coats containing medication out of sight. Parents and caregivers can take a pledge on the campaign website to keep medication up and away from children. Those who take the pledge are encouraged to share it with friends and family via social media and email. The website is also available in Spanish.

Public Health

- **Above the Influence**, created as part of the National Youth Anti-Drug Media Campaign, aims to help teens stand up to peer pressure and other influences that encourage the use of drugs and alcohol. Through television commercials, Internet advertising, and regular communication with teens via Facebook, this educational campaign encourages teens to be aware and critical of all messages they receive about drugs and alcohol. Acknowledging that the campaign provides one of many messages teens receive about alcohol and drug use, the website urges teens to review sources of information to check the facts and make informed decisions.

- **National Institute on Drug Abuse (NIDA) for Teens: The Science Behind Drug Abuse** is a campaign geared toward adolescents ages 11 to 15 years. It uses a blog, videos, and drug factsheets to educate youth, parents, and teachers about the science behind drug misuse. The campaign website contains information on a wide array of substances, including emerging drug trends. The blog contains celebrity stories about the dangers of substance misuse, answers to real questions from teens, and information about how the brain works and the effects of drugs on the brain.

Underage Drinking

- **SAMHSA's "Talk. They Hear You."** is a public-service-announcement campaign that encourages parents and caregivers to talk to their children about the dangers of alcohol. It is designed to increase parents' awareness and understanding of underage drinking and to help them engage in thoughtful conversations on the topic with the young people in their lives. Resources available in English and in Spanish include information on the consequences of underage drinking, advice for answering difficult questions that children may ask about alcohol, and sample text messages that parents can send to their children reminding them not to drink.

- **SAMHSA's Too Smart to Start** public-education initiative aims to stimulate conversations between youth and adults on the harms of underage alcohol use and to create an environment where youth, parents, and the general public see underage drinking as harmful. The Too Smart to Start website includes separate sections for youth and teens, and families, educators, and community leaders, each with its own set of information and engagement tools.

- **We Don't Serve Teens**, developed by the U.S. Federal Trade Commission (FTC), provides materials for high schools, colleges, social-services organizations, and alcohol-industry members to spread the message that providing alcohol to teens is unsafe, illegal, and irresponsible. Campaign materials include press releases, letters to the editor, radio public-service announcements, and buttons to add to websites. The campaign website also includes facts about underage drinking, alcohol laws by state, and media literacy tools.

Part Seven

Additional Help and Information

Chapter 55

Glossary of Terms Related to Drug Abuse

addiction: A chronic, relapsing disease, characterized by compulsive drug seeking and use accompanied by neurochemical and molecular changes in the brain.

agitation: A restless inability to keep still. Agitation is most often psychomotor agitation, that is, having emotional and physical components. Agitation can be caused by anxiety, overstimulation, or withdrawal from depressants and stimulants.

agonist: A chemical compound that mimics the action of a natural neurotransmitter and binds to the same receptor on nerve cells to produce a biological response.

amphetamine: A stimulant drug with effects similar to cocaine.

amyl nitrite: A yellowish oily volatile liquid used in certain diagnostic procedures and prescribed to some patients for heart pain. Illegally diverted ampules of amyl nitrite are called "poppers" or "snappers" on the street.

anabolic-androgenic steroids: Male hormones, principally testosterone, that are partially responsible for the tremendous developmental changes that occur during puberty and adolescence. Male hormones can

---

This glossary contains terms excerpted from documents produced by several sources deemed reliable.

accelerate growth of muscle, bone, and red blood cells; decrease body fat; enhance neural conduction (anabolic effects); and produce changes in primary and secondary sexual characteristics (androgenic effects).

anabolic effects: Drug-induced growth or thickening of the body's nonreproductive tract tissues—including skeletal muscle, bones, the larynx, and vocal cords—and a decrease in body fat.

analgesics: A group of medications that reduce pain.

analog: A chemical compound that is similar to another drug in its effects but differs slightly in its chemical structure

barbiturate: A type of central nervous system (CNS) depressant often prescribed to promote sleep.

behavioral treatments: A set of treatments that focus on modifying thinking, motivation, coping mechanisms, and choices made by individuals.

benzodiazepine: A type of CNS depressant often prescribed to relieve anxiety. Valium® and Xanax® are among the most widely prescribed benzodiazepine medications.

blackout: A blackout is a period of amnesia or memory loss, typically caused by chronic, high-dose substance abuse. The person later cannot remember the blackout period. Blackouts are most often caused by sedative-hypnotics such as alcohol and the benzodiazepines.

brainstem: The lower portion of the brain. Major functions located in the brainstem include those necessary for survival, e.g., breathing, heart rate, blood pressure, and arousal.

buprenorphine: A partial opioid agonist for the treatment of opioid addiction that relieves drug cravings without producing the "high" or dangerous side effects of other opioids.

cannabinoid receptor: The receptor in the brain that recognizes and binds cannabinoids that are produced in the brain (anandamide) or outside the body (for example, THC and cannabidiol).

cannabinoids: Chemicals that bind to cannabinoid receptors in the brain. They are found naturally in the brain (anandamide) and are also chemicals found in marijuana (for example, THC and CBD).

Cannabis: The botanical name for the plant that produces marijuana.

CD4 Cells: A type of cell involved in protecting against viral, fungal, and protozoal infections. These cells normally stimulate the immune response, signaling other cells in the immune system to perform their special functions.

CNS depressants: A class of drugs (also called sedatives and tranquilizers) that slow CNS function; some are used to treat anxiety and sleep disorders (includes barbiturates and benzodiazepines).

co-occurring disorders (COD): It refers to co-occurring substance use (abuse or dependence) and mental disorders. Clients said to have COD have one or more mental disorders as well as one or more disorders relating to the use of alcohol and/or other drugs.

cocaine: A highly addictive stimulant drug derived from the coca plant that produces profound feelings of pleasure.

cognitive: Pertaining to the mind's capacity to understand concepts and ideas.

comorbidity: The occurrence of two disorders or illnesses in the same person, either at the same time (co-occurring comorbid conditions) or with a time difference between the initial occurrence of one and the initial occurrence of the other (sequentially comorbid conditions).

constricted pupils (pinpoint pupils): Pupils that are temporarily narrowed or closed. This is usually a sign of opioid abuse.

convulsions: A symptom of a seizure, characterized by twitching and jerking of the limbs. A seizure is a sudden episode of uncontrolled electrical activity in the brain. If the abnormal electrical activity spreads throughout the brain, the result may be loss of consciousness and a grand mal-seizure

crack: Slang term for a smokeable form of cocaine.

craving: A powerful, often uncontrollable desire for drugs.

culturally: competent treatment Biopsychosocial or other treatment that is adapted to suit the special cultural beliefs, practices, and needs of a client.

dependence: A physiological state that can occur with regular drug use and results in withdrawal symptoms when drug use is abruptly discontinued.

depression: A disorder marked by sadness, inactivity, difficulty with thinking and concentration, significant increase or decrease in appetite and time spent sleeping, feelings of dejection and hopelessness, and, sometimes, suicidal thoughts or an attempt to commit suicide.

detoxification: A process of allowing the body to rid itself of a drug while managing the symptoms of withdrawal; often the first step in a drug treatment program.

dopamine: A neurotransmitter present in regions of the brain that regulate movement, emotion, motivation, and the feeling of pleasure.

drug: A chemical compound or substance that can alter the structure and function of the body. Psychoactive drugs affect the function of the brain.

drugged driving: Driving a vehicle while impaired due to the lingering, intoxicating effects of recent drug use.

euphoria: A feeling of well-being or elation

fentanyl: A medically useful opioid analog that is 50 times more potent than heroin.

hallucinogens: A diverse group of drugs that alter perceptions, thoughts, and feelings. Hallucinogenic drugs include LSD, mescaline, PCP, and psilocybin (magic mushrooms).

hepatitis C virus (HCV): A virus that causes liver inflammation and disease. Hepatitis is a general term for liver damage and hepatitis C is the most common type of hepatitis found among those with HIV.

heroin: A synthetic opioid related to morphine. It is more potent than morphine and is highly addictive.

highly active antiretroviral therapy (HAART): A combination of three or more antiretroviral drugs used in the treatment of HIV infection and AIDS.

hormone: A chemical substance formed in glands in the body and carried by the blood to organs and tissues, where it influences function, structure, and behavior.

hyperthermia: A potentially dangerous rise in body temperature.

hypothalamus: A part of the brain that controls many bodily functions, including feeding, drinking, body temperature regulation, and the release of many hormones.

inhalant: Any drug administered by breathing in its vapors. Inhalants commonly are organic solvents, such as glue and paint thinner, or anesthetic gases, such as ether and nitrous oxide.

injection drug use (IDU): Act of administering drugs directly into a vein using a hypodermic needle and syringe. Injection drug users (IDUs) are individuals that abuse drugs in this way.

lysergic acid diethylamide (LSD): A hallucinogenic drug that acts on the serotonin receptor.

major depressive disorder: A mood disorder having a clinical course of one or more serious depression episodes that last 2 or more weeks. Episodes are characterized by a loss of interest or pleasure in almost all activities; disturbances in appetite, sleep, or psychomotor functioning; a decrease in energy; difficulties in thinking or making decisions; loss of self-esteem or feelings of guilt; and suicidal thoughts or attempts.

mania: A mood disorder characterized by abnormally and persistently elevated, expansive, or irritable mood; mental and physical hyperactivity; and/or disorganization of behavior.

marijuana: A drug, usually smoked but can be eaten, that is made from the leaves of the *Cannabis* plant. The main psychoactive ingredient is THC.

medication: A drug that is used to treat an illness or disease according to established medical guidelines. If the medication contains one or more controlled substances, it must be prescribed by a licensed physician.

methadone: A long-acting opioid agonist medication shown to be effective in treating heroin addiction.

methamphetamine: An addictive, potent stimulant drug that is part of the larger class of amphetamines.

methylphenidate (Ritalin®/Concerta®): A CNS stimulant that has effects similar to, but more potent than, caffeine and less potent than amphetamines. It has a notably calming and "focusing" effect on patients with ADHD, particularly children.

motivational enhancement therapy (MET): A systematic form of intervention designed to produce rapid, internally motivated change. MET does not attempt to treat the person, but rather mobilize his or her own internal resources for change and engagement in treatment.

naloxone: An opioid receptor antagonist that rapidly binds to opioid receptors, blocking heroin from activating them.

naltrexone: An opioid antagonist medication that can only be used after a patient has completed detoxification. Naltrexone is not addictive or sedating and does not result in physical dependence; however, poor patient compliance has limited its effectiveness.

neonatal abstinence syndrome (NAS): NAS occurs when heroin from the mother passes through the placenta into the baby's bloodstream during pregnancy, allowing the baby to become addicted along with the mother. NAS requires hospitalization and treatment with medication (often a morphine taper) to relieve symptoms until the baby adjusts to becoming opioid-free.

neuron (nerve cell): A unique type of cell found in the brain and throughout the body that specializes in the transmission and processing of information.

neurotransmitter: A chemical that acts as a messenger to carry signals or information from one nerve cell to another.

nicotine: The addictive drug in tobacco. Nicotine activates a specific type of acetylcholine receptor.

nitrites: A special class of inhalants that act primarily to dilate blood vessels and relax the muscles. Whereas other inhalants are used to alter mood, nitrites are used primarily as sexual enhancers.

noradrenaline: A neurotransmitter that is made in the brain and influences, among other things, the function of the heart.

norepinephrine: A neurotransmitter present in regions of the brain that affect heart rate and blood pressure.

opioid: A natural or synthetic psychoactive chemical that binds to opioid receptors in the brain and body.

opioid use disorder: A problematic pattern of opioid drug use, leading to clinically significant impairment or distress that includes cognitive, behavioral, and physiological symptoms as defined by the new *Diagnostic and Statistical Manual of Mental Disorders, 5th edition (DSM-V)* criteria.

partial agonist: A substance that binds to and activates the same nerve cell receptor as a natural neurotransmitter but produces a diminished biological response.

physical dependence: An adaptive physiological state that occurs with regular drug use and results in a withdrawal syndrome when drug use is stopped; usually occurs with tolerance.

placebo: An inactive substance (pill, liquid, etc.), which is administered to a comparison group, as if it were therapy, but which has no therapeutic value other than to serve as a negative control.

polydrug abuse: The abuse of two or more drugs at the same time, such as CNS depressants and alcohol.

posttraumatic stress disorder (PTSD): A disorder that develops after exposure to a highly stressful event (e.g., wartime combat, physical violence, or natural disaster). Symptoms include sleeping difficulties, hypervigilance, avoiding reminders of the event, and re-experiencing the trauma through flashbacks or recurrent nightmares.

prescription drug abuse: The use of a medication without a prescription; in a way other than as prescribed; or for the experience or feeling elicited.

propofol: A common type of anesthetic used for surgery.

psychedelic drug: A drug that distorts perception, thought, and feeling. This term is typically used to refer to drugs with actions like those of LSD.

psychoactive: Having a specific effect on the brain.

psychosis: A mental disorder (e.g., schizophrenia) characterized by delusional or disordered thinking detached from reality; symptoms often include hallucinations.

psychotherapeutics: Drugs that have an effect on the function of the brain and that often are used to treat psychiatric/neurologic disorders; includes opioids, CNS depressants, and stimulants.

relapse: In drug abuse, relapse is the resumption of drug use after trying to stop taking drugs. Relapse is a common occurrence in many chronic disorders, including addiction, that require behavioral adjustments to treat effectively.

route of administration: The way a drug is put into the body. Drugs can enter the body by eating, drinking, inhaling, injecting, snorting, smoking, or absorbing a drug through mucous membranes.

rush: A surge of euphoric pleasure that rapidly follows administration of a drug.

salvia: An herb in the mint family native to southern Mexico that is used to produce hallucinogenic experiences.

schizophrenia: A psychotic disorder characterized by symptoms that fall into two categories: (1) positive symptoms, such as distortions in thoughts (delusions), perception (hallucinations), and language and thinking and (2) negative symptoms, such as flattened emotional responses and decreased goal-directed behavior.

sedatives: Drugs that suppress anxiety and promote sleep; the NSDUH classification includes benzodiazepines, barbiturates, and other types of CNS depressants.

self-medication: The use of a substance to lessen the negative effects of stress, anxiety, or other mental disorders (or side effects of their pharmacotherapy). Self-medication may lead to addiction and other drug- or alcohol-related problems.

serotonin: A neurotransmitter used in widespread parts of the brain, which is involved in sleep, movement and emotions

Spice/K2: Dried plant material containing synthetic (or designer) cannabinoid compounds that produce mind-altering effects as well as other compounds that vary from product to product.

stimulants: A class of drugs that elevates mood, increases feelings of well-being, and increases energy and alertness. These drugs produce euphoria and are powerfully rewarding. Stimulants include cocaine, methamphetamine, and methylphenidate (Ritalin).

tetrahydrocannabinol (THC): Delta-9-tetrahydrocannabinol; the main psychoactive ingredient in marijuana, which acts on the brain to produce marijuana's psychoactive effects.

tobacco: A plant widely cultivated for its leaves, which are used primarily for smoking; the tabacum species is the major source of tobacco products.

withdrawal: A variety of symptoms that occur after use of an addictive drug is reduced or stopped.

Chapter 56

Glossary of Street Terms for Drugs of Abuse

Abyssinian Tea: Khat

Acid: LSD

Adam: Ecstasy (MDMA)

African Salad: Khat

Ah-pen-yen: Opium

Amidone: Methadone

Angel Dust: PCP

Aunti Emma: Opium

Aunti: Opium

Barbs: Barbiturates

barbs: Depressants

Beans: Ecstasy (MDMA)

Beautiful: 2,5-Dimethoxy-4-(n)-propylthiophenethylamine

Bennies: Amphetamines

Benzos: Benzodiazepines

This glossary contains terms excerpted from documents produced by several sources deemed reliable.

Big H: Narcotics

Big O: Opium

Black Beauties: Amphetamines

Black Beauties: Stimulants

Black Mamba: K2/"Spice"

Black Pill: Opium

Black Tar: Heroin

Black Tat: Narcotics

Block Busters: Barbiturates

Blotter Acid: LSD

Blue: Morphine

Blue Mystic: 2,5-Dimethoxy-4-(n)-propylthiophenethylamine

Blunts: Marijuana

Boat: PCP

Bold: Inhalants

Bombay Blue: K2/"Spice"

Boom: Marijuana

Bromo: 4-Bromo-2,5-dimethoxyphenethylamine

Brown Sugar: Narcotics

Bud: Marijuana

Buttons: Peyote and mescaline

Cactus: Peyote and mescaline

candy: Depressants

Cat Tranquilizer: Ketamine

Cat Valium: Ketamine

Catha: Khat

CCC: Dextromethorphan

Chalk: Methamphetamine

Chandoo: Opium

Chandu: Opium

Chat: Khat

Chinese Molasses: Opium

Chinese Tobacco: Opium

Chocolate Chip Cookies: Methadone

Christmas Trees: Barbiturates

Chronic: Marijuana

Circles: Rohypnol

Clarity: Ecstasy (MDMA)

Cloud Nine: Bath salts (synthetic cathinones)

Coca: Cocaine

Coke: Cocaine

Crack: Cocaine

Crank: Amphetamines or methamphetamine

Crystal: Phencyclidine (PCP)

D: Hydromorphone

Dex: Dextromethorphan

Dillies: Hydromorphone

Dopium: Opium

Dots: LSD

Dover's Powder: Opium

Downers: Depressants

Dream Gun: Opium

Dream Stick: Opium

Dreamer: Morphine

Dreams: Opium

Drone: Bath salts (synthetic cathinones)

Dust: Hydromorphone

DXM: Dextromethorphan

E: Ecstasy (MDMA)

Easing Powder: Opium

Easy Lay: Gamma-hydroxybutyric acid (GHB)

Embalming Fluid: PCP

Emsel: Morphine

Fake Weed: K2/"Spice"

Fi-do-nie: Opium

First Line: Morphine

Fizzies: Methadone

Flake: Cocaine

Footballs: Hydromorphone

Forget Pill: Rohypnol

Forget-Me-Pill: Rohypnol

Foxy: 5-methoxy-N,N-diisopropyltryptamine

Foxy methoxy: 5-methoxy-N,N-diisopropyltryptamine

G: Gamma-hydroxybutyric acid (GHB)

Gangster: Marijuana

Ganja: Marijuana

Gee: Opium

Genie: K2/"Spice"

Georgia Home Boy: Gamma-hydroxybutyric acid (GHB)

GHB: Gamma-hydroxybutyric acid

Glass: Methamphetamine

God's Drug: Morphine

God's Medicine: Opium

Go-Fast: Methamphetamine

Gondola: Opium

Goof Balls: Barbiturates

Goop: Gamma-hydroxybutyric acid (GHB)

Goric: Opium

Grass: Marijuana

Great Tobacco: Opium

Grievous Bodily Harm: Gamma-hydroxybutyric acid (GHB)

Guma: Opium

Hash: Marijuana

Hashish: *Cannabis*

Herb: Marijuana

Hillbilly Heroin: Narcotics

Hop/hops: Opium

Horse: Heroin

Hows: Morphine

i: 4-Iodo-2,5-dimethoxyphenethylamine

Ice: Amphetamines or methamphetamine

Jet K: Ketamine

Joint: Marijuana

Joy Plant: Opium

Juice: Hydromorphone or steroids

Junk: Narcotics

Kat: Khat

Kicker: Oxycodone

Kif: Marijuana

Kit Kat: Ketamine

La Rocha: Rohypnol

laughing gas: Inhalants

lean: Narcotics

Liquid Ecstasy: Gamma-hydroxybutyric acid (GHB)

Liquid X: Gamma-hydroxybutyric acid (GHB)

Lover's Speed: Ecstasy (MDMA)

Lunch Money Drug: Rohypnol

M.S.: Morphine

Magic Mushrooms: Psilocybin

Maria Pastora: *Salvia divinorum*

Maria: Methadone

Mary Jane: Marijuana

MDMA: Ecstasy

Mellow Yellow: LSD

Meow Meow: Bath salts (synthetic cathinones)

Mesc: Peyote and mescaline

Meth: Methamphetamine

Mexican Valium: Rohypnol

MPTP (New Heroin): Narcotics

Midnight Oil: Opium

Mira: Opium

Mister Blue: Morphine

Morf: Morphine

Morpho: Morphine

Mud: Narcotics

Mushrooms: Psilocybin

O: Opium

Oat: Khat

OC: Oxycodone

O.P.: Opium

Ope: Opium

Ox: Oxycodone

Oxy: Oxycodone

Oxycotton: Narcotics

Pastora: Methadone

Pen Yan: Opium

Perc: Oxycodone

Peyoto: Peyote and mescaline

phennies: Depressants

Pin Gon: Opium

Pingus: Rohypnol

Pinks: Barbiturates

Poor Man's PCP: Dextromethorphan

poppers: Inhalants

Pot: Marijuana

Pox: Opium

Purple: Ketamine

R2: Rohypnol

red birds: Depressants

Red Devils: Barbiturates

reds: Depressants

Reds and Blues: Barbiturates

Reefer: Marijuana

Reynolds: Rohypnol

Roach: Rohypnol

Roach 2: Rohypnol

Roaches: Rohypnol

Roachies: Rohypnol

Roapies: Rohypnol

Robo: Dextromethorphan

Robutal: Rohypnol

Rochas Dos: Rohypnol

Rocket Fuel: PCP

Roids: Steroids

Rojo: Dextromethorphan

Roofies: Rohypnol

Rophies: Rohypnol

Ropies: Rohypnol

Roples: Rohypnol

Row-Shay: Rohypnol

Roxy: Oxycodone

Ruffies: Rohypnol

Rush: Inhalants

Sally-D: *Salvia divinorum*

Scoop: Gamma-hydroxybutyric acid (GHB)

Shermans: PCP

Shrooms: Psilocybin

Sinsemilla: Marijuana

Sippin Syrup: Narcotics

Ska: Heroin

Skee: Opium

Skittles: Dextromethorphan

Skunk: Marijuana

Smack: Heroin or hydromorphone

Snow: Cocaine

Special K: Ketamine

Special La Coke: Ketamine

Spectrum: 4-Bromo-2,5-dimethoxyphenethylamine

Speed: Amphetamines or methamphetamine

Spice: K2

Street Methadone: Methadone

Super Acid: Ketamine

Super K: Ketamine

Supergrass: PCP

Tic Tac: PCP

Tina: Methamphetamine

tooies: Depressants

Toonies: 4-Bromo-2,5-dimethoxyphenethylamine

Toxy: Opium

Toys: Opium

Triple C: Dextromethorphan

Tripstay: 2,5-Dimethoxy-4-(n)-propylthiophenethylamine

Tweety-Bird Mescaline:
2,5-Dimethoxy-4-(n)-propylthiophenethylamine

2C-B, Nexus: 4-Bromo-2,5-dimethoxyphenethylamine

2C-I : 4-Iodo-2,5-dimethoxyphenethylamine

2C-T-7: 2,5-Dimethoxy-4-(n)-propylthiophenethylamine

2's: 4-Bromo-2,5-dimethoxyphenethylamine

T7: 2,5-Dimethoxy-4-(n)-propylthiophenethylamine

Unkie: Morphine

Uppers: Amphetamines

Vanilla Sky: Bath salts (synthetic cathinones)

Velvet: Dextromethorphan

Venus: 4-Bromo-2,5-dimethoxyphenethylamine

Vitamin K: Ketamine

Wafer: Methadone

Weed: Marijuana

When-shee: Opium

Whippets: Inhalants

White Lightning: Bath salts (synthetic cathinones)

Window Pane: LSD

Wolfies: Rohypnol

Yellow Jackets: Barbiturates

yellows: Depressants

Ze: Opium

Zero: Opium

Zohai: K2/"Spice"

Zoom: PCP

Chapter 57

Directory of State Substance-Abuse Agencies

Alabama
Division of Mental Health and
Substance Abuse Services
Alabama Department of Mental
Health
P.O. Box 301410
Montgomery, AL 36130-1410
Phone: 334-242-3454
Toll-Free TTY: 844-307-1760
Fax: 334-242-0725
Website: www.mh.alabama.gov/
sa
E-mail: Alabama.DMH@
mh.alabama.gov

Alaska
Division of Behavioral Health
Alaska Department of Health
and Social Services
P.O. Box 110620
Juneau, AK 99811-0620
Toll-Free: 877-266-4357
(Hotline)
Phone: 907-465-5808
Fax: 907-465-2185
Website: dhss.alaska.gov/dbh/
Pages/default.aspx
E-mail: randall.burns@alaska.
gov

Resources in this chapter were compiled from several sources deemed reliable;
all contact information was verified and updated in January 2019.

Arizona
Behavioral Health Services
Arizona Department of Health
Services
150 N. 18th Ave.
Phoenix, AZ 85007
Phone: 602-542-1025
Fax: 602-542-0883
Website: www.azdhs.gov
E-mail: DCW@azahcccs.gov

Arkansas
Division of Behavioral Health
Services
Arkansas Department of Human
Services
305 S. Palm St.
Little Rock, AR 72205
Phone: 501-686-9164
Toll-Free TDD: 501-686-9176
Fax: 501-686-9182
Website: humanservices.
arkansas.gov/dbhs/Pages/
default.aspx
E-mail: tommie.waters@
arkansas.gov

Colorado
Office of Behavioral Health
Department of Human Services
3824 W. Princeton Cir.
Denver, CO 80236-3111
Phone: 303-866-7400
Fax: 303-866-7428
Website: www.colorado.
gov/cs/Satellite/CDHS-
BehavioralHealth/
CBON/1251578892077
E-mail: cdhs.communications@
state.co.us

Connecticut
Department of Mental Health
and Addiction Services
P.O. Box 341431
410 Capitol Ave.
Hartford, CT 06134
Toll-Free: 800-446-7348
Phone: 860-418-7000
Toll-Free TDD: 860-418-6707
Website: www.ct.gov/dmhas

Delaware
Division of Substance Abuse and
Mental Health (DSAMH)
Community Mental Health and
Addiction Services
1901 N. DuPont Hwy main Bldg.
New Castle, DE 19720
Toll-Free: 800-652-2929
(Helpline—Delaware Only)
Phone: 302-255-9399
Fax: 302-255-4427
Website: www.dhss.delaware.
gov/dsamh/index.html

District of Columbia
Department of Health
Addiction Prevention and
Recovery Administration
(APRA)
64 New York Ave.
N.E., Third Fl.
Washington, DC 20002
Phone: 202-673-2200
Toll-Free TTY: 202-673-7500
Fax: 202-673-3433
Website: dbh.dc.gov/page/apra
E-mail: dbh@dc.gov

Florida
Substance Abuse Program Office
Florida Department of Children and Families
1317 Winewood Blvd.
Bldg. 6, Rm. 200
Tallahassee, FL 32399-0700
Phone: 850-487-2920
Fax: 850-414-7474
Website: www.myflfamilies.com/service-programs/substance-abuse
E-mail: samh@myflfamilies.com

Georgia
Division of Addictive Diseases
Department of Behavioral Health and Developmental Disabilities
Two Peachtree St. N.W.
24th Fl.
Atlanta, GA 30303-3171
Toll-Free: 800-715-4225 (Hotline)
Phone: 404-657-2331
Fax: 678-717-5812
Website: dbhdd.georgia.gov/addictive-diseases
E-mail: David@dbhdd.ga.gov

Hawaii
Alcohol and Drug Abuse Division
Hawaii Department of Health
601 Kamokila Blvd., Rm 360
64 New York Ave.
Kapolei, HI 96707
Phone: 808-692-7506
Fax: 808-692-7521
Website: health.hawaii.gov/substance-abuse
E-mail: ATRINFO@doh.hawaii.gov

Idaho
Division of Behavioral Health
Department of Health and Welfare
P.O. Box 83720
Boise, ID 83720-0036
Toll-Free: 800-922-3406 (Screening/Referral)
Phone: 208-334-5500
Fax: 208-334-6558
Website: www.healthandwelfare.idaho.gov
E-mail: DPHInquiries@dhw.idaho.gov

Illinois
Division of Alcoholism and Addiction
Department of Human Services
100 W. Randolph
Ste. 5-600
Chicago, IL 60601-3297
Toll-Free:800-843-6154 (Help Line)
Phone: 312-814-3840
Toll-Free TTY: 800-447-6404 (Help Line)
Fax: 312-814-2419
Website: www.dhs.state.il.us/page.aspx?item=29725
E-mail: DHSWebBits@illinois.gov

Indiana
Division of Mental Health and
Addiction
Family and Social Services
Administration
402 W. Washington St.
P.O. Box 7083
Indianapolis, IN 46207-7083
Toll-Free: 800-901-1133
Phone: 317-233-4454
Fax: 317-233-4693
Website: www.in.gov/fssa/dmha/
index.htm
E-mail: pla8@pla.in.gov

Iowa
Division of Behavioral Health
Department of Public Health
Lucas State Office Building
321 E. 12th St.
Des Moines, IA 50319-0075
Toll-Free: 866-227-9878
Phone: 515-281-7689
Fax: 515-281-4535
Website: www.idph.iowa.gov
E-mail: PLPublic@idph.iowa.gov

Kansas
Community Services and
Programs
Department for Aging and
Disability Services New England
State Office Building
503 S. Kansas Ave.
Topeka, KS 66603-3404
Phone: 785-296-4986
Fax: 785-296-0557
Website: www.dcf.ks.gov/Pages/
Default.aspx
E-mail: Amy.Neuman@dcf.
ks.gov

Kentucky
Cabinet for Health and Family
Services
Department for Behavioral
Health, Developmental, and
Intellectual Disabilities
275 E. Main St. 4WF
Frankfort, KY 40621
Phone: 502-564-4527
Toll-Free TTY: 502-564-5777
Fax: 502-564-5478
Website: chfs.ky.gov/dbhdid
E-mail: Sherry.Carnahan@
ky.gov

Louisiana
Office of Behavioral Health
Department of Health and
Hospitals
P.O. Box 629
Baton Rouge, LA 70821-0629
Toll-Free: 855-229-6848
Phone: 225-342-9500
Fax: 225-342-5568
Website: www.dhh.louisiana.
gov/index.cfm/subhome/10/n/6
E-mail: healthy@la.gov

Maine
Substance Abuse and Mental
Health Services
Department of Health and
Human Services
41 Anthony Ave.
#11 State House Stn.
Augusta, ME 04333-0011
Phone: 207-287-2595
Fax: 207-287-4334
Website: www.maine.gov/dhhs/
samhs/osa
E-mail: osa.ircosa@maine.gov

Maryland
Alcohol and Drug Abuse
Administration
Department of Health and
Mental Hygiene Spring Grove
Hospital Center Vocational
Rehabilitation Building
201 W. Preston St.
Rm. 216
Baltimore, MD 21201-2399
Toll-Free: 877-463-3464
Phone: 410-767-6500
Fax: 410-402-8601
Website: dhmh.maryland.gov
E-mail: adaainfo@dhmh.state.
md.us

Massachusetts
Bureau of Substance Abuse
Services
Health and Human Services
250 Washington St.
Boston, MA 02108-4609
Toll-Free: 800-327-5050
(Helpline)
Phone: 617-624-6000
Toll-Free TTY: 617-624-6001
Fax: 617-624-5206
Website: www.mass.gov/dph/
bsas
E-mail: DLSfeedback@state.
ma.us

Michigan
Office of Recovery Oriented
Systems of Care
Department of Community
Health
333 S. Grand Ave.
P.O. Box 30195
Lansing, MI 48909
Phone: 517-373-3740
Toll-Free TTY: 800-649-3777
Fax: 517-335-2121
Website: www.michigan.gov/mdhhs
E-mail: MDCH-BSAAS@
michigan.gov

Minnesota
Alcohol and Drug Abuse Division
Department of Human Services
P.O. Box 64977
Saint Paul, MN 55164-0977
Phone: 651-431-2460
Toll-Free TTY: 800-627-3529
Fax: 651-431-7449
Website: mn.gov/dhs
E-mail: dhs.adad@state.mn.us

Mississippi
Bureau of Alcohol and Drug
Services
Mississippi Department of
Mental Health
1101 Robert E. Lee Bldg.
239 N. Lamar St.
Jackson, MS 39201
Toll-Free: 877-210-8513 (Helpline)
Phone: 601-359-1288
Toll-Free TDD: 601-359-6230
Fax: 601-359-6295
Website: www.dmh.ms.gov/
alcohol-and-drug-services
E-mail: kimela.smith@dmh.
state.ms.us

Missouri
Division of Behavioral Health
Missouri Department of Mental
Health
1706 East Elm St.
Jefferson City, MO 65101
Toll-Free: 800-575-7480
Phone: 573-751-4942
Fax: 573-751-7814
Website: www.dmh.mo.gov/ada
E-mail: dbhmail@dmh.mo.gov

Montana
Addictive and Mental Disorders
Division
Department of Public Health
and Human Services
P.O. Box 202905
Helena, MT 59620-2905
Phone: 406-444-3964
Fax: 406-444-4435
Website: www.dphhs.mt.gov/
amdd
E-mail: hhsamdemail@mt.gov

Nebraska
Division of Behavioral Health
Department of Health and
Human Services
P.O. Box 95026
Lincoln, NE 68509-5026
Toll-Free: 888-866-8660
(Helpline)
Phone: 402-471-8553
Fax: 402-471-9449
Website: www.dhhs.ne.gov/
Behavioral_Health
E-mail: DHHS.
BehavioralHealthDivision@
Nebraska.Gov

Nevada
Substance Abuse Prevention and
Treatment Agency
Department of Health and
Human Services
4126 Technology Way
Second Fl.
Carson City, NV 89706
Phone: 775-684-4190
Fax: 775-684-4185
Website: www.hhs.gov/asl
E-mail: MHDS@mhds.nv.gov

New Hampshire
Bureau of Drug and Alcohol
Services
Department of Health and
Human Services
105 Pleasant St.
Concord, NH 03301
Toll-Free: 800-804-0909
Phone: 603-271-6738
Fax: 603-271-6105
Website: www.dhhs.nh.gov/
dcbcs/bdas/index.htm

New Jersey
Division of Addiction Services
Department of Human Services
222 S. Warren St.
Trenton, NJ 08625
Toll-Free: 800-238-2333
(Hotline)
Phone: 609-292-5760
Fax: 609-292-3816
Website: www.state.nj.us/
humanservices/das/home
E-mail: dmhas@dhs.state.nj.us

New Mexico

Behavioral Health Services
Division
Human Services Department
P.O. Box 2348
Santa Fe, NM 87504
Toll-Free: 800-362-2013
Phone: 505-476-9266
Toll-Free TTY: 855-227-5485
Fax: 505-476-9277
Website: www.hsd.state.nm.us/
bhsd
E-mail: kylerb.nerison@state.nm.us

New York

New York State Office of
Alcoholism and Substance Abuse
Services
1450 Western Ave.
Albany, NY 12203-3526
Toll-Free: 877-846-7369 (Hotline)
Phone: 518-473-3460
Fax: 518-457-5474
Website: www.oasas.ny.gov
E-mail: communications@oasas.
ny.gov

North Carolina

Department of Health and
Human Services
Division of Mental Health,
Developmental Disabilities, and
Substance Abuse Services
2001 Mail Service Center
Raleigh, NC 27699-2001
Toll-Free: 800-662-7030
Phone: 919-733-4670
Fax: 919-733-4556
Website: www.dhhs.state.nc.us/
mhddsas
E-mail: david.aaron@dhhs.
nc.gov

North Dakota

Division of Mental Health and
Substance Abuse Services
Department of Human Services
Prairie Hills Plaza 1237 W.
Divide Ave., Ste. 1C
Bismarck, ND 58501-1208
Toll-Free: 800-755-2719 (North
Dakota only)
Phone: 701-328-8920
Fax: 701-328-8969
Website: www.nd.gov/dhs/
services/mentalhealth
E-mail: dhsmhsas@nd.gov

Ohio

Ohio Department of Mental
Health and Addiction Services
30 E. BRd. St.
Eighth Fl.
Columbus, OH 43215-3430
Toll-Free: 877-275-6364
Toll-Free TTY: 888-636-4889
Fax: 614-752-9453
Website: mha.ohio.gov
E-mail: askODMH@mh.ohio.gov

Oklahoma

Oklahoma Department of
Mental Health and Substance
Abuse Services
P.O. Box 53277
Oklahoma City, OK 73152-3277
Toll-Free: 800-522-9054
Phone: 405-522-3908
Toll-Free TDD: 405-522-3851
Fax: 405-522-3650
Website: ok.gov/odmhsas
E-mail: Kendale.Williams@bbhl.
ok.gov

Oregon

Addictions and Mental Health
Division
Oregon Health Authority
500 Summer St. N.E.

Salem, OR 97301-1079
Phone: 503-945-5763
Toll-Free TTY: 800-375-2863
Fax: 503-378-8467
Website: www.oregon.gov/oha/
amh/Pages/index.aspx
E-mail: Amh.web@state.or.us

Pennsylvania

Department of Drug and Alcohol
Programs
Pennsylvania Department of
Health
132 Kline Plaza
Ste. A
Harrisburg, PA 17104-1579
Phone: 717-783-8675
Fax: 717-787-6285
Website: www.health.state.
pa.us/bdap
E-mail: ancatalano@pa.gov

Rhode Island

Department of Behavioral
Healthcare
Developmental Disabilities and
Hospitals
Barry Hall Bldg. 14 Harrington
Rd.
Cranston, RI 02920
Phone: 401-462-2339
Fax: 401-462-3204
Website: www.bhddh.ri.gov
E-mail: linda.reilly@bhddh.ri.gov

South Carolina

Department of Alcohol and
Other Drug Abuse Services
P.O. Box 8268
Columbia, SC, 29202
Phone: 803-896-5555
Fax: 803-896-5557
Website: www.daodas.org

South Dakota

Division of Community
Behavioral Health
Department of Social Services
c/o 700 Governor's Dr.
Pierre, SD 57501
Toll-Free: 800-265-9684
Phone: 605-773-3163
Fax: 605-773-7076
Website: dss.sd.gov/
behavioralhealth
E-mail: infoMH@state.sd.us

Tennessee

Division of Substance Abuse
Services
Department of Mental Health
and Substance Abuse Services
601 Mainstream Dr.
Nashville, TN 37243
Toll-Free: 800-560-5767
Phone: 615-532-6500
Website: www.tn.gov/mental
E-mail: OC.TDMHSAS@tn.gov

Texas
Mental Health and Substance
Abuse Division
Department of State Health
Services
P.O. Box 149347
Austin, TX 78714-9347
Toll-Free: 866-378-8440
Phone: 512-206-5000
Fax: 512-206-5714
Website: www.dshs.state.tx.us/
MHSA
E-mail: contact@dshs.state.tx.us

Utah
Division of Substance Abuse and
Mental Health
Utah Department of Human
Services
195 N. 1950 W.
Second Fl.
Salt Lake City, UT 84116
Phone: 801-538-3939
Fax: 801-538-9892
Website: www.dsamh.utah.gov
E-mail: dsamhwebmaster@utah.
gov

Vermont
Division of Alcohol and Drug
Abuse Programs
Department of Health
108 Cherry St.
Burlington, VT 05402-0070
Phone: 802-863-7200
Fax: 802-651-1573
Website: healthvermont.gov/
adap/adap.aspx
E-mail: AHS.VDHADAP@state.
vt.us

Virginia
Office of Substance Abuse
Services
Department of Behavioral
Health and Developmental
Services
P.O. Box 1797
Richmond, VA 23218-1797
Phone: 804-786-3906
Toll-Free TDD: 804-371-8977
Fax: 804-786-9248
Website: www.dbhds.virginia.gov
E-mail: OIG@oig.sc.gov

Washington
Division of Behavioral Health
and Recovery Services
Department of Social and Health
Services
P.O. Box 45330
Olympia, WA 98504-5330
Toll-Free: 877-301-4557
Toll-Free TTY: 800-833-6384
Fax: 360-586-0341
Website: www.dshs.wa.gov/bha
E-mail: DASAInformation@dshs.
wa.gov

West Virginia
Division of Alcoholism and Drug
Abuse
Bureau for Behavioral Health
and Health Facilities
350 Capitol St., Rm. 350
Charleston, WV 25301
Phone: 304-356-4811
Fax: 304-558-1008
Website: www.dhhr.wv.gov/
bhhf/Sections/programs/
ProgramsPartnerships/
AlcoholismandDrugAbuse/
Pages/default.aspx
E-mail: WVDUI@wv.gov

Wisconsin

Department of Health Services
Bureau of Prevention,
Treatment, and Recovery
P.O. Box 7851
One West Wilson St.
Madison, WI 53707-7851
Phone: 608-266-1865
Fax: 608-266-1533
Website: www.dhs.wisconsin.
gov/aoda/index.htm
E-mail:dhswebmaster@dhs.
wisconsin.gov

Wyoming

Behavioral Health Division
Mental Health and Substance
Abuse Services Department of
Health
6101 Yellowstone Rd., Ste. 220
Cheyenne, WY 82002
Toll-Free: 800-535-4006
Phone: 307-777-7656
Fax: 307-777-7439
Website: www.health.wyo.gov/
mhsa
E-mail: wdh@state.wy.us

Chapter 58

Directory of Organizations Providing Information about Drug Abuse

Government Organizations

Centers for Disease Control and Prevention (CDC)
1600 Clifton Rd.
Atlanta, GA 30333
Toll-Free: 800-CDC-INFO
(800-232-4636)
Toll-Free TTY: 888-232-6348
Toll-Free TDD: 800-232-4636
Website: www.cdc.gov
E-mail: cdcinfo@cdc.gov

National Criminal Justice Reference Service (NCJRS)
P.O. Box 6000
Rockville, MD 20849-6000
Toll-Free: 800-851-3420
Toll-Free TTY: 301-240-6310
Toll-Free TDD: 202-836-6998
Fax: 301-240-5830
Website: www.ncjrs.gov
E-mail: askojp@ncjrs.gov

Resources in this chapter were compiled from several sources deemed reliable; all contact information was verified and updated in January 2019.

National Institute on Alcohol Abuse and Alcoholism (NIAAA)
Toll-Free: 888-MY-NIAAA
(888-696-4222)
Phone: 301-443-3860
Website: www.niaaa.nih.gov
E-mail: niaaaweb-r@exchange.
nih.gov

National Institute on Drug Abuse (NIDA)
6001 Executive Blvd.
Rm. 5213, MSC 9561
Bethesda, MD 20892-9561
Phone: 301-443-1124
Website: www.drugabuse.gov
E-mail: media@nida.nih.gov

New York State Office of Alcoholism and Substance Abuse Services (OASAS)
1450 Western Ave.
Albany, NY 12203-3526
Phone: 518-473-3460
Website: www.oasas.ny.gov
E-mail: communications@oasas.
ny.gov

Office of Juvenile Justice and Delingquency Prevention (OJJDP)
810 Seventh St. N.W.
Washington, DC 20531
Toll-Free: 800-638-8736
Fax: 301-240-5830
Website:www.ojjdp.gov
E-mail: askojjdp@ncjrs.gov

Office of National Drug Control Policy (ONDCP)
Toll-Free: 800-851-3420
Website: www.whitehouse.gov/
ondcp

Substance Abuse and Mental Health Services Administration (SAMHSA)
5600 Fishers Ln.
Rockville, MD 20847-2345
Toll-Free: 877-SAMHSA-7
(877-726-4727)
Toll-Free TTY: 800-487-4889
Fax: 240-221-4292
Website: www.samhsa.gov
E-mail: SAMHSAInfo@samhsa.
hhs.gov

U.S. Department of Education (ED)
400 Maryland Ave. S.W.
Washington, DC 20202-6450
Toll-Free: 800-872-5327
Toll-Free TTY: 800-730-8913
Fax: 202-485-0013
Website: www2.ed.gov/about/
offices/list/oese/oshs/index.html
E-mail: oese@ed.gov

U.S. Department of Labor (DOL)
200 Constitution Ave., N.W.
Washington, DC 20210
Toll-Free: 866-487-2365
Website: webapps.dol.gov/elaws/
drugfree.htm
Email: webmaster@dol.gov

**U.S. Drug Enforcement
Administration (DEA)**
Office of Diversion Control
8701 Morrissette Dr.
Springfield, VA 22152
Toll-Free: 800-882-9539
Toll-Free TTY: 800-882-9539
Website: deadiversion.usdoj.gov
E-mail: DEA.Registration.Help@
usdoj.gov

Private Organizations

**American Society of
Addiction Medicine (ASAM)**
11400 Rockville Pike
Ste. 200
Rockville, MD 20852
Phone: 301-656-3920
Fax: 301-656-3815
Website: www.asam.org
E-mail: email@asam.org

Center on Addiction
Columbia University
633 Third Ave., 19th Fl.
New York, NY 10017-6706
Phone: 212-841-5200
Website: www.casacolumbia.org
E-mail: KKeneipp@
casacolumbia.org

**Co-Anon Family Groups
World Services**
P.O. Box 3664
Gilbert, AZ 85299
Toll-Free: 800-898-9985
Phone: 480 442-3869
Website: www.co-anon.org
E-mail: info@co-anon.org

**Cocaine Anonymous World
Services (CAWSO)**
P.O. Box 492000
Los Angeles, CA 90049-8000
Phone: 310-559-5833
Fax: 310-559-2554
Website: www.ca.org
E-mail: cawso@ca.org

**Community Anti-Drug
Coalitions of America
(CADCA)**
625 Slaters Ln., Ste. 300
Alexandria, VA 22314
Toll-Free: 800-542-2322
Fax: 703-706-0565
Website: www.cadca.org
E-mail: sadyanthaya@cadca.org

Narconon International
Phone: 877-445-7113
Website: www.narconon.org
E-mail: info@
narcononarrowhead.org

Narcotics Anonymous (NA)
P.O. Box 9999
Van Nuys, CA 91409
Phone: 818-773-9999
Fax: 818-700-0700
Website: www.na.org
E-mail: fsmail@na.org

National Council on Alcoholism and Drug Dependence, Inc. (NCADD)
217 Bdwy.
Ste. 712
New York, NY 10007
Toll-Free: 800-NCA-CALL
(800-622-2255)
Phone: 212-269-7797
Fax: 212-269-7510
Website: www.ncadd.org
E-mail: national@ncadd.org

National Families in Action (NFIA)
P.O. Box 133136
Atlanta, GA 30333-3136
Phone: 404-248-9676
Website: www.nationalfamilies.
org
E-mail: nfia@nationalfamilies.
org

The Partnership at Drugfree Kids
352 Park Ave. S.
9th Fl.
New York, NY 10010
Phone: 212-922-1560
Fax: 212-922-1570
Website: www.drugfree.org
E-mail: webmail@drugfree.org

Students Against Destructive Decisions (SADD)
1440 G St.
Washington, DC 20005
Toll-Free: 877-SADD-INC
(877-723-3462)
Phone: 508-481-3568
Fax: 508-481-5759
Website: www.sadd.org
E-mail: info@sadd.org

Index

Index